W9-CBA-862

Current Topics in Cardiovascular Medicine

General Editors:

Dr David K Brooks
Consultant Physician, St Mary's Hospital; Sub Dean, St Mary's Hospital Medical School, London; Formerly, Associate Professor of Medicine, Baylor College, Houston, Texas and University of Texas in Houston

Dr Everett Price
Clinical Associate Professor of Medicine, Baylor College of Medicine, Houston, Texas

Clinical Electrophysiology of the Heart

David E. Ward MD

Consultant in Cardiology,
Regional Cardiothoracic Unit,
St George's Hospital,
London,
England

A. John Camm MD

Professor of Clinical Cardiology,
Department of Cardiological Sciences,
St George's Hospital Medical School,
London,
England

With a Foreword by **Albert L. Waldo MD**

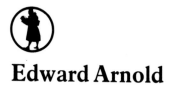

Edward Arnold

© David E. Ward and A. John Camm 1987

First published in Great Britain 1987 by
Edward Arnold (Publishers) Ltd, 41 Bedford Square, London WC1B 3DQ

Edward Arnold (Australia) Pty Ltd, 80 Waverley Road, Caulfield East,
Victoria 3145, Australia

Edward Arnold, 3 East Read Street, Baltimore, Maryland 21202, U.S.A.

Reprinted 1987

British Library Cataloguing in Publication Data

Ward, David E.
   Clinical electrophysiology of the heart.
   1. Arrhythmia 2. Electrophysiology
   I. Title II. Camm, A. John
   616.1'2807   RC685.A65

ISBN 0 7131 4507 2

Text set in 10pt Plantin
by 𝄖 Tek-Art Ltd, Croydon, Surrey
Printed and bound in Great Britain
by Butler & Tanner Ltd, Frome

Foreword

It was most flattering and a considerable honor for me to be asked to write the foreword to this book by Drs Ward and Camm. It is all the more so after having read the book. Without question, there has long been a need for a 'single'-authored monograph on the subject of clinical electrophysiology of the heart. This book meets that need enormously well. First, it is carefully written by two knowledgeable and sophisticated cardiac electrophysiologists who have used their considerable personal experience and command of the literature to produce a clear, integrated, up-to-date, and comprehensive monograph on this subject. Second, the breadth of the subjects covered in this fashion, including basic cardiac electrophysiology, arrhythmia mechanisms, diagnostic techniques with emphasis on invasive electrophysiologic studies, and *all* available antiarrhythmic therapies for both brady and tachyarrhythmias makes this monograph unique. Third, while this monograph largely reflects the considered approach of the authors, it presents a most balanced view, and clearly identifies areas that still remain clouded or controversial. For all these reasons, this book will well serve the student, the clinician, the investigator, and the teacher. In short, this book is a *tour de force* on the subject, and will serve as the standard reference in the field for years to come.

1987   Albert L. Waldo, M.D.
The Walter H. Pritchard Professor of Cardiology
and Professor of Medicine
Case Western Reserve University
University Hospitals of Cleveland
Cleveland, Ohio

Preface

Interest in the electrical activity of the heart began towards the end of the nineteenth century with experimental observations and the development of electrocardiography. Clinical electrophysiology became possible after the invention of cardiac catheterization and reliable methods of stimulating the heart. In the 20 years since stimulation was first applied to study clinical arrhythmias clinical cardiac electrophysiology has become a standard investigative method.

Although there are many texts about the subject, most of these are edited symposia, compilations of papers, progress reviews and such like. Since the method was introduced the indications for electrophysiological investigations have changed. For example, we have learned that the information gleaned in certain clinical settings (such as complete atrioventricular block) does not usually influence management. Electrophysiological studies have strengthened the foundations of electrocardiographic interpretation and we now realize that much of the information needed to make an accurate diagnosis is contained within the standard surface ECG. New methods of treatment (such as prevention or termination of tachycardia by pacemakers, surgical ablation and exclusion of tachycardia foci, transvascular electrical ablation and serial drug testing) have developed directly from information gained from these investigative clinical studies. Thus, the emphasis of clinical electrophysiology is changing from diagnosis to treatment. In this volume we have attempted to describe the place of modern clinical electrophysiology in the investigation and management of cardiac arrhythmias. In so doing we have included much of the information gained from early studies which is not now directly relevant to clinical decision-making. We believe this to be important because it provides the link between clinical electrocardiography and electrophysiology to which we have already referred. It is assumed that the reader will have a basic knowledge of clinical electrocardiography.

The book is divided into four sections: (1) a general introduction describing basic methods and practical techniques and measurements; (2) their application to the diagnosis and assessment of bradycardias; (3) their application to the diagnosis and assessment of tachycardias; (4) their place in the treatment of tachycardias using drugs, electrical methods and surgery. Greater emphasis has been given to the 'tachycardia' section because this aspect of clinical electrophysiological studies has become the dominant one. No attempt has been made to describe in detail the treatment of specific arrhythmias. On the contrary, we have endeavoured to discuss certain general principles of the investigation and management of clinical arrhythmias, as in Chapter 11, entitled 'Strategies', to illustrate the context within which clinical electrophysiological studies may be useful. At the end of each chapter a list of references and further reading is given. This list is not intended to be exhaustive but should enable the reader to refer, in detail, to the literature. Each list includes selected references of historical interest or importance, review articles, original reports and recent important communications. In the body of the text we have provided detailed references only in those sections which discuss topics of a controversial nature. The references at the end of the introductory chapter incorporate a general bibliography of books and symposia relating to clinical electrophysiology which may be useful to the reader.

The traces used to illustrate various phenomena have not always been selected to show 'ideal' examples. Thus, many traces, although illustrating the point being discussed, also have an added 'twist' or an additional detail making interpretation less straightforward. We have chosen this approach because such events are frequent and reflect actual clinical situations. The legends to the illustrations are detailed and substantive, not requiring the reader to refer to the main text.

Clinical electrophysiology has often been regarded as esoteric and complicated but we hope to show that this need not be so. It is becoming an increasingly important aspect of clinical cardiology and we trust that this book will be useful to all those involved in the management of patients with cardiac rhythm disturbances.

Acknowledgements

We would like to thank our many friends, colleagues and patients who contributed to the clinical studies, the information from which made this volume possible.

1987   DEW
                                                                              AJC

Contents

Part I

General Principles

1

Introductory Notes

Clinical cardiac electrophysiology has developed as a result of the merging of several different lines of investigation over the last 25 years. In 1958 the potentials from the His bundle of isolated hearts of cats and dogs were recorded by Alanis and colleagues and reported in the *Journal of Physiology*. The clinical importance of this discovery was not appreciated at this time. The first human recordings were made in 1960 by Giraud and colleagues. They also described the atrioventricular (AV) nodal electrogram but it is now recognized that consistent recording of such potentials is improbable. Some years later, Watson et al. (1966) reported His potentials from a patient with Ebstein's anomaly. However, in only 1 of 700 patients were they able to detect these potentials. The first description of a simple method of recording His potentials in man came from Scherlag et al. (1969). Using a multipolar catheter they could consistently and reliably record the His potential. They also noted changes in the AV nodal conduction time during carotid sinus massage with the heart rate fixed by atrial placing. Thus, a method for investigating the dynamic behaviour of the AV conduction pathway was established. In a later communication the same group investigated the effects of pacing and drugs on atrioventricular conduction.

Another line of investigation led to the development of a method of testing AV conduction using premature atrial stimulation. This method was devised in Moe's laboratory to investigate the functional properties of the conduction system of animals. This group was able to show reliable induction and termination of junctional tachycardia using the extrastimulus method in the dog (Moe et al., 1963). In 1967, Durrer and colleagues investigated the Wolff–Parkinson–White syndrome using the premature extrastimulus method. They observed that appropriately timed premature beats could initiate sustained tachycardia which in turn could be terminated by premature stimulation, strongly suggesting a re-entrant basis for these arrhythmias. Coumel had already provided evidence for circus movement as the mechanism of the permanent form of AV 'nodal' tachycardia (Coumel et al., 1967). Damato and associates (1969) combined the methods of intracardiac His bundle recording and premature stimulation to investigate the frequency-dependent properties of the human AV conduction system.

In 1971, Wellens published a detailed monograph on the use of the combined techniques of recording and stimulation in the clinical investigation of supraventricular tachycardias. He also observed that ventricular tachycardias in certain patients could be initiated and terminated by extrastimuli. The clinical study of ventricular tachycardia, now such an important element of the clinical method, was further advanced by Rosen's group in Chicago (Denes et al., 1976) and later by Josephson, Horowitz and their colleagues in Philadelphia (Josephson et al., 1978) in a long series of papers covering all aspects of clinical ventricular tachycardias. Although the initial emphasis was placed upon the experimental and investigative aspects of these technniques, this began to change as physiological and pathological mechanisms were unravelled. Thus, the importance of the technique as a diagnostic tool diminished but it became the foundation for the development of all forms of treatment of arrhythmias. Several investigators, most notably Rosen's laboratory (Wu et al., 1977) and Fisher and colleagues (1977), introduced the concept of serial drug testing in patients with recurrent tachycardias. Spurrell et al. (1973) used programmed stimulation to study ventricular tachycardias prior to surgical treatment of the arrhythmia. Until recently, the concept of re-entry in the clinical setting was based largely on indirect evidence relating to mode of initiation and termination of the arrhythmias. In an important series of publications, Waldo et al. (1977) developed a method of defining re-entry by 'entrainment' of the tachycardia circuit. This method, originally applied to the investigation of atrial flutter, is now accepted as an important clinical tool for identifying re-entrant tachycardia mechanisms (see Chapter 7).

The application of these methods to patients over the last decade has greatly enriched our understanding of a wide variety of complex conduction disorders and tachycardias. Furthermore, the development of specific therapeutic strategies for all types of tachycardias has been based largely on the wealth of information provided by cardiac electrophysiological studies. Although these studies have clarified the mechanisms of conduction delay and block and provided useful information about the nature and quality of escape rhythms in the presence of significant bradycardias, they have not emerged as important clinical tools in the investigation of patients with these disorders. Thus, the main clinical application of intracardiac electrophysiological techniques is in the investigation of patients with documented or suspected tachycardias of all types (Table 1.1), particularly those of a re-entrant nature. Nevertheless, there are instances when additional information from intracardiac studies may be of value

Table 1.1 INDICATIONS FOR ELECTROPHYSIOLOGICAL TESTING

Investigation of symptoms	Elucidation of abnormal ECG
Palpitations, etc.	Narrow complex tachycardias
Syncope and presyncope	Broad complex tachycardias
Sudden death syndrome	Bradycardia
Design of therapy	**Assessment of risk**
Serial drug testing	Ventricular arrhythmias
Pacemaker prescription	Wolff–Parkinson–White (or other
Consideration for surgery	forms of anomalous conduction)
Suitability for ablation	AV conduction block
	Escape rhythms

Relative contraindications include left main stem coronary artery disease (eg >75% stenosis), acute myocardial infarction (within 4 days), hypertrophic cardiomyopathy, severe aortic stenosis, electrolyte abnormality such as hypokalaemia, significant coexistent disease, etc.

in assessing a patient with documented or suspected bradycardia. The main applications of the method are:

1. Assessment of sinus node function (Chapter 4).
2. Assessment of atrioventricular conduction (Chapters 5 and 6).
3. Investigation of atrial, junctional and ventricular tachycardias (Chapters 8, 9 and 10).
4. Evaluation of methods of treatment (drugs, pacemakers, ablation, etc.) (Chapters 12, 13, 14 and 15).
5. Assessment of symptoms possibly caused by arrhythmias; e.g. syncope (suspected arrhythmia) (Chapter 10).
6. Assessment of the risk of developing an arrhythmia (spontaneous activation of a known substrate) or the presence of a suspected but latent substrate for an arrhythmia; e.g. ventricular tachycardia, complete AV block, sudden death, etc. (see, for example, Chapters 5, 10 and 16).
7. Application of therapeutic methods (control of tachycardias by drugs, pacing and ablation of tachycardia or conduction tissue) (see Chapters 11–15).

There are innumerable texts describing the electrocardiographic appearances of arrhythmias and many of these enumerate the various treatments, but there are relatively few which consider in detail the clinical electrophysiology of cardiac arrhythmias. Those volumes currently available are largely compilations of individual contributions discussing selected problems and controversies, or are large reference works which are not entirely suited to the needs of the non-specialist. Considering that the major advances in the investigation and treatment of clinical arrhythmias during the last decade have predominantly developed from electrophysiological methods, this deficiency is surprising. This volume is intended to provide an introduction to clinical cardiac electrophysiology with practical advice about the method.

References and further reading including a general bibliography

Alanis J, Gonzalez H, Lopez E. (1958) Electrical activity of the bundle of His. *Journal of Physiology* **142**, 127

Bircks W, Loogen F, Schulte HD, Seipel L. (1980) *Medical and Surgical Management of Tachyarrhythmias*. Springer Verlag: Heidelberg

Camm AJ, Ward DE. (1983) *Pacing for Tachycardia Control*. Telectronics: Sydney

Castellanos A. (1980) (Editor) *Cardiac Arrhythmias: Mechanisms and Management*. FA Davies: Philadelphia, Pa

Coumel P, Cabrol C, Fabiato A, Gourgon R, Slama R. (1967) Tachycardie permanente par rhythme reciproque. I. Preuves du diagnostic par stimulation auriculaire et ventriculaire. *Archives des Maladies du Couer* **20**, 1830

Cranefield PF. (1975) *The Conduction of the Cardiac Impulse. The Slow Response and Cardiac Arrhythmias*. Futura: Mount Kisco, NY

Damato AN, Lau SH, Patton RD, Steiner C, Berkowitz W. (1969) A study of atrioventricular conduction in man using premature atrial stimulation and His bundle recordings. *Circulation* **40**, 61

Davies MJ, Anderson RH, Becker AE. (1983) *The Conduction System of the Heart*. Butterworths: London

Denes P, Wu D, Dhingra RC, Amat-y-Leon F, Wyndham C, Mautner RK, Rosen KM. (1976) Electrophysiological studies in patients with chronic recurrent ventricular tachycardia. *Circulation* **54**, 229

Dreifus LS, Likoff W (Editors). (1973) *Cardiac Arrhythmias*. The Twentyfifth Hahnemann Symposium. Grune & Stratton: New York

Durrer D, Schoo L, Schuilenberg RM, Wellens HJJ. (1967) The role of premature beats in the initiation and termination of supraventricular tachycardia in the Wolff-Parkinson-White syndrome. *Circulation* **36**, 644

Fisher JD, Cohen HL, Mehra R, Altschuler H, Escher DJW, Furman S. (1977) Cardiac pacing and pacemakers. II. Serial electrophysiologic–pharmacologic testing for control of recurrent tachyarrhythmias. *American Heart Journal* **93**, 658

Fisher JD. (1981) Role of electrophysiologic testing in the diagnosis and treatment of patients with known and suspected bradycardias and tachycardias. *Progress in Cardiovascular Diseases* **24**, 25

Gillette PC, Garson A (Editors). (1981) *Pediatric Cardiac Dysrhythmias*. Grune & Stratton: New York

Giraud G, Puech P, Latour H. (1960) L'activite electrique physiologique du noeud de Tawara et du faisceau de His chez l'homme. Enregistrement electrocardiographique endocavitaire. *Bulletin de l'Academie Nationale de Medecine* **144**, 363

Harrison DC, Mason JW, Miller HA, Winkle RA (Editors). (1981) *Cardiac Arrhythmias. A Decade of Progress*. GK Hall Medical Publishers: Boston, Mass

Harthorne JW. (1981) Historic milestones of electrotherapy and cardiac pacing. *Progress in Cardiovascular Diseases* **23**, 389

Josephson ME, Horowitz LN, Farshidi A, Kastor JA. (1978) Recurrent sustained ventricular tachycardia. 1. Mechanisms. *Circulation* **57**, 431

Josephson ME, Seides SF. (1979) *Clinical Cardiac Electrophysiology: Techniques and Interpretations*. Lea & Febiger: Philadelphia, Pa

Josephson ME (Editor). (1982) *Ventricular Tachycardia: Mechanisms and Management*. Futura: Mount Kisco, NY

Josephson ME, Wellens HJJ (Editors). (1984) *Tachycardias: Mechanisms, Diagnosis, Treatment*. Lea & Febiger, Philadelphia, Pa

Katz, LN, Pick A. (1956) *Clinical Electrocardiography*. Part I. *The Arrhythmias*. Lea & Febiger, Philadelphia, Pa

Kelly DT (Editor). (1978) *Advances in the Management of Arrhythmias*. Telectronics: Sydney

Krikler DM, Goodwin JF (Editors). (1975) *Cardiac Arrhythmias: The Modern Electrophysiologic Approach*. WB Saunders: London

Kulbertus HE (Editor). (1977) *Re-entrant Arrhythmias: Mechanisms and Treatment*. MTP Press: Lancaster

Levy M, Vassalle M (Editors). (1982) *Excitation and Neural Control of the Heart*. American Physiological Society: Bethesda, Md

Levy S, Gerard R (Editors). (1983) *Recent Advances in Cardiac Arrhythmias*. I. *Antiarrhythmic Agents and Cardiac Pacing*. John Libbey: London

Levy S, Scheinman MM (Editors). (1984) *Cardiac Arrhythmias: From Diagnosis to Therapy*. Futura: Mount Kisco, NY

Lewis T. (1925) *The Mechanism and Graphic Registration of the Heart Beat*, 3rd edition Shaw: London

Mandel WJ (Editor). (1980) *Cardiac Arrhythmias: Their Mechanisms, Diagnosis and Management*. JB Lippincott: Philadelphia, Pa

Masoni A, Alboni P (Editors). (1982) *Cardiac Electrophysiology Today*. Academic Press: London

Michelson EL, Dreifus LS. (1984) Present status of clinical electrophysiologic studies: introduction–what studies are needed? *Pacing and Clinical Electrophysiology* **7**, 421

Moe GK, Preston JB, Burlington H. (1956) Physiological evidence for a dual AV transmission system. *Circulation Research* **4**, 357

Moe GK, Cohen W, Vick RL. (1963) Experimentally induced paroxysmal A–V nodal tachycardia in the dog. A 'case report'. *American Heart Journal* **65**, 87

Narula OS (Editor). (1975) *His Bundle Electrocardiography and Clinical Electrophysiology*. FA Davis: Philadelphia, Pa

Narula O (Editor). (1980) *Cardiac Arrhythmias: Electrophysiology, Diagnosis and Management*. Williams & Wilkins: Baltimore, Md

Noble D. (1979) *The Initiation of the Heartbeat*. Clarendon Press: Oxford

Pick A, Langendorf R. (1979) *Interpretation of Complex Arrhythmias*. Lea & Febiger: Philadelphia, Pa

Puech P, Slama R (Editors). (1979) *The Cardiac Arrhythmias*. Arrhythmia Working Group of the French Cardiac Society. Corbiere RMDP and Roussel-Uclaf: Paris

Reiser, HJ, Horowitz LN (Editors). (1985) *Mechanisms and Treatment of Cardiac Arrhythmias: Relevance of Basic Studies to Clinical Management*. Urban & Schwarzenberg: Baltimore, Md

Roberts NK, Gelband H (Editors). (1977) *Cardiac Arrhythmias in the Neonate, Infant and Child*. Appleton-Century-Crofts: New York

Rosen KM. (1980) Clinical cardiac electrophysiology. Key references. *Circulation* **61**, 1262

Rosenbaum M, Elizari MV (Editors). (1983) *Frontiers of Cardiac Electrophysiology*. Martinus Nijhoff: The Hague

Sandoe E, Flensted-Jensen E, Olsen KH (Editors). (1970) *Symposium on Cardiac Arrhythmias*. AB Astra: Sodertalje, Sweden

Sandoe E, Julian DG, Bell JW (Editors). (1978) *Management of Ventricular Tachycardia – Role of Mexilitine*. Excerpta Medica: Amsterdam

Scheinman MM, Morady F. (1983) Invasive cardiac electrophysiologic testing: the current state of the art. *Circulation* **67**, 1169

Scherf D, Schott A. (1973) *Extrasystoles and Allied Arrhythmias*. Heinemann Medical: London

Sherf L, Neufeld HN. (1978) *The Preexcitation Syndrome: Facts and Theories*. Yorke Medical Books: New York

Scherlag BJ, Lau SH, Helfant RH, Berkowitz W, Stein E, Damato AN. (1969). Catheter technique for recording His bundle activity in man. *Circulation* **39**, 13

Spurrell RAJ, Sowton E, Deuchar D. (1973) Ventricular tachycardia in four patients evaluated by programmed electrical stimulation of heart and treated in 2 patients by surgical division of anterior radiation of left bundle-branch. *British Heart Journal* **35**, 1014

Surawicz B. (1982) Intracardiac extrastimulation studies: how to? where? by whom? *Circulation* **65**, 428

Surawicz B, Reddy CP (Editors). (1984) *Tachycardias*. Martinus Nijhoff: Boston, Mass

Waldo AL, Kaiser GA. (1973). Study of ventricular arrhythmias associated with acute myocardial infarction in the canine heart. *Circulation* **47**, 1222

Waldo AL, MacLean WAH, Karp RB, Kouchokos NT, James TN. (1977) Entrainment and interruption of atrial flutter with atrial pacing. Studies in man following open heart surgery. *Circulation* **56**, 737

Waldo AL, MacLean WAH. (1980) *Diagnosis and Treatment of Arrhythmias following Open Heart Surgery. Emphasis on the Use of Atrial and Ventricular Epicardial Wire Electrodes*. Futura: Mount Kisco, NY

Waldo AL, Wells JL, Cooper TB, MacLean WAH. (1981) Temporary cardiac pacing: applications and techniques in the treatment of cardiac arrhythmias. *Progress in Cardiovascular Diseases* **23**, 451

Waldo AL, Plumb V, Arciniegas JG, MacLean WAH, Cooper TB, Priest MF, James TN. (1983) Transient entrainment and interruption of the atrioventricular bypass type of paroxysmal atrial tachycardia. A model for understanding and identifying re-entrant arrhythmias. *Circulation* **67**, 73

Watson H, Emslie-Smith D, Lowe KG. (1966) The intracardiac electrogram of human atrioventricular conducting tissue. *American Heart Journal* **74**, 66

Wellens HJJ. (1971) *Electrical Stimulation of the Heart in the Study and Treatment of Tachycardias*. University Park Press: Baltimore, Md

Wellens HJJ, Lie KI, Janse MJ (Editors). (1976) *Conduction System of the Heart: Structure, Function and Clinical Implications*. Lea & Febiger: Philadelphia, Pa

Wellens, HJJ. (1978) Value and limitations of programmed electrical stimulation of the heart in the study and treatment of tachycardias. *Circulation* **57**, 845

Wiener I. (1982) Current applications of clinical electrophysiologic study in the diagnosis and treatment of cardiac arrhythmias. *American Journal of Cardiology* **49**, 1287

Wu D, Wyndham CR, Denes P, Amat-y-Leon F, Miller RH, Dhingra RC, Rosen KM. (1977) Chronic electrophysiological study in patients with recurrent paroxysmal tachycardia: a new method for developing successful oral antiarrhythmic therapy. In: *Re-entrant Arrhythmias: Mechanisms and Treatment*, p. 294. Ed. by H Kulbertus. MTP Press: Lancaster

Zipes DP. (1971) The contribution of artificial pacemaking to understanding the pathogenesis of arrhythmias. *American Journal of Cardiology* **28**, 211

Zipes, DP, Bailey JC, Elharrar V (Editors). (1980) *The Slow Inward Current and Cardiac Arrhythmias*. Martinus Nijhoff: The Hague

Zipes DP (Editor), (1983) Symposium on Electrophysiology and Electrocardiography in honor of Alfred Pick and Kenneth M Rosen. *Pacing and Clinical Electrophysiology* **6**, 993

Zipes D, Jalife J (Editors). (1985) *Cardiac Electrophysiology and Arrhythmias*. Grune & Stratton: Orlando, Fla

2

Clinical Electrophysiological Methods

The aim of clinical electrophysiological methods is to record electrical activity from within the heart cavities and to stimulate the heart when appropriate. The general objectives of the investigation are to achieve a diagnosis and to establish a rational basis for treatment. These aims and the nature of the procedure should be clearly explained to the patient in a form of words appropriate to the patient's level of understanding (in this sense, this approach differs from the principle of 'informed consent'). This alleviates anxiety and enhances patient confidence and co-operation. Further explanations and reassurances should be given at all stages of the procedure.

Table 2.1 ELECTRODE CATHETERS FOR ELECTROPHYSIOLOGY STUDY

Description	Type	Purpose
Multipole	Bipolar, quadripolar hexapolar	General pacing and sensing; coronary sinus mapping
Multipole with remote indifferent pole	J-shaped, straight	Atrial, AV and ventricular pacing
Multipole with curved tip	Tripolar	His bundle recording
	Josephson (4-pole)	His bundle recording and mapping; ventricular mapping
	J-shaped	Atrial appendage location for atrial sensing and pacing
Active fixation	Screw-in tip	Repeat studies where stable electrode position is essential
Multipole with stylet	Malleable stylet	Introduction into difficult positions
	Gallagher (stiff curved stylet)	Right AV ring mapping
Multipole with lumen	Zucker, Gorlin	Pacing and sensing plus infusion or pressure recording
Oesophageal	Unipolar, bipolar	Left atrial sensing and pacing via oesophagus
Monophasic action potential	Suction, contact	Repolarization studies; drug studies

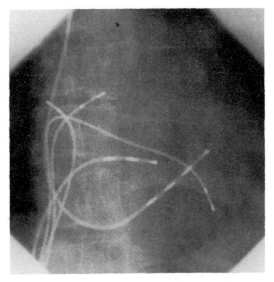

Fig. 2.1 The placement of electrode catheters for an electrophysiological study of a patient with junctional tachycardias. There are two bipolar electrode catheters in the right atrium (one of which is used for activation mapping and the other for pacing), a coronary sinus quadripolar catheter, a right ventricular bipolar catheter, and a tripolar electrode for recording from the His bundle region.

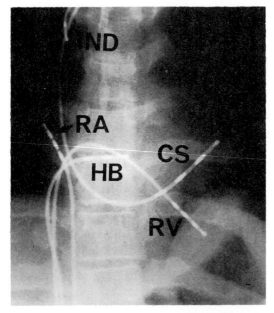

Fig. 2.2 An alternative arrangement of electrodes with an indifferent pole (IND) positioned in the superior vena cava to allow 'unipolar' endocardial recordings. CS = coronary sinus quadripolar electrode; HB = His bundle tripolar electrode; RA = right atrial quadripolar electrode; RV = right ventricular quadripolar electrode.

Cardiac electrical activity is recorded from the endocardium using standard bipolar pacing electrodes or purpose-built bipolar or multipolar catheters. One or more electrode catheters (Table 2.1) are inserted under X-ray screening and connected to appropriate recording and stimulation devices. The most commonly used are 5F or 6F woven Dacron, polyethylene or polyurethane catheters with 5 mm or 10 mm interelectrode distances. The number and types of electrode catheters used depend on the purpose of the investigation. Thus, in studies of atrioventricular (AV) conduction it is necessary to have a minimum of two electrodes, one positioned near the sinus node or in the atrial appendage and another across the tricuspid valve to monitor the His potential. In studies of junctional tachycardia additional electrodes are required to be positioned (Figs. 2.1 and 2.2) in the right ventricle and coronary sinus (see Chapter 8). The study itself is usually conducted with the patient in the supine position for convenience but a tilting table may be of value on occasions. For example, in patients with junctional tachycardias, sustained tachycardia may only be inducible in the upright position. Furthermore, symptoms due to induced arrhythmias may not be apparent in the supine position (Hammill et al., 1984).

Introduction of electrodes

The studies are performed in aseptic conditions. The patients are fasting and usually unsedated or lightly sedated. In young children a general anaesthetic is often necessary. Anticholinergic premedications should be avoided if possible, as they will affect cardiac electrophysiology. For initial or baseline studies all relevant cardioactive medications, particularly antiarrhythmic drugs, should have been discontinued for at least five drug elimination half-lives before the study is undertaken.

There are several commonly used methods for the insertion of electrode catheters but only one (used by the authors) will be described here. Up to four electrodes may be introduced via the femoral vein. The guide-wire method is used to puncture the vein after infiltration with a local anaesthetic (1% lignocaine is usually sufficient but should not be used too liberally because it may interfere with cardiac excitability). A single puncture of the vein is all that is required to introduce several electrodes. Using a percutaneous needle, a guide wire is introduced into the vein. After removal of the needle the introducer sheath and obturator are then advanced over the guide wire. The guide wire and obturator are removed and a further one, two or three guide wires (as required and depending on the size of the sheath) are inserted into the vein via the sheath (Fig. 2.3). The sheath is removed leaving the guide wires in the vein. Introducer sheaths can then be advanced over each guide wire in turn to allow introduction of the electrodes without the need for further venous punctures. The lead used for recording His bundle activity is positioned last and the introducer sheath is left in the vein to allow easier manipulation of the lead by preventing friction with the other leads in the femoral vein. To reduce the risk of thromboembolism some investigators prefer to heparinize the patient when all electrode catheters are in place. This is more important when electrode catheters are positioned in the left ventricle or when many catheters remain *in situ* for prolonged periods.

In patients undergoing studies of junctional tachycardia it may be necessary

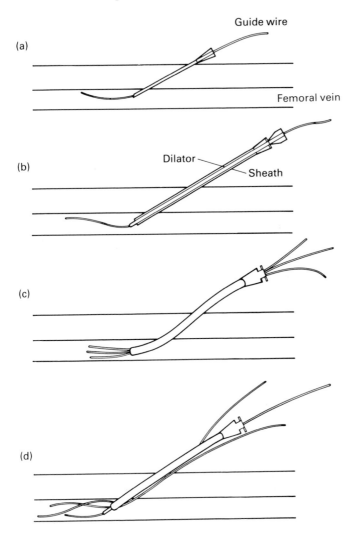

Fig. 2.3 Method of introduction of multiple catheters into a large vein. (*a*) Introduction of a guide wire through a needle. A dilator and sheath are passed over the guide wire (*b*) and, following withdrawal of the obturator, additional wires can be introduced (*c*). The sheath is removed and each wire is used in turn to introduce a separate sheath for the catheters (*d*). It is important to withdraw each sheath after the electrode catheter is in position to minimize bleeding and trauma. The His bundle catheter is introduced last of all and, if appropriate, the sheath may be left in the vein to allow easier manipulation of the catheter.

to position additional catheters in the coronary sinus or right atrium. Since many of these patients will also undergo serial drug testing (see Chapter 12) it is appropriate to insert the relevant electrode catheter(s) via a site which is comfortable for the patient, at the same time providing ease of access and a reduced risk of displacement. For this purpose, a direct puncture of the subclavian vein or jugular vein can be performed (the subclavian is preferable, especially using the infraclavicular method of puncture which is less likely to cause a pneumothorax). This approach is especially useful for positioning electrodes in the coronary sinus but right atrial and ventricular catheters can also be inserted using this route. Catheters inserted in this way may be left *in situ* for several days, allowing further studies. Additional electrodes may be required in patients investigated for ventricular tachycardia. These can be introduced via the other femoral vein. If left ventricular electrodes are needed, they can be introduced by direct femoral artery puncture using the method described above.

Positioning of electrodes

As each electrode is introduced it is manoeuvred into position under fluoroscopic guidance. For studies of sinus node function, both recording and stimulating electrodes should be positioned close to the expected site of the sinus node at the junction of the superior vena cava with the right atrium. To provide stability this catheter is usually placed against the lateral wall. In doing this, care must be taken to avoid stimulation of the phrenic nerve which lies against the lateral aspect of the right atrium. Most investigators now use a quadripolar electrode such that two poles may be used for pacing and two poles for recording the atrial electrogram. We prefer to use the distal and proximal pole for pacing and the central poles for recording.

The His bundle potential ('spike') is located by careful manipulation of the electrode across the septal leaflet of the tricuspid valve. As the catheter is advanced the amplitude of the atrial electrogram gradually diminishes and a small spike should appear between the atrial and the ventricular signals. The catheter is then withdrawn with some clockwise torque until a good sized atrial electrogram is recorded whilst preserving the His potential as much as possible. Because the His potential is an important marker for activation of the His bundle it is essential to obtain a clear recording, particularly in studies of AV conduction and tachycardias involving the AV junction. Many investigators use a multipolar catheter and record several simultaneous channels in order to preserve the His potential during catheter movement (Fig. 2.4). Occasionally it may be necessary to record the His potential from a catheter introduced from above (Fig. 2.5).

Manipulation of an electrode into the coronary sinus is most easily accomplished from a subclavian entry site. However, it is also possible to enter the coronary sinus from the femoral vein by forming a loop in the right atrium (Fig. 2.6). When the electrode has entered the coronary sinus it should be possible to record distinct left atrial and left ventricular electrograms (Fig. 2.7). In most cases the catheter can be advanced well into the coronary sinus, thus facilitating coronary sinus mapping studies. A quadripolar catheter is usually selected for coronary sinus recording and, by convention, is positioned with the most proximal pole at the ostium of the sinus (see Fig. 2.1). Occasionally it is possible to record left atrial activity directly via a persistent foramen ovale. In instances where it is not possible to enter the left atrium or the coronary sinus, left atrial activity can sometimes be recorded from an electrode in the main or right pulmonary artery. The signals recorded from the pulmonary artery are often of low voltage and indistinct.

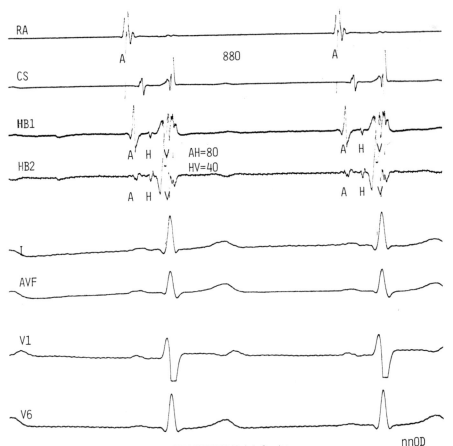

Fig. 2.4 Recordings from the His bundle region using a multipolar catheter. The proximal poles (HB1) record good-sized low right atrial (A) and His (H) potentials with an AH of 80 msec and HV of 40 msec. The distal poles (HB2) are further across the tricuspid valve and show a low amplitude atrial signal and a larger His potential. Paper speed 100 mm/sec. CS = coronary sinus; RA = right atrium.

For stability of pacing and sensing, the right ventricular electrode is usually placed at the apex. Occasionally, pacing at this site may also stimulate the diaphragm, in which case the pacing energy can be reduced or the lead resited. For ventricular tachycardia studies it is often necessary to move this electrode to the outflow region or to insert an additional lead.

Rarely, a left ventricular electrode is required for investigation of ventricular tachycardia or left-sided anomalous pathways. The electrode is introduced via the femoral artery and manipulated retrogradely across the aortic valve. Fine positioning of the electrode tip within the left ventricular cavity requires considerable manual dexterity. A long introducer sheath may be positioned

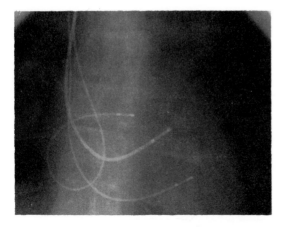

Fig. 2.5 A method of positioning the catheter for His bundle recording using the subclavian vein approach. The catheter is looped against the free wall of the right atrium in a clockwise direction and advanced toward the tricuspid valve. Coronary sinus and right ventricular electrodes are also shown.

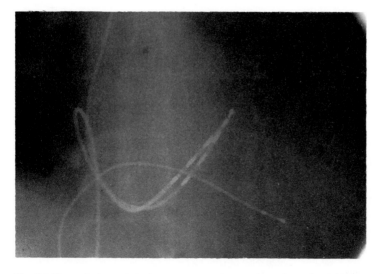

Fig. 2.6 The technique of placing a coronary sinus catheter from the right femoral vein approach and the left subclavian vein approach. From the leg, the catheter is looped against the free wall of the right atrium and advanced toward the ostium of the coronary sinus (both catheters are shown in position for demonstration purposes only – for the study, one was withdrawn).

within the left ventricle to permit easier manipulation. For detailed mapping studies of ventricular tachycardia, biplane fluoroscopy is useful.

For certain types of study, additional catheters are sometimes used. For example, a fine (4F) flexible bipolar electrode catheter or angioplasty guide wire can be passed down the right coronary artery to increase the accuracy of

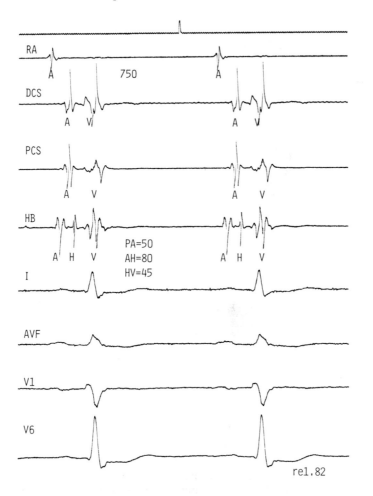

Fig. 2.7 Normal sinus rhythm. The atrial activation sequence is shown by the atrial electrograms (A). In this example the earliest activity is in the high right atrium (RA) synchronous with the onset of the P wave in the surface ECG (occasionally it is possible to record preatrial activity which is thought to reflect sinus node depolarization – see Chapter 4). The proximal coronary sinus (PCS), low right atrial (His bundle (HB) region) electrograms and distal coronary sinus signals follow. Paper speed 100 mm/sec.

localization of right AV free wall anomalous pathways (see Chapter 9). For 'unipolar' recordings, an indifferent electrode may be placed in the superior vena cava.

Complications

The complications of invasive electrophysiological studies are related to the insertion of the electrode catheters and the nature of the procedure itself (Table 2.2). The recognized complications of cardiac catheterization include venous

Table 2.2 COMPLICATIONS OF ELECTROPHYSIOLOGY STUDIES

	Horowitz (1986)*		Camm and Ward (unpublished)†	
	Patients		Patients	
Complication	No.	%	No.	%
Cardiac perforation	19	0.47	1	0.14
Venous thrombosis	20	0.49	4	0.58
Haemorrhage	4	0.10	3	0.43
Arterial injury	8	0.20	2	0.29
Pulmonary embolus	NA		2	0.29
Pneumothorax	NA		11	1.59
Death	5	0.12	2	0.29

* 8545 studies in 4015 patients.
† 787 studies in 690 patients.
NA = not available

problems (uncontrollable bleeding, thrombosis, embolism, thrombophlebitis and AV fistula formation). Fortunately, the incidence of these problems is less than 2 per cent. Repeated studies involving several punctures and catheter insertions at a single site (especially the femoral veins) is probably not wise, as venous irritation may predispose to thrombophlebitis. Heparin administration is advised if many catheters are to be inserted or if a long procedure time is anticipated, especially if a left ventricular electrode is inserted. The use of left ventricular electrodes requires arterial puncture with the recognized risks of retrograde arterial catheterization. Careful consideration should be given to the necessity of left ventricular studies before they are performed. When catheters are introduced via a jugular or subclavian vein, there is a risk of pneumothorax which should be excluded by fluoroscopy after insertion and before return to the ward. A portable chest X-ray should be performed within 2 hours of the procedure.

Manipulation of any catheter within the heart can result in trauma to the specialized conduction system. It is not uncommon to see right bundle branch block appear during positioning of catheters within the right ventricle. This usually subsides within minutes or hours. The effect is of little consequence in most instances. However, ventricular tachycardias dependent on anterograde right bundle branch conduction to sustain tachycardia (a rare entity) will no longer be inducible. The left bundle branch is much less susceptible when catheters are manipulated within the left ventricle. Anomalous pathways are also subject to traumatic block which interferes with initiation of sustained atrioventricular re-entrant tachycardia (see Chapters 6 and 9).

In many cases initiation of tachycardias is an integral part of the procedure. The risk of inducing unwanted arrhythmias is in part determined by the stimulation protocol used. In patients investigated for manifest or suspect ventricular tachycardias, however, the initiation protocol becomes progressively more likely to induce unwanted ventricular arrhythmias including ventricular fibrillation (see Chapter 9). This is an accepted risk, the danger from which is virtually zero in skilled hands. Nevertheless, this potentially dangerous risk emphasizes the need for properly trained staff and well-maintained equipment during electrophysiological investigation.

In a small proportion of patients the use of rapid atrial pacing to induce or terminate junctional tachycardias may initiate atrial fibrillation. In most it is transient, terminating spontaneously after several seconds or minutes. In some, arrhythmia may persist and prevent completion of the study. If this occurs the patient may be cardioverted so that the study can proceed. Cardioversion, which produces only transient electrophysiological effects, obviates the need to administer a drug which may cause sustained electrophysiological changes. External cardioversion should be regarded as a possible part of the clinical electrophysiological study and the patient should be so informed.

Equipment

A schematic diagram of the equipment for clinical cardiac electrophysiological studies is shown in Fig. 2.8. Each electrode is connected to an isolation amplifier via a junction box of the matrix type. This permits any input to be connected

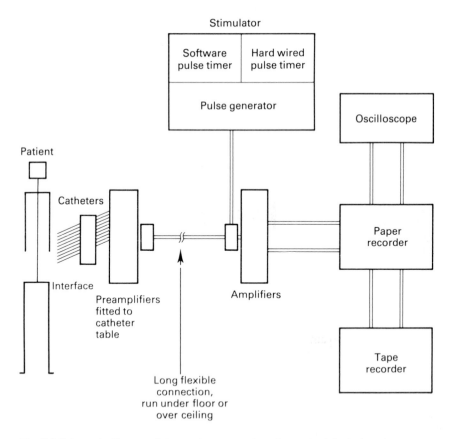

Fig. 2.8 Schematic diagram of the equipment used at electrophysiological study.

to any output providing a flexible system. The amplifiers should be electrically isolated for safety reasons. The intracardiac signals are amplified (approximately 1 cm/mV), filtered and recorded on a high fidelity recorder. The high pass band filter should be 40–50 Hz and the low pass filter is usually approximately 500 Hz. These settings are optimal for recording the His potential.

The electrograms are recorded with three roughly orthogonal surface electrocardiographic leads (e.g. I, aVF, V1). Some investigators also record lead V6 routinely, and during the investigation of patients with ventricular tachycardia as many simultaneous leads as possible are recorded. A high speed ink-jet or photographic recorder is suitable for this purpose. Paper speeds of up to 250 mm/sec are necessary for accurate measurement of intervals. Ideally, all recordings should be stored on magnetic tape. If continuous recording on magnetic tape is not possible, it is advisable to record the entire study directly onto paper using the most appropriate recording speeds. If magnetic tape recording is preferred, a triggered storage oscilloscope can be used to observe events more closely.

Several purpose-built stimulators are available. Some of these are controlled by software but simple manually operated devices are adequate for most clinical purposes. The stimulator should have an adjustable voltage output, with a range of stimulation frequences from 0.5 to 25 Hz (30 to 1500 pulses per minute). It

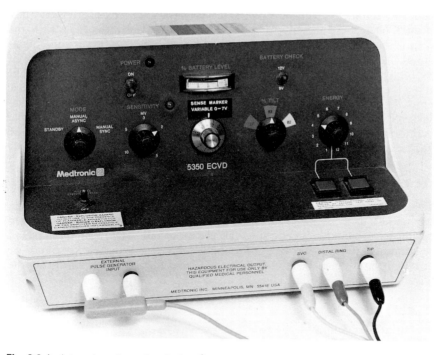

Fig. 2.9 An internal cardioversion device. The energy delivered can be controlled by a rotary knob. Other adjustable features include sensitivity, waveform and mode of response. Special catheters are needed to use this device (see Chapter 13). This type of equipment is especially useful in the study of patients with haemodynamically unstable ventricular tachycardia.

should have two or more independent pacemakers capable of delivering not less than three extrastimuli linked to a paced sequence or to the intrinsic heart rhythm. Thus, it must be able to sense from any recording channel. The sensitivity of the receiver amplifier must be adjustable.

The study should be performed in a catheter laboratory or other area equipped with facilities for full resuscitation. An external defibrillator must be available. Recently, a low energy (less than 5 W–s) internal cardiovertor (Fig. 2.9) has been employed for the repeated cardioversions which may be necessary, particularly during the study of ventricular tachycardias.

Costs

The costs of electrophysiological studies are difficult to estimate and, naturally, vary according to the institute and the country in which they are performed. It is prudent, however, to pay attention to this aspect of electrophysiological testing, especially in the current climate of economic restraint. Ross et al. (1980) estimated that in Holland the total cost of an electrophysiological study in 1980 was around US$800. This included disposable items and salaries at $550. Hospitalization costs and treatment of complications were not included in the analysis. The average time taken to introduce catheters was 1 hour, with additional time for programmed stimulation (83 minutes) and research drug studies (43 minutes). From 360 to 2100 feet of paper were recorded at each study (mean 1260 feet). This study did not attempt to offset these costs with the potential or actual benefit to the patient or community (e.g. fewer subsequent admissions, less time off work, etc.) Saksena (1985) has studied this aspect of electrophysiological studies in some detail and estimates that the cost/benefit ratio of electrophysiologically guided treatment compared to the empirical approach is 10:1 for patients with recurrent supraventricular tachycardias (Saksena, 1985) and 18:1 for patients with recurrent ventricular tachycardias (Ferguson et al., 1984). Thus, although the initial cost of electrophysiological studies can be high, it is recouped within a short time.

Measurement of intervals

For ease of interpretation, we arrange the recordings as shown in Fig. 2.5. This gives an idea of the sequence of cardiac activation during normal sinus rhythm and illustrates how conduction intervals are measured. The relative timings of the stimulus artefact, the atrial, His bundle and ventricular electrograms are dependent on catheter positions, and excessive catheter movement during the course of the study will introduce errors. Ranges of normal intervals are given in Table 2.3

Intra-atrial conduction

The intra-atrial conduction time is reflected by the PA interval. This is measured from the earliest point of atrial activation on any intracardiac or surface lead to the intrinsic deflection of the low right atrial electrogram recorded from the His bundle electrode (see Fig. 2.7). Intra-atrial conduction time is determined by the

Table 2.3 NORMAL VALUES (in msec) OF CONDUCTION INTERVALS, REFRACTORY PERIODS AND SINUS NODE FUNCTION

	Infants	Children	Adults	Elderly
PA	0 – 35	0 – 40	25 – 55	30 – 65
AH	40 – 95	40 – 120	60 – 120	55 – 110
HV	15 – 55	30 – 55	35 – 55	35 – 55
A ERP*	—	160 – 210	170 – 300	200 – 350
AVN ERP*	—	150 – 390	230 – 430	160 – 400
AVN FRP*	—	285 – 500	330 – 500	—
V ERP*	170 – 210	180 – 220	180 – 280	—
SNRT	<1280	<1075	<1600	<1700
CSNRT	—	<275	<550	<650
SACT	—	50 – 200	50 – 150	50 – 250

These values are derived from a variety of papers from different laboratories. The majority of studies were performed in normal or near normal subjects.
* Major variations with cycle length.
A = atrium; AH, HV and PA = anterograde conduction intervals during sinus rhythm; AVN = atrioventricular node; CSNRT = corrected sinus node recovery time; ERP = effective refractory period; SACT = sinoatrial conduction time; SNRT = sinus node recovery time; V = ventricle.

complex geometry of the atria as well as the properties of the atrial myocardium. Thus the PA interval is a measure of the conduction time over the fastest pathway from the high to the low right atrium.

Intranodal conduction

Conduction time through the AV node cannot be measured directly because there is no consistent marker of AV nodal depolarization. The atrio–His (AH) interval reflects AV nodal conduction time and can be measured from the recordings from the electrode positioned near to the AV node–His bundle. The AH interval is measured from the intrinsic deflection of the low right atrial electrogram in that recording to the onset of the His potential. The measurement may also be taken from the onset of the atrial electrogram but this point is dependent on far-field effects which are more obvious at higher gains.

The AH interval is variable. This variability is determined by sympathetic and vagal tone, heart rate and local structural and functional influences. Thus the AH interval is prolonged if vagal tone increases but the effect may be countered by a slowing of heart rate which tends to shorten the AV nodal conduction time. The AH interval changes if the origin of the atrial impulse changes. For example, pacing from the distal coronary sinus will result in a shorter AH interval than when pacing originates from the high right atrium (Fig. 2.10). This does not

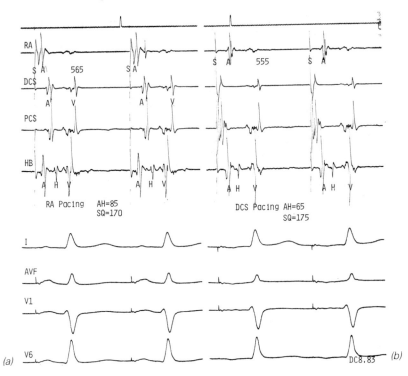

Fig. 2.10 Changes in the AH interval with change of atrial pacing site. During right atrial (RA) pacing (*a*) at a cycle length of 565 msec there is a normal atrial activation pattern (A) and the AH interval is 85 msec. The stimulus (S) to Q (SQ) interval is 170 msec. Pacing from the distal coronary sinus (DCS) at a similar cycle length results in an abnormal atrial activation pattern with delayed right atrial activation (A) in shortening of the AH interval to 65 msec which is not reflected in a change in the SQ interval. This effect is not due to changes in AV nodal conduction time but reflects the altered geometry of the atrial depolarization wavefront which enters the AV node from different sites during right and left atrial pacing. Thus, during left atrial pacing the AV node is activated earlier relative to the low right atrium which is delayed. Paper speed 100 mm/sec. HB = His bundle region; PCS = proximal coronary sinus.

necessarily reflect changes in intranodal conduction (although a different wavefront morphology does alter AV nodal transit time in experimental animal studies) but rather the difference between conduction time from the stimulation site (S) to the low right atrium (LRA) and that to the His bundle:

$$AH = (S–His) - (S–LRA).$$

This is because the low right atrial electrode is activated later during left atrial pacing than during right atrial pacing and the wavefront may enter the AV node without traversing the low right atrium. This source of AH variability should be taken into consideration, especially during drug studies. Similarly, during junctional tachycardias, especially intranodal re-entrant tachycardias (see Chapter 9), the AH interval does not reflect intra-AV nodal conduction time but, rather, the relative activation time of the His bundle compared to the low right atrium.

Intraventricular conduction

Intraventricular conduction is reflected by the HV interval and the QRS duration. The HV interval represents the shortest conduction time from the His bundle to the myocardium over the specialized multifascicular intraventricular conduction system. Thus this interval is not prolonged unless there is conduction delay in *all* the branches of the system or in the His bundle prior to its division. This concept is important in the assessment of AV conduction defects (see Chapter 5). The HV interval is measured from the onset of the His potential to the earliest onset of ventricular activation in any intracardiac or surface ECG lead. The normal value of the HV interval ranges from 35 to 55 msec in adults but is shorter in children. It exhibits no significant variation in the absence of important disease or drug treatment. The QRS duration is the time taken to activate the myocardial mass.

McAnulty et al. (1986) have assessed the reliability of measurement of the AH interval, the HV interval and the His potential duration between one observer and another and for the same observer on two different occasions. They found good intraobserver and interobserver agreement for both the AH and the HV interval measurement but poor agreement in both comparisons for His potential duration. As there is no accepted range of normal values for this measurement, perhaps the result is not surprising.

The QT interval

The QT interval is a measure of the duration of ventricular repolarization. It incorporates the QRS duration. There are no universally accepted criteria for the measurement of this interval. If absolute measurements are required the durations of these intervals should be from the earliest onset in any ECG lead, usually lead II (ideally a simultaneous 12-lead ECG should be used but a minumum of three orthogonal leads is necessary), to the latest offset in any lead, usually an anterior precordial lead. If only changes in the duration of the QT interval are to be assessed (e.g. during a drug study), a single lead showing a clear QT onset and offset will probably suffice, provided that the T wave amplitude and vector are not much changed by the procedure.

These are the basic intervals which can be derived at electrophysiological study. Whether or not it is necessary to measure these intervals at any particular investigation depends upon the clinical and research content of the study. It is important to appreciate, however, that an understanding of these intervals and skills in their accurate measurement are essential in the evaluation and appreciation of the dynamic responses of cardiac conduction tissue to change in heart rate and drug interventions (e.g. estimation of refractory periods, construction of conduction curves, etc.).

Electrophysiological studies using oesophageal catheters

The oesophagus passes immediately posterior to the left atrium and therefore it acts as a natural conduit to the posterior aspect of the heart. Recordings from oesophageal electrodes were used in the early part of this century to investigate the electrocardiographic findings in posterior myocardial infarction and the origin of ventricular premature beats. The method fell into decline as the surface ECG improved and was better understood. It reappeared as a method of discerning hidden atrial activity, especially during tachycardia, and as clinical electrophysiology has developed there has been a resurgence of interest in this non-invasive method for both diagnosis and treatment.

Electrograms from the oesophagus can be recorded using bipolar temporary pacing catheters or purpose-built leads. Permanent bipolar pacing leads are also useful because they are floppy and less likely to cause damage. They are particularly suitable for use in infants and children. The optimal interelectrode distance in adults is about 3–5 cm and in children about 1–2 cm. The lead is introduced like any nasogastric tube. The lubricated catheter can be passed through the nasopharynx with little difficulty. Both atrial and ventricular signals can be detected and recorded on a multichannel recorder (unipolar or bipolar) or on a standard ECG machine by connecting one pole to the chest lead. Specially constructed amplifiers and filters, designed to improve the quality of the signal, are available for use with conventional ECG machines. The advantages of the method include its simplicity, avoidance of intracardiac trauma (especially relevant to studies of anomalous pathway conduction where catheter trauma can alter the properties of the pathway – see above) and general safety.

The lead is gently moved up and down in the oesophagus until a large amplitude atrial signal is recorded. This process is made easier by recording the oesophageal signal together with at least one surface ECG lead. In this way the signals can be timed against the P wave and QRS complexes. Although not a problem during sinus rhythm, timing of the oesophageal electrogram may sometimes be difficult when rapid tachycardias are present.

The lead may also be used for pacing the atria. The lowest threshold for stimulation is usually obtainable at the site of the maximal atrial electrogram and especially at the site of maximum rate of upstroke of the electrogram (dV/dT). Thresholds are in the range of 10–20 mA with a pulse width of 10 msec (cf. direct myocardial thresholds) but many times more with conventional pacing pulse widths of 1–2 msec. High voltage oesophageal stimulation is painful and a special wide pulse width is therefore needed.

The oesophageal recording and pacing method has been usefully applied to a wide variety of clinical electrophysiological problems.

1. The differentiation of ventricular tachycardia from supraventricular tachycardia with wide QRS complexes due to aberration can sometimes be difficult. Atrioventricular dissociation can easily be detected using this method. When 1:1 retrograde VA conduction exists, however, interpretation can be more difficult.
2. Junctional tachycardias can be studied by this method. Oesophageal atrial pacing can be used to initiate and terminate many junctional tachycardias (Fig. 2.11) in the same way as intratrial pacing. Thus, serial drug studies (see Chapter 12) can be performed in this way. The method can also provide some information about the type of junctional tachycardia. A short interval between the QRS and the subsequent A wave (VA interval of less than 70 msec) implies an intranodal re-entrant tachycardia whereas an interval of more than 100

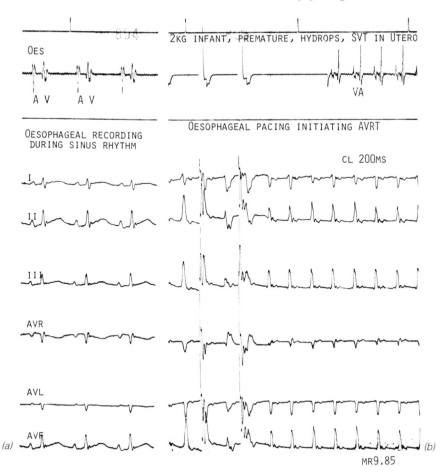

Fig. 2.11 Electrophysiological study using an oesophageal lead (1) to diagnose the arrhythmia and (2) to test the efficacy of drug treatment in a neonate with refractory tachycardia causing hydrops fetalis. During sinus rhythm (*a*) the oesophageal recording shows clearly the atrial (A) and ventricular (V) electrograms. Rapid pacing (*b*) via the oesophageal lead (Oes) initiates tachycardia with a cycle length of 200 msec and a VA interval of 70 msec. After propranolol therapy oesophageal pacing resulted in only short-lived episodes of tachycardia (<3 sec). Paper speed 50 mm/sec.

msec implies an atrioventricular re-entrant tachycardia of the type due to re-entrant anomalous retrograde conduction (see Chapter 9). Termination of tachycardia by transoesophageal atrial pacing can also be used for short-term control of refractory junctional tachycardias (Fig. 2.12).

3. Atrial flutter can usually be terminated by rapid atrial pacing (see Chapter 8). This can also be achieved occasionally by rapid transoesophageal atrial pacing.
4. Atrial fibrillation can be produced by rapid transoesophageal atrial pacing. In patients with the Wolff–Parkinson–White syndrome in whom atrial fibrillation may be a dangerous arrhythmia (see Chapter 6), serial studies

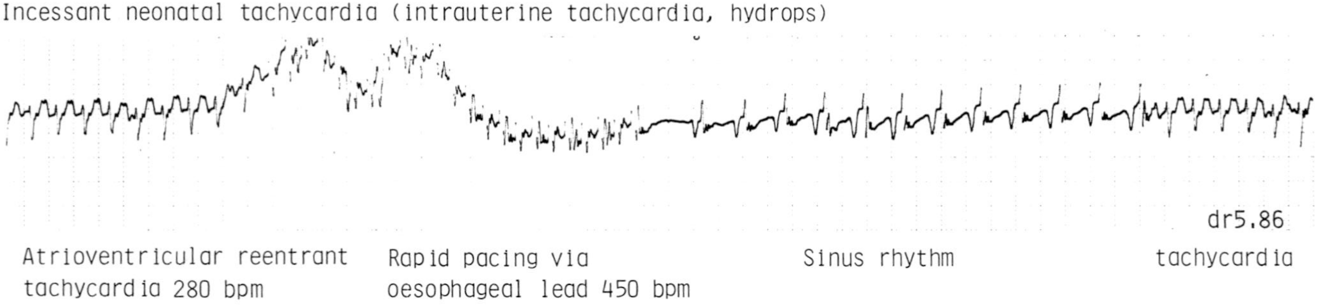

Incessant neonatal tachycardia (intrauterine tachycardia, hydrops)

Atrioventricular reentrant tachycardia 280 bpm

Rapid pacing via oesophageal lead 450 bpm

Sinus rhythm

tachycardia

dr5.86

Fig. 2.12 Oesophageal pacing used to terminate an episode of tachycardia in a neonate.

assessing the effects of different manoeuvres (e.g. exercise, posture) and drugs can be performed with relative ease with transoesophageal atrial pacing at rates of 400–1200 b.p.m.

5. Short-term emergency control of sinus bradycardias by atrial pacing.
6. Emergency control of refractory ventricular arrhythmias associated with the long QT syndrome by increasing the heart rate.
7. Oesophageal pacing and recording can be useful in electrophysiological studies (both diagnostic and therapeutic) in small children.

It is important to appreciate that oesophageal stimulation cannot be used reliably for ventricular pacing.

Monophasic action potential recordings

There has been considerable interest in the use of this method as an adjunct to the conventional electrophysiological recording methods. Monophasic action potentials (MAPs) are injury potentials obtained by direct contact of an electrode with the myocardium. Their shape resembles that of an intracellular transmembrane action potential. They can be recorded from the endocardium using specially constructed electrodes. Recordings can be made using suction electrodes which maintain contact by drawing in a small volume of endocardial cells. The signal therefore represents the combined electrical activity of all the cells within this volume.

Studies of these electrical recordings began in the early part of this century but the emphasis was on the method of recording and physiological information provided by a single recording rather than information from the heart as a whole unit. It was then shown that the duration of these potentials accurately reflected the duration of the intracellular action potential. Interest in the application of suction-electrode MAP recordings to humans began in the 1950s with the studies of effects of drugs and other interventions on the duration of repolarization. A simpler catheter system depending on contact (silver wire) rather than suction has been devised by Miller et al. (1980). The electrogram is the potential difference between the distal 'contact' electrode and a second electrode 2 mm proximal to the first. The signals are filtered between DC and 50–100 Hz and amplified. They can be recorded on a conventional multichannel machine of the type used for conventional electrophysiological recordings.

Recent clinical experimental applications of the MAP method have included:

1. Investigation of drug-induced effects on repolarization.
2. Investigation of time-dependent characteristics of repolarization (see Fig. 3.1 and Chapter 3).
3. Detection of endocardial ischaemia.
4. Detection of inhomogeneities of repolarization, especially in patients with the long QT syndrome (Fig. 2.13).
5. Detection of afterdepolarizations in prolonged repolarization syndromes.
6. Stability of repolarization at the onset of ventricular tachycardia.

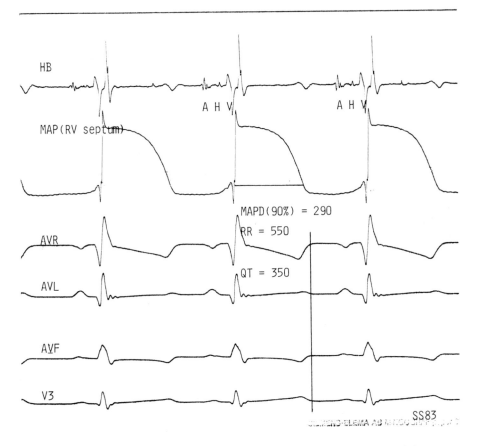

Fig. 2.13 Use of the monophasic action potential catheter in a patient with congenital prolongation of the QT interval and deafness. The silver–silver chloride electrode is mounted in a standard woven Dacron catheter and no suction is required. The monophasic action potential (MAP) is clearly inscribed. The catheter can be used to investigate local repolarization at various different locations. The duration of the monophasic action potential when the amplitude is 10 per cent from the baseline (MAPD 90) is 290 msec. Paper speed 100 mm/sec.

Non-invasive recording of intracardiac conduction intervals

High-resolution signal-averaged surface ECG recordings have become readily available through rapid advances in recording and processing technology in

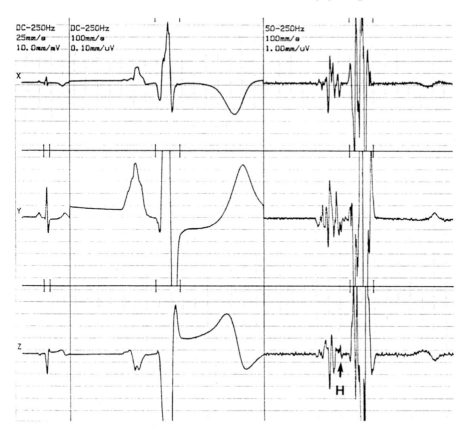

Fig. 2.14 Non-invasive recordings of the His potential (arrowed) using signal-averaged high-resolution electrocardiography. The XYZ orthogonal lead configuration was used in this example. The left panel shows the conventional ECG recording. The centre panel is recorded at higher gain (0.10 mm/μV) and at 100 mm/sec. The right panel is a greatly amplified recording (1.0 mm/μV) and the high-pass filter is set at 50 Hz. The His potential is most clearly inscribed in the highly amplified Z lead, illustrating an advantage of an orthogonal system of recording. The HV interval is normal at 40 msec. The filtering, paper speed and amplification of each recording are shown in the upper part of each panel.

recent years. These electrocardiograms are obtained by recording and averaging a large number of beats to remove random noise and amplifying the recording too observe periodic events (e.g. the His potential as in Fig. 2.14). The applications of the technique (Hombach et al., 1982) include:

1. Recording of sinus node activity.
2. Recording of AV nodal potentials.
3. Recording of His bundle potentials.
4. Recording of late potentials in the QRS complex (see Chapter 10).

The reproducibility of sinus node and AV nodal electrical activity using this method is poor and these applications of high resolution electrocardiography have not been widely utilized. Furthermore, there has been no adequate validation of these surface potentials. Surface His bundle potentials can be obtained in about 70 per cent of recordings. Background noise and atrial overlap may obscure the His spike. Atrioventricular blocking agents or atrial (oesophageal) pacing can be used to prolong the AH interval to overcome atrial overlap in some instances. The HV interval can thus be obtained non-invasively. However, because this information is of little clinical value in the assessment of AV conduction (see Chapter 5), the method has yet to find a clinically useful application. Areas of potential value may be: (1) assessment of antiarrhythmic drug effects; and (2) non-invasive evaluation of AV conduction in infants and children with postoperative conduction defects (Ward et al., 1984). The investigation of late potentials in the QRS complex has been more fruitful (see Chapter 10).

References and further reading

Akhtar M, Damanto, AN, Gilbert-Leeds CJ, Batsford WP, Reddy CP, Gomes JA, Calon AH, Dhatt MS. (1977) Induction of iatrogenic electrocardiographic patterns during electrophysiologic studies. *Circulation* 56, 60

Ahktar M, Fisher JD, Gillette PC, Josephson ME, Prystowsky EN, Ruskin JN, Saksena S, Scheinman MM, Waldo AL, Zipes DP. (1985) NASPE ad hoc committee on guidelines for cardiac electrophysiological studies. *Pacing and Clinical Electrophysiology* 8, 611

American Heart Association. (1980) Standards and guidelines for cardiopulmonary resuscitation and emergency cardiac care. *Journal of the American Medical Association* 244, 453

Anderson JL, Mason JW. (1986) Criteria for selection of patients for programmed electrical stimulation. *Circulation* 73, suppl. 119, II–50

Benson DW, Dunnigan A, Benditt DG, Pritzker MR, Thompson TR. (1983). Transesophageal study of infant supraventricular tachycardia: electrophysiologic characteristics. *American Journal of Cardiology* 52, 1002

Benson DW, Sanford M, Dunnigan A, Benditt DG. (1984) Transesophageal pacing threshold: role of interelectrode spacing, pulse width and catheter insertion depth. *American Journal of Cardiology* 53, 63

Binkley PF, Bush CA, Fleishman BL, Leier CV. (1986) In vivo validation of the origin of the esophageal electrogram. *Journal of the American College of Cardiology* 7, 813

Bonatti V, Rolli A, Botti G. (1983) Recording of monophasic action potentials of the right ventricle in the long QT syndrome complicated by severe ventricular arrhythmias. *European Heart Journal* 4, 168

Campbell RWF, Gardiner P, Amos PA, Chadwick D, Jordan RS. (1985) Measurement of the QT interval. *European Heart Journal* 6, suppl. D, 81

Curry PVL, Rowland E, Fox KM, Krikler DM. (1978) The relationship between posture, blood pressure and electrophysiological properties in patients with paroxysmal supraventricular tachycardia. *Archives des Maladies du Coeur* 71, 293

Ferguson D, Saksena S, Greenberg E, Craelius W. (1984) Management of recurrent ventricular tachycardia: economic impact of therapeutic alternatives. *American Journal of Cardiology* 53, 531

Franz M. (1983) Long-term recording of monophasic action potentials from human endocardium. *American Journal of Cardiology* 51, 1629

Franz M, Flaherty JT, Platia EV, Bulkley BH, Weisfeldt ML. (1984) Localization of myocardial ischemia by recording of monophasic action potentials. *Circulation* **69**, 593

Gallagher JJ, Smith WM, Kasell J, Smith WM, Grant AO, Benson DW. (1980) Use of esophageal leads in the diagnosis of reciprocating supraventricular tachycardia. *Pacing and Clinical Electrophysiology* **3**, 336

Gallagher JJ, Smith WM, Kerr CR, Kassell J, Cook L, Reiter M, Sterba R, Harte M. (1982) Esophageal pacing: a diagnostic and therapeutic tool. *Circulation* **65**, 336

Grossman W. (1986 (New Edition)) *Cardiac Catheterization and Angiography*. Kimpton: London

Hamill SC, Pritchett ELC, Klein GJ, Gallagher JJ. (1981) A comparison of clinical electrophysiological studies in different institutions. *American Heart Journal* **101**, 263

Hammill SC, Holmes DR, Wood DL, Osborn MJ, McLaren C, Sugure DD, Gersh BJ. (1984) Electrophysiologic testing in the upright position: improved evaluation of patients with rhythm disturbances using a tilt table. *Journal of the American College of Cardiology* **4**, 65

Hombach V, Braun V, Hopp HW, Gil-Sanchez D, Scholl H, Behrenbeck DW, Tauchert M, Hilger HH. (1982) The applicability of the signal averaging technique in clinical cardiology. *Clinical Cardiology* **5**, 107

Horowitz L. (1986) Safety of electrophysiologic studies. *Circulation* **73**, suppl. II, 28

Josephson ME, Seides SF. (1979) *Clinical Cardiac Electrophysiology: techniques and interpretations*. Lea & Febiger: Philadelphia, Pa

McAnulty JH, Nichol P, Morris C, Nichol L, Rahimtoola S. (1986) Measurement of the AH and HV interval and His bundle duration: interobserver and intraobserver variation. *American Journal of Cardiology* **57**, 970

Miller GAH, Noble MIM, Papadoyannis D, Pidgeon J, Seed WA. (1980) A catheter-tip method for recording monophasic action potentials from the canine or human endocardium. *Journal of Physiology* **305**, 7–8P

Narula OS. (1975). *His Bundle Electrocardiography and Clinical Electrophysiology*. FA Davis: Philadelphia, Pa

Nattel S, Rinkenberger RL, Lehrman LL, Zipes DP. (1979) Therapeutic blood concentrations after local anesthesia for cardiac electrophysiologic studies. *New England Journal of Medicine* **301**, 418

Nishimura M, Katoh, T, Hanai S, Watanabe Y. (1986) Optimal mode of transesophageal atrial pacing. *American Journal of Cardiology* **57**, 791

Prystowsky EN, Pritchett ELC, Gallagher JJ. (1980) Origin of the atrial electrogram recorded from the esophagus. *Circulation* **61**, 1017

Ross DL, Farré J, Bar FWHM, Vanagt EJ, Dassen WRM, Weiner I, Wellens HJJ. (1980) Comprehensive clinical electrophysiologic studies in the investigation of documented or suspected tachycardias. Time, staff, problems and costs. *Circulation* **61**, 1010

Saksena S. (1985) Electrophysiological evaluation for recurrent tachycardias: a financially endangered technique. *International Journal of Cardiology* **7**, 431

Schnittger I, Rodriguez IM, Winkle R. (1986) Esophageal electrocardiography: new technology revives an old technique. *American Journal of Cardiology* **57**, 604

Shabetai R, Surawicz B, Hammill W. (1968) Monophasic action potentials in man. *Circulation* **38**, 341

Ward DE, Camm AJ. (1980) Methodologic problems in the use of atrial pacing studies for the assessment of AV conduction. *Clinical Cardiology* **3**, 155

Ward DE, Makinen L, Carter S, Shinebourne EA. (1984) Signal-averaged electrocardiography in infants and children with congenital heart disease. *International Journal of Cardiology* **6**, 699

3

Conduction Dynamics and Refractory Periods

Clinical electrophysiology of cardiac tissue

Decremental and non-decremental conduction

The basis of many electrophysiological deductions is the distinction between so-called decremental and non-decremental conduction characteristics (Table 3.1). Normal atrial myocardium and ventricular myocardium respond to stimulation by conduction at a velocity which changes very little if the rate of stimulation is changed. With very rapid large changes in rate (e.g. a very short RR interval preceded by a series of much longer ones) there may be some slowing of intramyocardial conduction and disorganized conduction spread as shown by recordings of fragmentation and delay of the propagated response. Similarly, the conduction velocity of the intraventricular conduction system in the absence of disease does not change significantly with changes in stimulation frequency. This type of response may be described as non-decremental. Another cardiac tissue which possesses this property in its usual manifestations is that which is found in anomalous atrioventricular conduction pathways of the type seen in the Wolff–Parkinson–White syndrome (see Chapter 6). Decremental conduction properties are most obviously manifest by the AV node. In response to higher frequences of stimulation the AH interval gradually increases until AV block occurs, usually in the form of second degree Mobitz type I block (Wenckebach pattern). Thus, conduction velocity decreases as rate of stimulation increases. Some types of anomalous pathway may also demonstrate decremental characteristics (see Chapter 9).

The clinical view of 'decremental' AV nodal conduction is almost certainly an oversimplification and, possibly, not entirely accurate. Rosenblueth (1958) suggested an alternative explanation for decremental conduction. He proposed that conduction delay occurred at a single refractory barrier within the node rather than throughout an extensive region with homogeneous properties. Thus, during AV nodal Wenckebach periods, it is proposed that the single-step delay progressively increases and block occurs when the effective refractory period (see later in this chapter) of distal tissue exceeds the coupling interval of the input to the barrier. This hypothesis contrasts with the classic view in which impulses are progressively delayed until propagation fails completely. The Rosenblueth model explains many of the AV nodal conduction phenomena seen in humans (Young et al., 1986a, b). It may also account for decremental phenomena in tissue not typically possessing this property; for example, anomalous pathways.

A physiological basis for Rosenblueth's hypothesis in the intact AV node has

Table 3.1 ELECTROPHYSIOLOGICAL CHARACTERISTICS OF DECREMENTAL VERSUS NON-DECREMENTAL TISSUE

	Decremental	Non-decremental
Conduction velocity	Slow	Fast
Response to premature stimulation	Delay	No delay
Dependence of refractory period on cycle length	Inverse	Direct
Dependence of conduction velocity on cycle length	Inverse	None
Form of conduction block	Mobitz I	Mobitz II
Concealed conduction	Easily demonstrated	Not easily demonstrated
Drug sensitivity	Verapamil Adenosine	Ajmaline Other class 1C agents

not been clearly demonstrated. The phenomenon may be modelled by representing the AV node as a matrix of elements (each of a certain refractory period) each connected to its four neighbouring elements, with a single element in the centre of the matrix whose refractory period is much shorter than the others. An essential property of this model is 'anisotropic' conduction (conduction between neighbouring elements in the transverse direction is much slower than in the longitudinal direction; see Chapter 7).

Recovery of excitability

Recovery of excitability is also frequency dependent. In tissues exhibiting decremental conduction characteristics, recovery of excitability is prolonged at higher rates of stimulation. The opposite is true for tissue showing non-decremental conduction (e.g. ventricular myocardium; Fig. 3.1). Thus the effective refractory period (see later in this chapter) of the atrial myocardium shortens gradually as the frequency of stimulation at which it is estimated is increased.

The AV node appears to behave in the opposite manner; that is, refractoriness increases as frequency of the drive is increased. This classic view of the AV node has been challenged by Young et al (1986b). Using the Rosenblueth hypothesis (see above) of a single AV nodal refractory barrier, Young and colleagues derived an index of refractoriness at the single barrier which is directly (rather than inversely) related to drive cycle length. The study was based on data derived from children in whom it is known that conventional measures of AV nodal refractoriness (e.g. effective refractory period) may shorten with increased rates (DuBrow et al., 1975). However, whereas this relationship was variable in the children in their study, the modified index of refractoriness bore a direct relationship to drive cycle length in all cases.

The characteristic decremental conduction properties exhibited by the AV node may be regarded teleologically as those which might be expected of a filter.

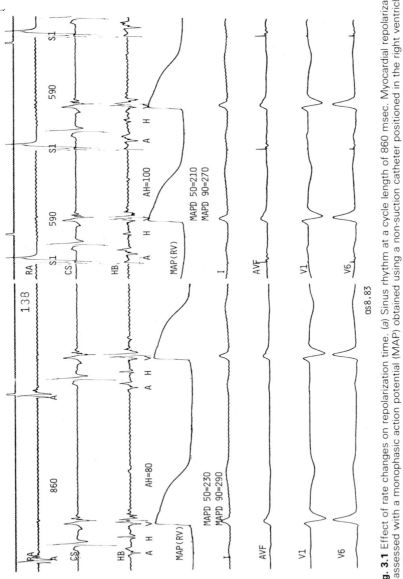

Fig. 3.1 Effect of rate changes on repolarization time. (a) Sinus rhythm at a cycle length of 860 msec. Myocardial repolarization is assessed with a monophasic action potential (MAP) obtained using a non-suction catheter positioned in the right ventricle (RV). The duration of the MAP measured at 50 and 90 per cent of full repolarization is 230 and 290 msec, respectively. Several minutes after the pacing rate has been increased, the MAPD is shortened. This reflects the normal reduction in myocardial repolarization time when rate is increased. Paper speed 100 mm/sec; CS =coronary sinus; RA = right atrium.

This filtering mechanism is a property of specialized cells in the mid-nodal (NH) region.

Although healthy myocardial conduction tissue does not show decremental properties, they may appear in the presence of disease which reduces the transmembrane potential. This effect is especially important in the production of slowed conduction necessary for the initiation of re-entrant arrhythmias (see Chapter 7).

Stimulation protocols

Using pacing techniques the heart rate may be controlled in a predictable manner. Thus it is possible to estimate the effect of controlled changes in rate on conduction and recovery characteristics of excitable tissue. The pacing methods most commonly employed for this purpose are:

1. Incremental pacing.
2. Extrastimulation methods:
   (a) isolated extrastimulation;
   (b) pacing combined with extrastimulation.

These pacing sequences (protocols) may be used at the atrial level to assess anterograde (from atrium to ventricle) conduction characteristics or at ventricular level to assess retrograde (from ventricle to atrium) conduction. There are various modifications of these protocols which are discussed in their relevant context in later chapters.

Incremental pacing

Incremental pacing consists of stimulating a particular site and observing the rate-dependent changes in the conduction intervals and the myocardial response. The endpoint of this type of study is usually the development of conduction delay or block. During atrial pacing at progressively faster rates (either stepwise increases or a gradual increase or 'ramp') there is very little myocardial delay (the PA interval remains unchanged) but AV nodal conduction delay is indicated by a gradually increasing AH interval (Fig. 3.2) until second degree Mobitz type I or II AV block occurs. The degree to which the AH interval increases and the point at which AV block develops (Wenckebach point) are determined by a variety of factors. These include autonomic influences, rate of change of stimulation frequency, local structural and physiological factors within the AV node and the presence of junctional pathways (within or anatomically closely associated with the AV node) which possess attenuated decremental conduction properties and therefore conceal the normal AH delay (Fig. 3.3). This type of response is usually associated with a higher Wenckebach point and shortened AV nodal refractory periods. (Rather confusingly, some investigators have recently introduced the term 'decremental pacing' to describe progressive decreases of the cycle length of pacing. We prefer the term 'incremental' in this setting to distinguish the investigational protocol from some pacing modes of tachycardia termination.)

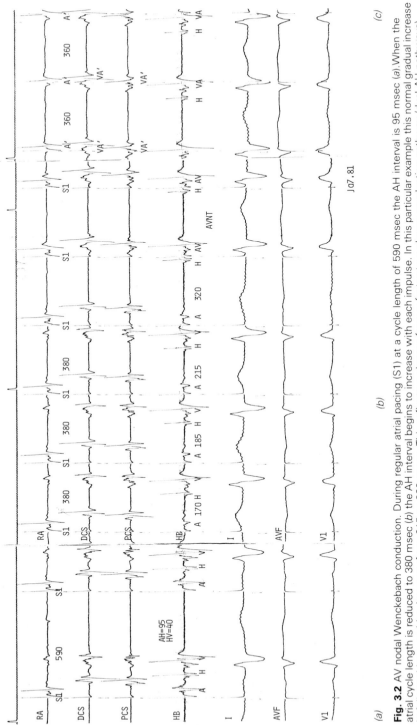

Fig. 3.2 AV nodal Wenckebach conduction. During regular atrial pacing (S1) at a cycle length of 590 msec the AH interval is 95 msec (a). When the atrial cycle length is reduced to 380 msec (b) the AH interval begins to increase with each impulse. In this particular example this normal gradual increase is followed by a sudden increase from 215 to 320 msec. This reflects a change from a faster to a slower conduction pathway (dual AH pathways). Coincident with this is the initiation of AV nodal re-entrant tachycardia (AVNT) with a change in atrial activation (A') shown more clearly in (c) (see Chapter 9). Paper speed 100 mm/sec. DCS = distal coronary sinus; HB = His bundle; PCS = proximal coronary sinus; RA = right atrium.

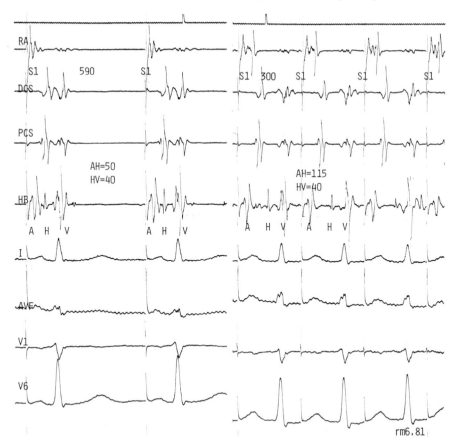

Fig. 3.3 Response of the AV node to incremental right atrial pacing (S1S1) in a patient with the Lown–Ganong–Levine syndrome. The AH interval during sinus rhythm (cycle length 690 msec) was 50 msec. Atrial pacing at a cycle length of 590 msec caused no change in the AH intervaL. At a cycle length of 300 msec the AH interval increased to 115 msec. Wenckebach AH conduction was induced at a cycle length of 235 msec. Paper speed 100 mm/sec. HB = His bundle; PCS = proximal coronary sinus; RA = right atrium.

Extrastimulation methods

Extrastimulation techniques are used to examine dynamic conduction characteristics in a controlled manner. Thus, using a specified pacing protocol, it is possible to examine the response of the stimulated tissue by plotting a graph of the response interval against the stimulation interval. From such a graph it is possible to derive refractory periods.

Isolated extrastimulation (Fig. 3.4)

The technique of isolated extrastimulation involves the repeated introduction of single stimulus during the patient's intrinsic rhythm—usually sinus rhythm. The

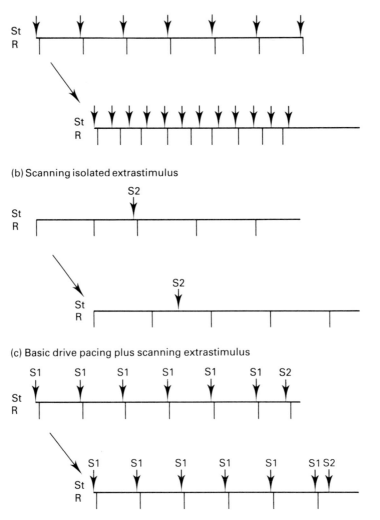

(a) Incremental pacing

(b) Scanning isolated extrastimulus

(c) Basic drive pacing plus scanning extrastimulus

Fig. 3.4 Schematic diagram of pacing protocols used at electrophysiological study. In each diagram the upper level shows the stimulus (St) and the lower level the response (R). (a) Incremental pacing. The pacing rate is increased until block develops. (b), An isolated extrastimulus (S2); the coupling interval is reduced until block develops. (c) extrastimulus (S2) delivered after a train of regular pacing (S1). The extrastimulus coupling interval (S1S2) is reduced until block develops.

sensing amplifiers are used to detect incoming signals during sinus rhythm – or any intrinsic rhythm – and the timing of extrastimulation is coupled to the sensed event. The method is useful in the estimation of sinoatrial conduction (see Chapter 4), tachycardia initiation and termination, and the study of tachycardias by extrastimulus methods (see Chapters 7, 8, 9 and 10).

Pacing and extrastimulation (Fig. 3.4)

Because conduction time and refractory periods are frequency dependent (especially in the AV node), small variations in the sinus cycle length may introduce variations in these measurements. If the heart rate is controlled by regular pacing sequences (referred to as the 'basic drive'), these variations are prevented. The technique of pacing combined with extrastimulation is therefore most suitable for the investigation of conduction properties. It is also important in the investigation of tachycardias because the conduction delay induced by, for example, extrastimulation is a necessary requirement for the initiation of 're-entrant excitation' (see Chapter 9).

In the extrastimulus method, a premature stimulus is introduced after a regular sequence of paced beats. With each successive sequence the interval between the last paced impulse (S1) and the premature stimulus (S2, which is referred to as the 'test' stimulus) is gradually reduced in small decrements of 10–50 msec. The response to the decreasing coupling interval (S1S2) of the test stimulus is best demonstrated in the form of a conduction curve (see below).

Refractory periods

Refractoriness is a measure of the inability of depolarized tissue to be re-excited by premature stimulation. The concept of refractoriness in the intact heart where several cells are stimulated together, and where recordings of the response to stimulation are made at some distance from the point of stimulation, must be distinguished from refractoriness of individual cells where stimulation and recording are made within the same cell and the element of propagation of an impulse from one cell or group of cells to another is absent. Thus, clinical refractoriness applies to propagated responses. In the clinical setting three measures of refractoriness are commonly used:

1. The effective refractory period.
2. The functional refractory period.
3. The relative refractory period.

The derivation of these measurements in relation to the AV node is shown in the anterograde conduction curve illustrated in Fig. 3.5. Because conduction times and refractory periods are rate dependent, the basic drive cycle length at which they are estimated must be stated. In clinical practice refractory periods are derived if possible (i.e. if the intrinsic sinus rate is less than 100 b.p.m.) at a drive cycle of 600 msec (100 b.p.m.) and at one or more higher rates.

The effective refractory period (ERP)

This is a measure of the inability of excited tissue to respond to early restimulation by a premature stimulus and is defined as 'the longest coupling interval of the input stimulus which does not produce a propagated response'. Thus, the ERP of the atrial myocardium is the longest coupling interval of the input stimulus (S1S2) which does not result in a propagated atrial response as evidenced by the absence of a local atrial electrogram at a nearby recording site (Fig. 3.6). The ERP

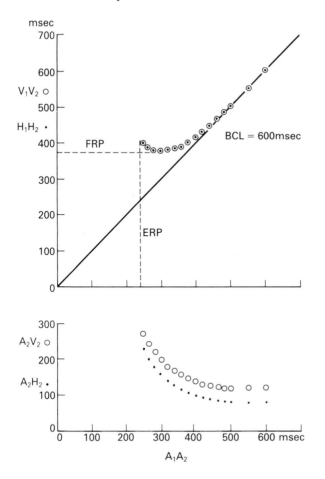

Fig. 3.5 Anterograde AV conduction curve. Conduction curves are devices which depict graphically the response of cardiac conduction tissue to stimulation (whether spontaneous or induced.). As the coupling interval of the test stimulus (A1A2) is reduced the AV nodal conduction time (AH interval) prolongs. Therefore, the H1H2 interval exceeds the A1A2 interval (above the line of identity). The typical curve is described as 'hockey-stick' in shape. The effective refractory period (ERP) and functional refractory period (FRP) of the AV node are indicated. The relative refractory period is the longest coupling interval (A1A2) at which the H1H2 interval exceeds the A1A2 interval. The ERP and FRP are also related to basic cycle length (BCL).

Fig. 3.6 Estimation of the atrial effective refractory period (AERP). After a regular right atrial pacing sequence (S1S2) at a cycle length of 470 msec 'test' atrial extrastimulus (S2) is introduced at gradually decreasing S1S2 intervals. (*a*) Some fragmentation and delay of the atrial electrogram (A) after S2. The atrial functional refractory period (FRP) was estimated at 210 msec. The test stimulus propagates through the AV node to the ventricles. (*b*) The test stimulus is introduced 10 msec earlier and atrial capture is not achieved. Thus the AERP is 170 msec and the AV nodal ERP cannot be estimated but is less than the atrial FRP. Paper speed 100 mm/sec.

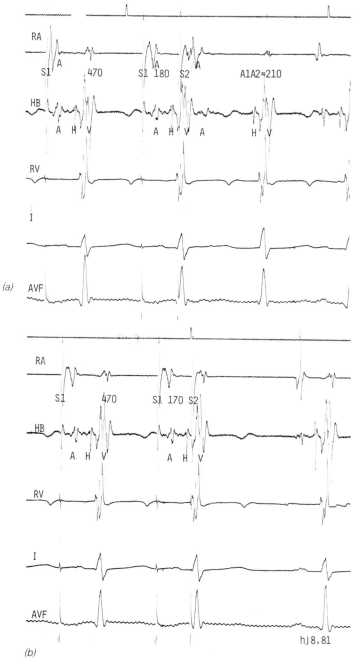

(a)

(b)

hj8.81

of the AV node is the longest interval between successive inputs which does not result in conduction to the His bundle. The low right atrial signal on the His bundle recording is taken as the input to the AV node. Thus the ERP of the AV node is the longest A1A2 interval which blocks above the His bundle within the AV node. The ERP of other tissues (ventricular myocardium, anomalous pathways, etc.) are defined by analogous statements.

It is evident from these definitions that the site of stimulation of excitation and the site of detecting the propagated response should be as close as possible to the structure or tissue whose refractoriness is being studied. Remote sites will not allow any account to be taken of conduction delay between the site of excitation and the structure under investigation. Thus, marked conduction delays between the site of stimulation in the high right atrium and the AV node will lead to a falsely short estimation of the AV nodal ERP unless these delays are accounted for by measuring the input coupling interval (A1A2) in the low right atrium.

The functional refractory period (FRP)

This is a measure of the ability of tissue to propagate repeated impulses and is defined as the shortest interval between propagated or conducted responses to any input interval. For example, the FRP of the AV node is the shortest interval between successive His depolarizations (H1H2) in response to any A1A2 interval (measured from the low right atrial recording on the His bundle channel). By definition the FRP of a structure (e.g. the AV node) exceeds the ERP (even in the absence of conduction delay) unless there is supernormal conduction. A small or no excess is characteristic of non-decremental conduction. A large excess is characteristic of decremental conduction, as in the case of the AV node itself. The FRP of the atrial myocardium is the shortest A1A2 interval in response to any S1S2 interval. The value of the FRP of a plane of tissue (as opposed to a specific pathway such as the AV node) depends on the site of stimulation and recording, which must therefore be specified. The atrial FRP is usually determined by high right atrial stimulation and low right atrial recording.

Simson et al. (1979) have pointed out that the FRP does not provide the same information about refractoriness as the ERP. The clinical definition of the FRP implies stable conduction of the basic drive beats (S1) and relative delay of test beats (S2). The FRP is inversely related to the conduction time of the control beats. In relation to the AV node, increasing the basic drive rate increases the control conduction time. Thus the ERP of the AV node may increase while the FRP decreases with a shortening of the drive cycle. If the FRP of the AV node is defined as the minimum output interval H1H2, it follows that increasing delay of H1 not paralleled by H2 results in a diminution of the H1H2 intervals and the FRP. This is precisely what happens during 'typical' AV nodal Wenckebach periods when the increment in the AH interval (and therefore the HH interval) decreases, causing progressive shortening of the RR interval.

The relative refractory period (RRP)

This is defined as the coupling interval of an input stimulus at which additional conduction delay emerges (i.e. when the output interval begins to exceed the input interval). For example, the RRP of the AV node is defined as the atrial coupling interval (A1A2 on the low right atrial recording) at which the interval between corresponding His spikes (H1H2) exceeds the A1A2 interval (see Fig. 3.5).

Clearly, in a complex conduction system comprising several sequentially arranged components the precise response to stimulation of the system as a whole unit will depend on the relationship between the effective and the functional refractory periods of one component and the next. Thus, if the ERP of the atrium exceeds that of the AV node, conduction cannot continue and the ERP of the AV node cannot be estimated. Similarly, if there is conduction delay within the atrium such that the atrial FRP always exceeds the AV nodal ERP, conduction through the AV node will always occur and the ERP of the AV node cannot be estimated. Usually, however, the FRP of the atrium is less than the ERP of the AV node. These interactions between components of the conduction system are important in the investigation of refractoriness of the intraventricular conduction system. Phenomena arising from longitudinal interaction of various components include distal block, aberrant conduction, 'gaps' in AV conduction and apparent 'supernormal' conduction. An example of interaction in parallel is 'dual pathways'. In one remarkable case (Ward, 1982), functional (phase 3 block) right or left bundle branch delay, type 1 gap phenomenon and dual AV nodal pathways were all manifest spontaneously during the complex interaction of sinus and junctional escape rhythms!

Functional distal block

The decremental properties of the AV node are such that the FRP of the AV node is almost always greater than the ERP of the His bundle and intraventricular conduction system. If atrial premature stimulation results in HV prolongation, 'relative' His–Purkinje refractoriness is said to exist. If the ERP of the His bundle is in excess of the FRP of the AV node, block occurs within or below the His bundle. This finding is extremely uncommon in patients with normal AV conduction. This response is more common in those with distal conduction system disease (see Chapter 5). In patients with enhanced AV nodal conduction the FRP of the AV node may be very short and can be exceeded by the refractoriness of the distal conduction system, thus causing infranodal block or delay. This effect may also be produced by lengthening the refractoriness of the distal tissue by using a long cycle prior to the test cycle (so-called long–short cycle testing; Fig. 3.7). The basis for this type of block is arrival of the impulse during the refractory period of distal tissue, in this example, the right or left bundle branch). The term 'phase 3 block' has been used to describe this and similar phenomena, because the impulse is blocked by tissue in the rapid repolarization phase (phase 3) of the action potential (see Fig. 7.1). One of the many possible consequences of these interplays in the conduction system is aberrant conduction.

Aberrant conduction

This phenomenon has been most extensively studied in relation to intraventricular conduction. The term describes the appearance of

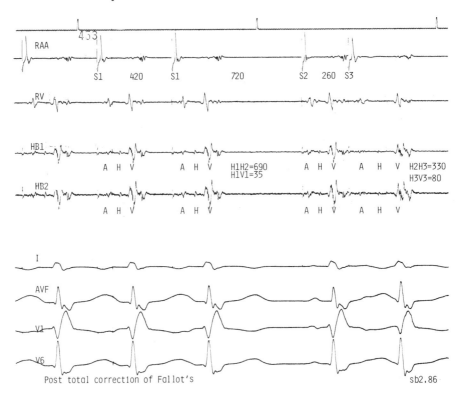

Fig. 3.7 Prolongation of intraventricular conduction time (HV interval) in response to atrial stimulation. This patient had had total correction of Fallot's tetralogy and presented with dizzy spells. At electrophysiological study atrial pacing (S1S1) at various rates did not induce any HV prolongation (HV = 35 msec). Atrial premature stimuli alone also conducted normally. However, when the pretest cycle (S1S2) was increased, thereby increasing intraventricular refractoriness, the test beat (S3) conducted with HV prolongation (HV = 80 msec). Paper speed 100 mm/sec. HB = His bundle; RAA = right atrial appendage; RV = right ventricle.

intraventricular conduction delay in response to a change in the cycle length of a supraventricular impulse. A classic example of functional bundle branch delay is the Gouaux–Ashman phenomenon during atrial fibrillation in which an impulse terminating a short ventricular cycle, which was preceded by a long ventricular cycle, conducts with a bundle branch block pattern (usually right bundle branch block).

Functional bundle branch block is common during sustained, regular supraventricular tachycardias of all types. The mechanism of sustained functional or aberrant bundle branch conduction was first described by Moe et al. (1965) in dogs, and later demonstrated in humans by Wellens and Durrer (1968). The initial bundle branch block is caused by supraventricular impulses reaching the His–Purkinje system before complete recovery (phase 3 block). Aberration is sustained by repetitive retrograde concealed conduction into the bundle branch. It can be removed by ventricular (and occasionally atrial) premature stimulation during tachycardia. This disturbs the critical timing necessary for the concealed conduction to be perpetuated and anterograde conduction is restored. Left bundle branch aberrant conduction is more easily initiated by right ventricular stimulation than right atrial stimulation because the retrograde refractory period of the left bundle is shorter than that of the right, allowing retrograde left bundle branch conduction which impairs subsequent anterograde conduction (Wellens et al., 1985).

Delay and block may also be dependent upon the development of slowed heart rates and are referred to as 'bradycardia-dependent block'. The mechanism of this type of block is thought to be due to a decrease in the resting diastolic potential due to spontaneous diastolic depolarization (phase 4 depolarization). Bradycardia-dependent bundle branch block and exit block from an ectopic focus are possible clinical manifestations of 'phase 4 block'.

Gap phenomena

Another consequence of interplay between proximal and distal conduction and refractoriness is the so-called 'gap phenomenon'. The term 'gap' refers to a gap in a formally constructed conduction curve; that is, a range of coupling intervals for which there is no response bracketed by zones of intact conduction. Gaps in conduction occur when distal refractoriness prevents conduction at longer coupling intervals. When proximal conduction delay at very short input coupling intervals allows distal refractoriness to be exceeded, block is relieved, conduction resumes and the gap is defined (Fig. 3.8).

Several different types of gaps have been described. The first classification devised by Gallagher et al. (1973) into types 1 and 2 was subsequently expanded by Damato and colleagues (1976), and is summarized in Table 3.2. The classification is based on the site of initial block and the mechanism of relief of conduction block. The most common type of gap has been mentioned above; if the FRP of the AV node is less than the ERP of the His bundle, block will occur. If the ERP of the AV node is sufficiently short allowing continued AV nodal conduction), distal conduction will resume when AV nodal delay increases such

Table 3.2 CLASSIFICATION OF GAP PHENOMENA

Type	Direction	Site of proximal delay	Site of distal block
1	Anterograde	AV node	His–Purkinje system
2	Anterograde	Proximal His–Purkinje system	Distal His–Purkinje system
3	Anterograde	His bundle	His–Purkinje system
4	Anterograde	Atrium His–Purkinje system	AV node or
5	Anterograde	Proximal AV node	Distal AV node
6	Anterograde	AV node (enhanced AV conduction)	His–Purkinje
1	Retrograde	His–Purkinje system	AV node
2	Retrograde	Distal His–Purkinje system	Proximal His–Purkinje system

Modified from Damato et al. (1976).

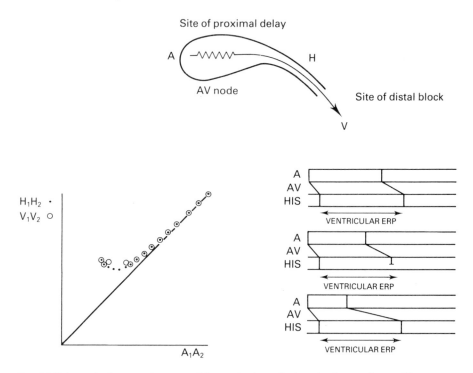

Fig. 3.8 Schematic diagram of one possible mechanism of a type I anterograde gap. The upper diagram of the AV node indicates the sites of proximal delay and distal block. The ladder diagrams show how further delay in AV nodal conduction allows distal tissue (the His–Purkinje system or ventricular myocardium) to recover. The typical anterograde conduction curve is shown on the left.

that the H1H2 interval exceeds the ERP of distal tissue (type 1 gap). Although rare, a gap in AV conduction can be produced by the interplay between fast and slow AV nodal pathways (Fig. 3.9). Conduction gaps may occur in the anterograde or retrograde direction. In the presence of anterogradely or retrogradely functioning anomalous atrioventricular pathways, gaps in AV or VA conduction in the normal conduction system may be concealed.

Dual pathways

Complex conduction patterns may also occur if two conduction pathways act in parallel. The phenomena resulting from such an interaction are best illustrated by referring to the duality of AV nodal conduction. The AV node is a complex network of specialized cells providing a substrate for numerous potential conduction pathways from the atria to the penetrating bundle of His. In most subjects there is a single dominant pathway. However, on occasions, two or more such potential pathways may be manifest either spontaneously or during the extrastimulus method. The two pathways are revealed only if the conduction times within the pathways are discernibly different. Sudden spontaneous changes

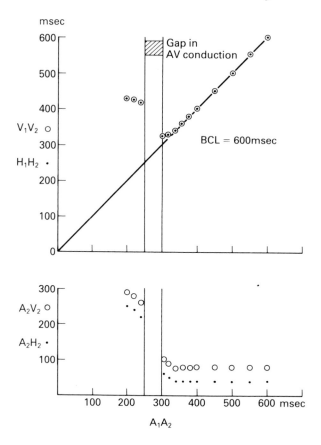

Fig. 3.9 Graphical representation (anterograde conduction curve) of a gap in AV conduction in a patient with the Lown–Ganong–Levine syndrome. As the coupling interval of the test beat (A1A2) is reduced there is attenuated prolongation of the AH interval such that the short H1H2 interval results in infranodal conduction block. Conduction resumes with shorter A1A2 intervals because of refractoriness in the fast pathway and a sudden jump in the AH interval (and therefore the H1H2 interval) due to continued conduction in a slow pathway. BCL = basic cycle length.

in the PR interval (Fig. 3.10) reflect change of conduction from one pathway to the other. Such events are rarely observed. They are, however, frequently seen in the setting of formal anterograde conduction studies using the extrastimulus test. Let us suppose that the faster of the two pathways has the longer ERP. Thus, when the coupling interval of A1A2 is less than the ERP of the faster pathway, this pathway fails to sustain conduction. Because the slower pathway has the shorter ERP, it continues to conduct but, since the conduction time is slower, there is a sudden increase in the AH interval at this point.

From the anterograde conduction curve shown in Fig. 3.11, it is easy to appreciate the dynamic concept of dual AV nodal pathways. It may also be seen that the effective and functional refractory periods of these pathways can be

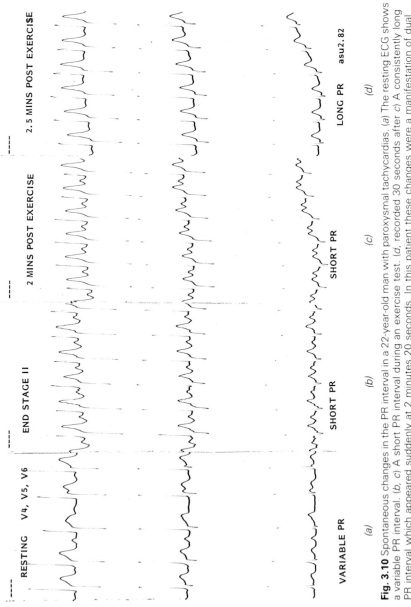

Fig. 3.10 Spontaneous changes in the PR interval in a 22-year-old man with paroxysmal tachycardias. (a) The resting ECG shows a variable PR interval. (b, c) A short PR interval during an exercise test. (d, recorded 30 seconds after c) A consistently long PR interval which appeared suddenly at 2 minutes 20 seconds. In this patient these changes were a manifestation of dual AV nodal pathways. Paper speed 25 mm/sec.

derived from the curve. The ERP of the fast pathway is the longest A1A2 interval which results in slow pathway conduction. The ERP of the slow pathway is the longest A1A2 interval which blocks that pathway. Clearly, if the ERP of the fast pathway is shorter than that of the slow pathway, conduction in the latter would always be concealed by faster conduction. The FRP of the fast pathway is the shortest H1H2 interval during fast pathway conduction. The FRP of the slower pathway is similarly defined as the shortest H1H2 interval during slow pathway conduction. This derivation is, however, less meaningful because it is determined to an unknown extent by the ERP of the faster pathway since slow pathway conduction is obscured until the fast pathway blocks at its ERP.

Duality of AV nodal conduction is a commonly observed electrophysiological response and may be found in patients with no other abnormality of conduction or associated rhythm disturbance. Its clinical significance, however, is its association with AV nodal re-entrant tachycardias for which it is probably the functional substrate. The generation of continuous re-entrant excitation by dual AV nodal pathways can be understood by further study of the anterograde conduction curve. When there is block in the faster pathway, delayed conduction in the slower pathway can allow re-entry of the impulse into the unexcited distal end of the faster pathway with retrograde conduction to the atria causing an atrial echo (see Chapter 7). Under certain conditions sustained re-entrant tachycardia can result. (The principles of re-entrant excitation are discussed in greater detail in chapter 7, and intranodal re-entrant tachycardias in chapter 9.) The anatomical and functional basis for dual AV nodal pathways is not known. Experimental 'reflected re-entry' (Chapter 7) may account for some of the features of duality.

Other manifestations of dual AV nodal pathways include:

1. Sudden spontaneous changes in the duration of the PR interval triggered by changes in heart rate, atrial or ventricular premature beats or without any obvious precipitating factor (Wu, 1982).
2. Complex patterns of AV conduction due to changes from fast to slow pathway conduction (and vice versa) (Ward and Valantine 1983), sustained slow pathway conduction with atrial rate increases (San-Jou et al., 1985) and spontaneous gap phenomenon (Ward, 1982).
3. Simultaneous conduction in both fast and slow pathways with a double ventricular response. This may be persistent, giving rise to a tachycardia (Csapo, 1979; Buss et al., 1985).

In clinical practice is is not necessary to measure refractory periods in great detail because they are usually of little direct relevance to the clinical problem (other than for purposes of comparison; e.g. during a drug study – see Chapter 12). A thorough understanding of the derivation of these measurements and their determinants is, however, essential for a proper appreciation of clinical electrophysiological phenomena and interpretation of complex rhythm disturbances whether induced in the laboratory or occurring spontaneously.

Concealed conduction

A phenomenon which can be readily demonstrated in tissue with decremental properties is 'concealed conduction' in which an impulse propagates in a part of

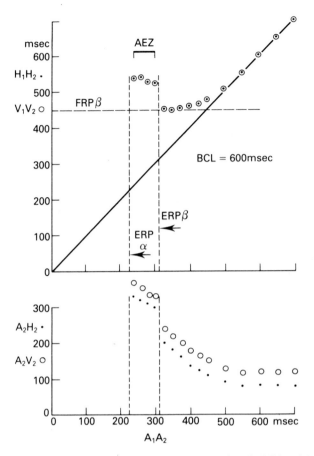

Fig. 3.11 Anterograde conduction curve showing dual AV nodal pathways in a patient with paroxysmal AV nodal re-entrant tachycardia (see Chapter 9). The graph shows the response of the AV node to atrial premature stimulation. The His potential is considered to reflect the output of the AV node. The input is the low right atrial electrogram (A). The data for construction of the curve are derived from the extrastimulus method (see Fig. 3.7). In this example the basic atrial drive cycle length is 610 msec. As A1A2 is reduced the AH interval increases, resulting in a relative delay of H2 (increasing H1H2 interval), the curve deviating from the line of identity. In this patient a sudden increase in the AH interval and the H1H2 interval occurred when the test beat was introduced at a coupling interval of 330 msec. This reflects a sudden transition of conduction from a faster to a slower AV nodal pathway. This is typical of 'dual AV nodal pathways'. Concomitantly with the sudden increase in the AH conduction time AV nodal re-entrant atrial echo beats and sustained tachycardia were observed (see also Chapter 9). The test beat blocks in the faster (beta) pathway but continues in the slower (alpha) pathway. The impulse re-enters the faster pathway at some point during its transit through the AV node and returns to the atria over the fast pathway.

   This curve illustrates the definition of the various AV nodal refractory periods. The effective refractory period (ERP) of the faster pathway (also known as the beta pathway) is the longest A1A2 interval which fails to conduct in this pathway (vertical line at A1A2 = 330 msec). The ERP of the slow pathway (alpha pathway) is the longest A1A2 interval which fails to conduct in this pathway. The functional refractory period (FRP) of the faster (beta) pathway is the shortest H1H2 interval during fast pathway conduction. The FRP of the slow pathway could be similarly derived but it would have less meaning because it is determined to some extent by the ERP of the fast pathway since continued fast pathway conduction obscures slow pathway conduction. BCL = basic cycle length. AEZ = atrial echo zone.

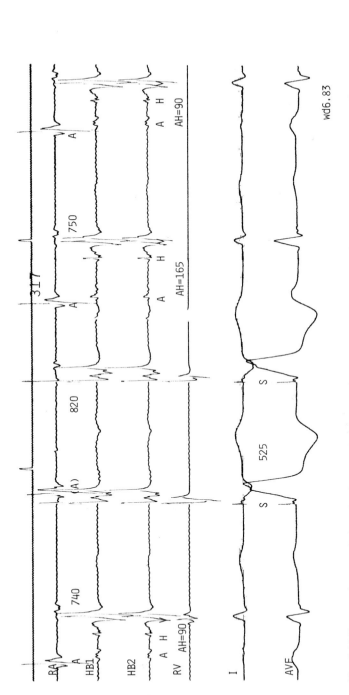

Fig. 3.12 Retrograde concealed conduction into the AV node. During regular sinus rhythm (A) the AH interval is 90 msec. Two ventricular stimuli (S) are delivered separated by an interval of 525 msec. These beats do not conduct to the atrium. The next sinus impulse conducts with prolongation of the AH interval which returns to normal with the following beat. The prolonged AH is a result of concealed retrograde conduction of the ventricular beats into the AV node rendering it relatively refractory and delaying the anterograde impulse. Paper speed 100 mm/sec. HB1 and HB2 = His bundle region; RA= right atrium; RV = right ventricle.

the AV conduction system (e.g. the AV node) but fails to complete its passage (partial penetration into the AV node). Electrocardiographers had deduced the existence of this effect by careful scrutiny and analysis of AV conduction patterns. The term 'concealed' was used to indicate that the impulse itself was not manifest on the surface ECG. Thus the deductive analysis was based on observations of the consequences of concealed conduction, of which the commonest include delay or block of subsequent impulses. The AV node has been the traditional model for both the electrocardiographic and the electrophysiological demonstrations of the phenomenon. Both anterograde and retrograde concealed conduction into the AV node can be demonstrated at electrophysiological study. It has been said that the term 'concealed' is no longer strictly appropriate because many of the surface electrocardiographic consequences of concealment can be 'revealed' during clinical electrophysiological studies. These studies, however, merely allow us to define the consequences of concealed conduction more clearly rather than reveal the concealed conduction itself. Thus the term is equally applicable to events recorded by intracardiac techniques. For example, a ventricular heart beat during sinus rhythm may incompletely penetrate the AV node retrogradely and cause a prolongation in the PR interval of the next sinus beat (Fig. 3.12). The site of this prolongation can be localized to the AV node because the AH interval is increased. The extrastimulus test can be used to demonstrate formally the concept of concealed AV nodal conduction (Fig. 3.13). Atrial fibrillation also provides a model of concealed conduction (see Chapter 8). The phenomenon can also be demonstrated in the atria, bundle branches and in anomalous AV pathways (see Chapter 6). An important clinical manifestation of concealed conduction is the perpetuation of functional bundle branch block during supraventricular tachycardia (see 'Aberrant conduction').

Supernormal conduction

Supernormal conduction has been defined in various ways depending on the setting in which it has been observed. In general, it describes an unexpected improvement (decreased conduction time) of normal or depressed conduction. (It is to be distinguished from 'supernormal excitability' where subthreshold stimuli, delivered in diastole, result in capture when delivered within a zone near to the end of repolarization.) It is now realized that many of these phenomena can be explained by interaction of the various longitudinal or parallel components of the AV conduction system. For example, gap phenomena of all kinds are responsible for unexpected improvement of delayed conduction or resumption of blocked conduction (see above). Interaction of parallel components of the conduction system may also cause apparent supernormal conduction. For example, a premature atrial stimulus (A2) which blocks in the faster of dual AV nodal pathways may conduct in the slow pathway. However, a third impulse delivered shortly after A2 may find the fast pathway recovered and reach the ventricles before A2 (Denes et al., 1975).

As yet, there is no convincing evidence for supernormal AV conduction as a distinct phenomenon. It would seem that all examples of so-called supernormal AV conduction may be adequately explained by interaction of the various

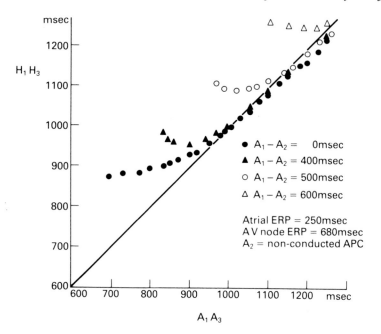

Fig. 3.13 Demonstration of concealed AV nodal conduction using the extrastimulus method in a patient with a long PR interval. In this study, two test stimuli were used. The stimulus A2 was coupled such that it failed to conduct to the His bundle. Four different coupling intervals (A1A2) were used. The test stimulus A3 was introduced at gradually decreasing coupling intervals for each of the settings of A1A2. When A1A2 was zero (i.e. A2 was not present) the curve was normal but with long AH intervals (solid circles). With A1A2 set at 400 msec (solid triangles) the FRP and ERP of the AV node were prolonged. This effect was more pronounced when A1A2 was increased to 500 msec (open circles) and 600 msec (open triangles) respectively. Thus, A3 encountered increasing AV nodal delay as A1A2 was lengthened, presumably allowing increased concealed penetration of A2 into the node. APC = atrial premature contraction.

components of the atrioventricular conduction system.

True supernormal conduction in the atrial and ventricular myocardium has been demonstrated in intact dog using intracardiac stimulation and recording methods. It has been shown that stimuli delivered close to the end of repolarization may propagate with a decreased conduction time compared to those delivered later in the cycle. These phenomena may be caused by the period of supernormal excitability (Spear and Moore, 1977; Puech et al., 1979). The clinical importance of true supernormal conduction is not known (Childers, 1984).

Retrograde conduction

The capacity for conduction from the ventricles to the atria (retrograde conduction) is present in about 60 per cent of subjects with normal, intact anterograde conduction (Akhtar, 1981b). In these cases, anterograde conduction capacity is better than retrograde conduction capacity (as reflected by higher rates

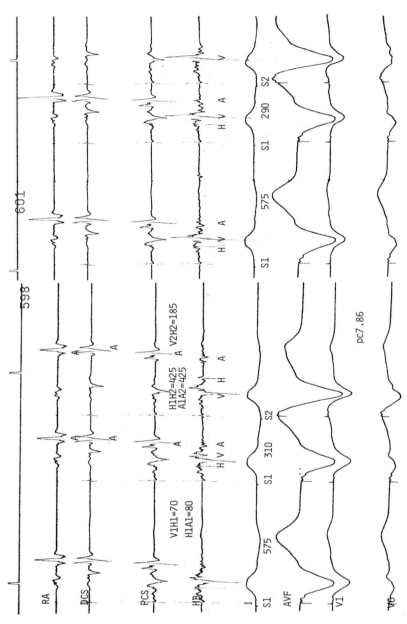

Fig. 3.14 Normal retrograde conduction pattern. Regular ventricular pacing (S1S2) at a cycle length of 575 msec results in retrograde conduction with a normal atrial activation pattern (A) beginning in the region of the His bundle (HB). The retrograde His potential (H) is clearly inscribed. After a premature stimulus (S2), retrograde conduction to the His bundle is delayed whereas the HA interval reflecting the intranodal component of retrograde conduction is unchanged (H1H2 = A1A2). Thus, retrograde delay in this instance is largely due to intraventricular conduction delay. Retrograde block in the His–Purkinje system occurred when the coupling interval of S2 was reduced to 290 msec. Paper speed 100 mm/sec. DCS = distal coronary sinus; HB = His bundle; PCS = proximal coronary sinus; RA = right atrium.

at which 1:1 conduction can occur and shorter Wenckebach cycle lengths). In patients with bundle branch block retrograde conduction may be impaired but this is due to delay or block within the His–Purkinje system (HPS) rather than the AV node itself.

Retrograde conduction can be examined by using the technique of incremental pacing of the right ventricle. The usual response of the VA conduction interval during gradually increasing ventricular paced rates is prolongation until VA block (second degree type I, 2:1 or higher) occurs. However, in about one-third of patients the reverse is true. As the stimulation rate increases, the refractoriness of the HPS decreases and retrograde conduction capacity (to the His bundle and AV node) is maintained. Often the degree of VA lengthening is minimal during incremental pacing. The site of retrograde delay may be within the AV node or the intraventricular conduction system. If no retrograde His potential is visible, it is not possible to localize the site of delay or block (if anomalous ventriculoatrial pathways are present the response of the normal pathway to ventricular pacing may be masked: see Chapter 6).

To examine further the dynamics of retrograde conduction, the extrastimulus method can be used. A ventricular extrastimulus is delivered at progressively shorter coupling intervals. A retrograde conduction curve can be constructed in a manner analogous to the anterograde curve (see above). As the interval of the test beat is decreased, it encounters relative refractoriness within the HPS and there is a progressive delay of His bundle depolarization (Fig. 3.14), often without any additional delay in the node itself (no change in the HA interval). Retrograde block with early extrastimuli occur within the HPS (Fig. 3.14) or the AV node. The former mechanism of block is the most common (Akhtar, 1981a, b).

An important aspect of retrograde conduction studies is the examination of the atrial activation sequence during retrograde VA conduction. In normal subjects in whom retrograde conduction is intact, the impulse emerges from the AV node and spreads to the right and left atria from that region (Fig. 3.14). This is detected by a suitable arrangement of recording electrodes in the atria. The selection of recording sites depends on the clinical indication for study. In patients with junctional tachycardias (see Chapter 9) it is essential to record left atrial activity, preferably from the coronary sinus in addition to the low right atrium and the high right atrium. A study of the changes in atrial activation during ventricular extrastimulus testing can provide useful information about the location and behaviour of anomalous VA conduction (see Chapter 6).

Analysis of retrograde conduction is an important factor when considering the use of DDD (dual chamber sensing and stimulation) pacemakers. Intact retrograde conduction may support circus movement tachycardias mediated by the pacing system (pacemaker-mediated tachycardia (PMT) or endless-loop tachycardia (ELT)). These arrhythmias are sustained because the atrial electrode senses the retrograde P waves and responds by activating the ventricular electrode. Thus retrograde conduction is essential for the continuation of the PMT. If the P wave falls within the postventricular atrial refractory period of the pacemaker, it will not be sensed and tachycardia cannot be sustained. Long retrograde conduction times are not uncommon, however, and the P wave may fall outside the pacemaker refractory period. Retrograde conduction may be

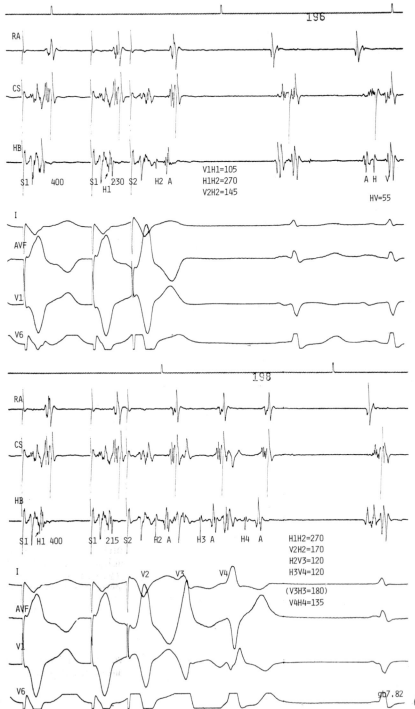

(a)

(b)

intermittent. Thus, VA conduction may be absent at the time of implantation but reappear days later (den Dulk et al., 1984). An important factor in this respect is variation in the level of autonomic tone. Mahmud et al. (1984) have shown that AV sequential pacing may facilitate retrograde conduction.

A phenomenon commonly observed during investigation of retrograde conduction by ventricular stimulation is 'repetitive ventricular responses' (Fig. 3.15). There are several mechanisms for these responses (Farshidi et al., 1980; Akhtar, 1981a)):

1. Macrore-entry within the His–Purkinje system or bundle branches (hence the term bundle branch re-entry).
2. Local re-entry at the site of stimulation (intraventricular re-entry).
3. Atrioventricular nodal re-entry due to the presence of dual AV nodal pathways.
4. Atrioventricular re-entry using a retrograde anomalous pathway.
5. 'Subjunctional' re-entry via a nodoventricular pathway (see Chapter 9).

In examples 3, 4 and 5, a wide QRS complex may be produced by aberrant conduction or ventricular pre-excitation (see Chapter 6).

Re-entry within the bundle branch system is caused by retrograde block of the stimulated beat in either one or other of the bundle branches and the development of sufficient retrograde delay to allow recovery of the retrogradely blocked bundle (Akhtar et al., 1974a). This permits anterograde conduction and a repetitive response of the same QRS type as the paced impulse (LBBB type) if retrograde block occurred in the right bundle (the commonest mechanism) or RBBB type if retrograde block occurred in the left bundle. The repetitive beat is often referred to as 'V3' and the response is also referred to as the 'V3 phenomenon'.

Fig. 3.15 Repetitive ventricular response. (*a*) After a regular right ventricular pacing sequence (S1S2) at a cycle length of 400 msec, an extrastimulus S2 is coupled at 230 msec. A clear retrograde His potential is seen with intraventricular conduction delay (H1H2 = 270 msec). Retrograde atrial activation (A) occurs normally. (*b*) When the extrastimulus is coupled at 215 msec the H1H2 remains at 270 msec but a repetitive response (V3) is seen. The QRS morphology of this beat is very similar to that of V1 and V2. This is followed by a His potential, H3, and a second response V4, with a narrower QRS of right bundle branch block pattern and superior axis. This is also followed by a His spike, H4. The V3 phenomenon occurred in association with V2H2 intervals of 170 msec or more. Were it not for V4, it would be tempting to suggest that V3 was a result of macrore-entry. In this explanation, V2 blocks retrogradely in the right bundle and conducts to the His bundle (H2) via the left bundle and back to the myocardium in the right bundle, producing a QRS complex (V3) with an LBBB pattern with H2V3 exceeding the HV interval during sinus rhythm. The His spike H3 is from retrograde conduction via the left bundle. The different morphology of V4 makes local intraventricular re-entry improbable. However, if V4 is macrore-entrant, it conducts anterogradely in the left bundle branch. If so, the His potential which preceded it (H3) cannot be a result of retrograde left bundle branch conduction. Thus V3 is probably an intraventricular re-entrant beat with incidental activation of the His bundle (H3) as a result of retrograde conduction through the right bundle, whereas V4 is macrore-entrant rather than intraventricular. The complex, V3, blocks retrogradely in the left bundle branch and retrograde conduction via the right bundle branch to the His bundle is followed by anterograde conduction in the left bundle branch resulting in V4 with an RBBB pattern. Therefore, H4 is due to retrograde right bundle branch conduction. Paper speed 100 mm/sec. CS = coronary sinus; HB = His bundle region; RA = right atrium.

It is always preceded by activation of the His bundle. The H2V3 interval exceeds the HV interval recorded during sinus rhythm. The critical retrograde delay (V2H2 intervals) required for this phenomenon can be measured if a retrograde His potential is observed. If it cannot be recorded, intramyocardial re-entry cannot be differentiated from bundle branch re-entry. Even if the His bundle spike is recorded, complex events may defy simple explanation (Fig. 3.15). Intramyocardial re-entry does not exhibit these features.

Repetitive responses occur in about 60 per cent of patients undergoing electrophysiological study, and are now regarded as physiological. Several years ago, however, such responses were thought to be harbingers of sudden death (Greene et al., 1978) or ventricular arrhythmias (Farshidi et al., 1980). Subsequent studies (Mason, 1980; Ruskin et al., 1981) have demonstrated that neither bundle branch re-entry nor intramyocardial re-entry indicates a susceptibility to more dangerous, pathological arrhythmias. This controversy was a forerunner of many others concerning the ventricular extrastimulus method (see Chapter 10).

References and further reading

Abella JB, Teixeira OHP, Misra KP, Hastrieter AR. (1972) Changes of atrioventricular conduction with age in infants and children. *American Journal of Cardiology* **30**, 876

Agha AS, Befeler B, Castellanos AM, Sung RJ, Castillo CA, Myerburg RJ, Castellanos A. (1976) Bipolar catheter electrograms for study of retrograde atrial activation pattern in patients without pre-excitation syndromes. *British Heart Journal* **38**, 641

Akhtar M, Damato AN, Batsford WP, Ruskin JN, Ogunkelu JB, Vargas G. (1974a) Demonstration of re-entry within the His–Purkinje system in man. *Circulation* **50**, 1150

Akhtar M, Damato AN, Batsford WP, Caracta AR, Vargas G, Lau SH. (1974b). Unmasking and conversion of gap phenomenon in the human heart. *Circulation* **49**, 624

Akhtar M, Damato AN, Batsford WP, Ruskin JN, Ogunkelu JB. (1975) A comparative analysis of antegrade and retrograde conduction patterns in man. *Circulation* **52**, 766

Akhtar M, Damato AN, Ruskin JN, Batsford WP, Reddy CP, Ticzon AR, Dhatt AR, Gomes JAC, Calon AH. (1978) Antegrade and retrograde conduction characteristics in three patterns of paroxysmal atrioventricular junctional re-entrant tachycardia. *American Heart Journal* **95**, 22

Akhtar M. (1981a) The clinical significance of the repetitive ventricular response. *Circulation* **63**, 773

Akhtar M. (1981b) Retrograde conduction in man. *Pacing and Clinical Electrophysiology* **4**, 548

Befeler B, Berkovits BV, Aranda JM, Sung RJ, Moleiro F, Castellanos A. (1979) Programmed simultaneous biventricular stimulation in man, with special reference to its use in the evaluation of intraventricular re-entry. *European Journal of Cardiology* **9**, 369

Buss J, Kraatz J, Stegaru B, Neuss H, Heene DL. (1985) Unusual mechanism of PR interval variation and nonre-entrant supraventricular tachycardia as a manifestation of simultaneous anterograde fast and slow conduction through dual atrioventricular nodal pathways. *Pacing and Clinical Electrophysiology* **8**, 235

Castellanos A, Embi A, Aranda J, Befeler B. (1976) Retrograde His bundle deflection in bundle-branch re-entry. *British Heart Journal* **38**, 301

Castillo C, Castellanos A. (1971) Retrograde activation of the His bundle in the human heart. *American Journal of Cardiology* 27, 264

Childers RW. (1984) Supernormality: recent developments. *Pacing and Clinical Electrophysiology* 7, 1115

Cranefield PF. (1975) *The Conduction of the Cardiac Impulse. The Slow Response and Cardiac Arrhythmias*. Futura: Mount Kisco, NY

Csapo G. (1979) Paroxysmal non-resistant tachycardias due to simultaneous conduction in dual atrioventricular nodal pathways. *American Journal of Cardiology* 43, 1033

Curry PVL. (1980) The hemodynamic and electrophysiological effects of paroxysmal tachycardia. In: *Cardiac Arrhythmias: Electrophysiology, Diagnosis and Management*, p. 364. Ed. by OS Narula, Williams & Wilkins, Baltimore, MD

Damato AN, Akhtar M, Ruskin J, Caracta AR, Lau SH. (1976) Gap phenomena: antegrade and retrograde. In: *Conduction System of the Heart: Structure, Function and Clinical Implications*, p. 504. Ed. by HJJ Wellens, KI Lie, MJ Janse. Lea & Febiger: Philadelphia, Pa

den Dulk K, Lindemans FW, Wellens HJJ. (1984) Noninvasive evaluation of pacemaker circus movement tachycardias. *American Journal of Cardiology* 53, 537

Denes P, Wu D, Dhingra R, Chuquimia R, Rosen KM. (1973) Demonstration of dual AV nodal pathways in patients with paroxysmal supraventricular tachycardia. *Circulation* 48, 549

Denes P, Wu D, Dhingra R, Pietras RJ, Rosen KM. (1974). The effects of cycle length on cardiac refractory periods in man. *Circulation* 49, 32

Denes P, Wyndham CRC, Wu D, Rosen KM. (1975) 'Supernormal conduction' of a premature impulse utilizing the fast pathway in a patient with dual AV nodal pathways. *Circulation* 51, 811

DuBrow IW, Fisher EA, Amat-y-Leon F, Denes P, Wu D, Rosen KM, Hastreiter AR. (1975) Comparison of cardiac refractory periods in children and adults. *Circulation* 51, 485

Farshidi A, Michelson EL, Greenspan AM, Spielman SR, Horowitz LN, Josephson ME. (1980) Repetitive responses to ventricular extrastimuli: incidence, mechanisms and significance. *American Heart Journal* 100, 59

Gallagher JJ, Damato AN, Caracta AR, Varghese PJ, Josephson ME, Lau, SH. (1973) Gap in AV conduction in man: types I and II. *American Heart Journal* 85, 78

Goldreyer B, Bigger JT. (1970) Ventriculo-atrial conduction in man. *Circulation* 41, 935

Greene HL, Reid PR, Scaeffer AH (1978) The repetitive ventricular response in man: a predictor of sudden death. *New England Journal of Medicine* 299, 729

Han J, Moe GK. (1969) Cumulative effects of cycle length on refractory periods of cardiac tissues. *American Journal of Physiology* 217, 106

Hoffman BF, Moore EN, Stuckey JH, Cranefield PF. (1963) Functional properties of the atrioventricular conduction system. *Circulation Research* 13, 308

Jalife J. (1983) The sucrose gap preparation as a model of AV nodal transmission: are dual pathways necessary for reciprocation and AV nodal 'echoes'? *Pacing and Clinical Electrophysiology* 6, 1106

Langendorf R. (1974) Concealed AV conduction: the effect of blocked impulses on the formation and conduction of subsequent impulses. *American Heart Journal* 35, 542

Lehmann MH, Denker S, Mahmud R, Akhtar M. (1984) Patterns of human atrioventricular nodal accommodation to a sudden acceleration of atrial rate. *American Journal of Cardiology* 53, 71

Levy S, Pouget B, Clementy J, Bemurat M, Bricaud H. (1979) Pacing-induced alternate Wenckebach periods: incidence and clinical significance. *Pacing and Clinical Electrophysiology* 2, 614

Levy S, Roudaut R, Bouvier E, Obel IWP, Clementy J, Bricaud H. (1980) Alternate ventriculoatrial Wenckebach conduction. *Circulation* 61, 648

Mahmud R, Lehmann M, Denker S, Gilbert CJ, Akhtar M. (1983) Atrioventricular sequential pacing: differential effect on retrograde impulse conduction related to level of impulse collision. *Circulation* **68**, 23

Mahmud R, Denker S, Lehmann M, Akhtar M. (1984) Effect of atrioventricular sequential pacing in patients with no ventriculoatrial conduction. *Journal of the American College of Cardiology* **4**, 273

Mason JW. (1980) Repetitive beating after single ventricular extrastimuli: incidence and prognostic significance in patients with recurrent ventricular tachycardia. *American Journal of Cardiology* **45**, 1126

Mehta AV, Wolff GS, Tamer D, Pickoff AS, Casta A. Garcia OL, Gelband H. (1981) Determinants of ventricular refractory periods in children with congenital heart disease: effects of cycle length and age. *American Heart Journal* **102**, 75

Moe GK, Preston JB, Burlington H. (1956) Physiological evidence for a dual AV transmission system. *Circulation Research* **4**, 357

Moe GK, Mendez C, Han J. (1965) Aberrant AV impulse propagation in the dog heart. A study of functional bundle branch block. *Circulation Response* **16**, 26

Moe GK, Mendez C. (1971) Functional block in the intraventricular conduction system. *Circulation* **43**, 949

Moore EN, Knoebel S, Spear JF. (1971) Concealed conduction. *American Journal of Cardiology* **28**, 406

Puech P, Guimond C, Nadeau R, Morena H, Molina L, Matina D. (1979) Supernormal conduction in the intact heart. In: *Cardiac Arrhythmias: Electrophysiology, Diagnosis and Management*, p. 41. Ed. by OS Narula. Williams & Wilkins: Baltimore, Md

Rosenblueth A. (1958) Mechanism of the Wenckebach–Luciani cycles. *American Journal of Physiology* **194**, 491

Ruskin JN, DiMarco JP, Garan H. (1981) Repetitive responses to single ventricular extrastimuli in patients with serious ventricular arrhythmias: incidence and clinical significance. *Circulation* **63**, 767

San-Jou Y, Yahn-Chyurn W, Fun-Chung L, Jui-Sung H, Wu D. (1985) Pseudosimultaneous fast and slow pathway conduction: a common finding in patients with dual atrioventricular nodal pathways. *Journal of the American College of Cardiology* **6**, 927

Simson M, Spear J, Moore EN. (1979) The relationship between atrioventricular nodal refractoriness and functional refractory period in the dog. *Circulation Research* **44**, 121

Spear JF, Moore EN. (1977) Effect of potassium on supernormal conduction in the bundle branch–Purkinje system of the dog. *American Journal of Cardiology* **40**, 923

Ward DE, Camm AJ. (1978) Gaps in anterograde conduction in patients with the short PR interval, normal QRS complex syndrome. *British Heart Journal* **40**, 1119

Ward DE, Camm AJ. (1980) Methodologic problems in the use of atrial pacing studies for the assessment of AV conduction. *Clinical Cardiology* **3**, 155

Ward DE. (1982) Unusual capture phenomena during interaction of dissociated sinus and junctional rhythms: spontaneous expression of intranodal duality and gap phenomenon. *Journal of Electrocardiology* **15**, 299

Ward DE, Valantine H. (1983) Spontaneous manifestation of dual AV nodal pathways resulting in complex patterns of AV conduction. *Pacing and Clinical Electrophysiology* **6**, 272

Watanabe Y. (1978a) Terminology and electrophysiologic concepts in cardiac arrhythmias. II. Aberrant conduction. *Pacing and Clinical Electrophysiology* **1**, 231

Watanabe Y. (1978b) Terminology and electrophysiologic concepts in cardiac arrhythmias. III. Concealed conduction. *Pacing and Clinical Electrophysiology* **1**, 345

Watanabe Y. (1979) Terminology and electrophysiologic concepts in cardiac arrhythmias. VI. Phase 3 and phase 4 block. *Pacing and Clinical Electrophysiology* **1**, 624

Wellens HJJ, Durrer D. (1968) Supraventricular tachycardia with left aberrant conduction due to retrograde invasion into the left bundle branch. *Circulation* **36**, 673

Wellens, HJJ, Durrer D. (1968) Supraventricular tachycardia with left aberrant during supraventricular tachycardia in man: observations on mechanisms and their incidence. In: *Cardiac Electrophysiology and Arrhythmias*, p. 435. Ed. by D Zipes, J Jalife. Grune & Stratton: Orlando, Fla

Wit AL, Weiss MB, Berkowitz WD, Rosen KM, Steiner C, Damato AN. (1970a) Patterns of atrioventricular conduction in the human heart. *Circulation Research* **27**, 345

Wit A, Damato AN, Weiss MB, Steiner C. (1970b) Phenomenon of the gap in atrioventricular conduction in the human heart. *Circulation Research* **27**, 679

Wu D, Denes P, Dhingra R, Rosen KM. (1974) Nature of the gap phenomenon in man. *Circulation Research* **34**, 682

Wu D, Denes P, Amat-y-Leon F, Wyndham CR, Dhingra R, Rosen KM. (1977) An unusual variety of atrioventricular nodal re-entry due to retrograde dual atrioventricular nodal pathways. *Circulation* **56**, 50

Wu D. (1982) Dual atrioventricular nodal pathways: a reappraisal. *Pacing and Clinical Electrophysiology* **5**, 72

Young M, Gelband H, Castellanos A, Wolff GS. (1985) Rapid atrial pacing-induced infra-His conduction block in children. *American Heart Journal* **110**, 652

Young M, Wolff GS, Castellanos A, Gelband H. (1986a) Application of the Rosenblueth hypothesis to assess atrioventricular nodal behaviour. *American Journal of Cardiology* **57**, 131

Young M, Wolff GS, Castellanos A, Gelband H. (1986b) Application of the Rosenblueth hypothesis to assess cycle length effects on the refractoriness of the atrioventricular node. *American Journal of Cardiology* **57**, 142

Part II

Investigation of Bradycardias

4

Sinus Node Abnormalities

Disorders of the natural automaticity of the sinus node present with a wide variety of symptoms varying from lethargy to dizziness and blackouts. Many patients are asymptomatic. The intermittent nature of the disorder makes clinical assessment difficult, and various clinical electrophysiological tests (Table 4.1) have been devised in an attempt to improve diagnostic accuracy. The two tests that have been most studied are: (1) Sinus node recovery time (SNRT); and (2) Sinoatrial conduction time (SACT).

Sinus node recovery time (SNRT)

Naturally automatic pacemaker cells are suppressed by a period of stimulation faster than their natural discharge rate. This is known as 'overdrive suppression'. The mechanism of suppression is related to complex biochemical and ionic changes in the pacemaker cells. A clinical estimation of SNRT is obtained by atrial pacing for a short period and recording the time taken for the sinus node to recover after the atrial pacemaker is switched off (as described by Mandel et al., 1971 and Rosen et al., 1971) (Fig. 4.1). To estimate the maximal recovery time in response to overdrive suppression, several different rates of stimulation are chosen. The slow rate should be just in excess of the intrinsic sinus rate. The fastest rate used is generally between 130 and 150 b.p.m. Most investigators pace for 1 minute although durations of 15 seconds and 30 seconds are also commonly used. This can result in a prolonged period of testing. The SNRT is derived by measuring the time taken for the sinus node to recover after pacing is turned off. Often the subsequent sinus rate is also markedly slowed, especially in patients

Table 4.1 ELECTROPHYSIOLOGICAL TESTS OF SINOATRIAL NODE FUNCTION

Intrinsic heart rate (after atropine and propranolol)
Sinus node recovery time
Corrected sinus node recovery time
Total sinus node recovery time
Sinus node recovery time after atropine
Sinus node recovery times after atropine and propranolol
Sinoatrial conduction time (Strauss method)
Sinoatrial conduction time (Narula method)
Sinoatrial conduction time (Tonkin method)
Sinoatrial conduction and recovery time (Satoh method)
Sinoatrial conduction and recovery time (direct method)
Sinus node suppression time

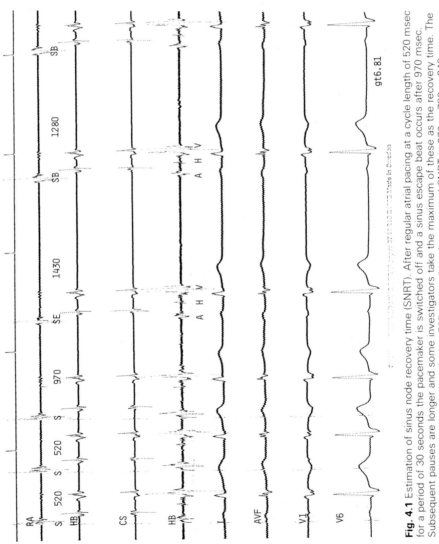

Fig. 4.1 Estimation of sinus node recovery time (SNRT). After regular atrial pacing at a cycle length of 520 msec for a period of 30 seconds the pacemaker is switched off and a sinus escape beat occurs after 970 msec. Subsequent pauses are longer and some investigators take the maximum of these as the recovery time. The control (prepacing) sinus cycle length was 730 msec; thus the corrected SNRT is 970 − 730 = 240 msec. Paper speed 50 mm/sec.

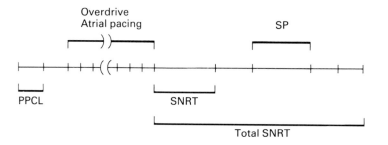

Fig. 4.2 Schematic diagram of estimation of the sinus node recovery time. The conventional sinus node recovery time (SNRT) is measured from the last paced atrial electrogram to the first escape atrial electrogram provided it is of sinus origin. The total SNRT is the time taken for the sinus cycle length to approximate the prepacing sinus cycle length (PPCL). Secondary pauses (SP) are accounted for using this method.

with sinoatrial disease. Thus some investigators also measure 'total recovery time' – that is, the time taken for the postpacing sinus cycle length to reach the prepacing value (Fig. 4.2). This is normally less than 5 seconds.

Because the SNRT varies with underlying intrinsic heart rate the sinus node recovery time may be corrected by subtracting the intrinsic sinus cycle length from the absolute SNRT. The normal SNRT value is generally taken as less than 1500 msec, with a corrected SNRT (CSNRT) of less than 550 msec. The published normal values have, however, varied widely (SNRT from <1200 to <1600 msec and CSNRT from <525 to <600 msec). The SNRT may also be expressed as a ratio of the value to the basic sinus cycle length (SNRT/SCL). Mandel et al. (1971) gave a normal value of this ratio of less than 130 per cent. Josephson and Seides (1979) have a higher figure of less than 150 per cent. The presence of a junctional escape beat before the sinus escape interferes with the test. Atrial electrogram recordings allow confirmation of sinus escape which should, of course, result in a normal P wave on the surface ECG. The test is rarely abnormal in patients without sinoatrial disease, but in patients with the disorder the SNRT can be several seconds in duration. In these patients, however, there is a high incidence of falsely negative tests (normal result in a patient with sinoatrial disease). Thus the test has a low sensitivity but high specificity.

Sinoatrial conduction time (SACT)

This is estimated by measuring the effect of premature atrial depolarizations on the duration and timing of the sinus cycle. The method, devised by Strauss, involves a complete scan of the sinus cycle (A1A1) with stimulated single atrial premature beats delivered to the high right atrium near the sinus node. The coupling interval (A1A2) of the premature beat (A2) is gradually decreased and the response in terms of the timing of the next sinus beat (A2A3) is recorded (Figs. 4.3 and 4.4). The results of this sequence are best expressed in the form of a graph (Fig. 4.5): the test beat interval (A1A2) is plotted as a percentage of the A1A1 interval on the abscissa and the result interval (A2A3) is similarly

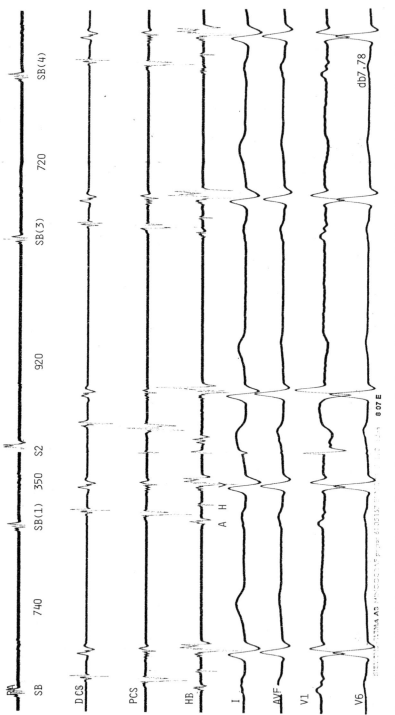

Fig. 4.3 Estimation of sinoatrial conduction time using the extrastimulus method of Strauss et al. (1974). During sinus rhythm (cycle length 740 msec) a test stimulus (S2) is introduced at gradually decreasing coupling intervals, shown in this example at a coupling interval of 350 msec. This enters the sinus node and resets the spontaneous diastolic mechanism such that the next sinus beat (SB3) is advanced. The sinoatrial conduction time is derived from responses which show sinoatrial reset (see Figs. 4.4 and 4.5).

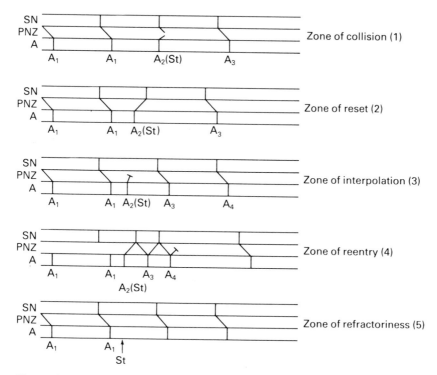

Fig. 4.4 Schematic ladder diagrams of the method of derivation of the sinoatrial conduction time (SACT) by the Strauss method. The responses to the sinus node may be classified into five types. (1) When the test stimulus (St) is delivered late in the sinus cycle it collides with the emerging sinus impulses and does not enter the sinus node (SN). The sinus impulse is not propagated through the perinodal zone (PNZ) to the atrium (A) because it encounters refractory tissue in the wake of the stimulated beat. The next expected sinus impulse appears at the predicted time (A1A3 = A1A1 × 2). The interval A2A3 increases by an amount equal to the reduction in A1A2. This response defines the 'collision zone'. (2) When the test beat is delivered earlier in the cycle the sinus node is depolarized and the next sinus impulse is advanced ('reset zone'). (3) Failure of the test beat to invade and reset the sinus node at early coupling intervals is reflected by the occurrence of the next sinus beat on time. This is the 'zone of interpolation'. (A1A3 = A1A2 + A2A2). (4) Occasionally there is a sudden transition from A2A3 intervals which exceed A1A1 to those which are very much shorter. This is thought to reflect sinoatrial re-entry (A3 and A4). (5) Very premature stimuli encounter atrial refractoriness and have no effect.

represented on the ordinate. The possible responses of the sinus node fall into five different zones (see Fig. 4.4):

1. The zone of collision.
2. The zone of reset.
3. The zone of entrance block or interpolation.
4. The zone of re-entry.
5. The zone of refractoriness.

When the test stimulus is delivered late in the sinus cycle, the sinus impulse collides with the atrial paced impulse at some point remote from the sinus

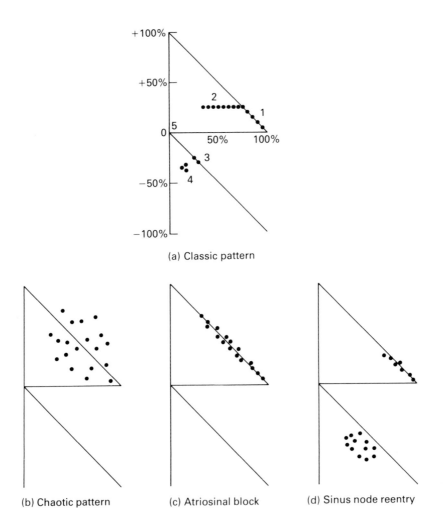

(a) Classic pattern

(b) Chaotic pattern   (c) Atriosinal block   (d) Sinus node reentry

Fig. 4.5 The response of the sinus node to atrial extrastimulation. The coupling interval of the test beat is expressed as a percentage of the basic sinus cycle length (A1A2/A1A1 or A1A2%). The return cycle (that immediately following the test beat (A2A3)) is plotted on the ordinate as a percentage of the basic sinus cycle length (A2A3/A1A1 or A2A3%). Zones 1–5 (see Fig. 4.4) are indicated on the upper graph. The conduction time of an impulse into the sinus node is derived from the responses during the zone of reset. The derivation is based on the notion that a finite interval is required for the test beat to enter and reset the sinus node and for the next sinus impulse to activate the atria. Thus the total atriosinus and sinoatrial conduction time may be expressed as A2A3 − A1A1. Division by 2 derives the sinoatrial conduction time. The classic pattern showing constant reset (horizontal reset zone in (a) may not always be observed. (b – d) Variations: (b), reset is chaotic and unpredictable; (c) failure of reset due to sinoatrial entrance block; (d) early development of sinoatrial re-entry with no reset zone.

pacemaker cells. Therefore the test impulse does not gain access to the pacemaker cells, and the sinus impulse is not propagated because it encounters depolarized atrial tissue. The next sinus impulse appears on time (A1A3 = 2 × A1A1). This is the collision zone. As the A1A2 interval is decreased, the sinus cells are depolarized by the invading test impulse and the pacemaker cells are reset. Reset continues as the A1A2 interval is progressively shortened. During this period the return cycle A2A3 remains relatively constant or gradually increases. Failure of the test impulse to invade the sinus pacemaker at early coupling intervals (entrance block) is reflected by appearance of the next expected sinus beat on time (i.e. A1A3 = A1A1). Occasionally the return cycle is considerably shorter than the sinus cycle (A1A3 < A1A1). This is thought to reflect sinoatrial re-entry. A similar phenomenon may be seen in patients with so-called sinoatrial re-entrant tachycardia (see Chapter 8).

The conduction time of the test impulse into the sinus node is derived from the responses during the zone of reset. The excess of the return cycle over the basic sinus cycle during the zone of reset is supposed to represent the combined atriosinus (retrograde conduction into the node) and sinoatrial conduction time which is, therefore:

Total SACT = (A2A3) − (A1A1)

Theoretically, division by 2 gives the value for conduction in one or the other direction. The value is derived by considering the mean value of all differences within the reset zone. Some investigators use only differences in the longest third or half of the zone.

There are several assumptions in this derivation (Fig. 4.6). Sinus node suppression occurs following atrial pacing, and it cannot be assumed that the excess of A2A3 over A1A1 is entirely accounted for by conduction into and out of the sinus node. The atriosinus conduction time may not be equal to the sinoatrial conduction time, and the conduction times to and from the stimulation and recording catheter will also contribute to the value. Narula et al. (1978) devised an alternative method for deriving sinoatrial conduction time which utilizes continuous atrial pacing. The rate of pacing is adjusted to exceed the sinus rate by about 5 b.p.m. in order to minimize sinus node suppression. The SACT is calculated by subtracting the mean of ten prepacing sinus cycles (mean SCL) from the first return cycle after eight beats of pacing (SCL1):

Total SACT = mean SCL − SCL1

This method has not been shown to be superior to the Strauss method in that suppression cannot be avoided and occasionally acceleration of the sinus rate to the pacing rate is observed.

Satoh et al. (1984) have developed a different method in which two atrial premature stimuli, delivered close to the atrial effective refractory period (ERP), are followed by a regular paced sequence, slightly faster than the sinus rate. The early stimuli reset the sinus node which is constantly reset thereafter during the regular sequence. The return cycle (A1Ar) and the next cycle (ArA3) after this sequence are measured several times and an average obtained. A test stimulus (A2) is then interposed between the end of the pacing sequence and the return cycle. The coupling interval (A1A2) is reduced to the atrial ERP. In this way a

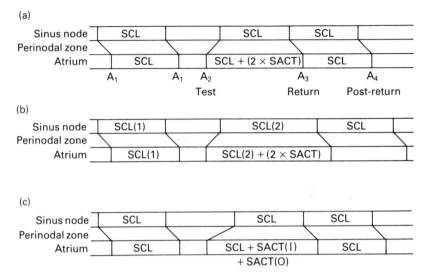

Fig. 4.6 Schematic ladder diagrams illustrating some of the limitations of the Strauss method for derivation of SACT. The coupling interval (A1A2) of the test stimulus is gradually reduced at successive trials until the atrium is refractory. The response of the sinus node (A2A3) is determined by various factors including the conduction time of the test beat into the node, the intrinsic automaticity of the sinus node, the conduction time of the next sinus impulse out of the node and the timing of the extrastimulus. (*a*) The theoretical response. (*b*) The effect of sinus suppression where SCL2 exceeds SCL1. (*c*) How unequal conduction times into and out of the sinus node may distort estimation of the true SACT. SCL = sinus cycle length.
(O) = impulse exit from node
(I) = impulse entry to node

reset and non-reset zone can be defined by plotting A2A3 against A1A2. The starting point is defined by plotting ArA3 against A1Ar. The coupling interval (A1A2) at the transition point between one zone and the other defines the sinus node return cycle. The difference between this value and A1Ar defines the sinoatrial conduction time (all values of A1A2 greater than that at the transition point fail to conduct into the node, by definition). The method assumes constant sinus reset during the regular paced sequence and equal anterograde and retrograde sinoatrial conduction times. It is a complex method and likely to be useful in a research application.

In summary, electrophysiological testing of sinus node function does not make an important contribution to the care of patients with sinus node disorders. Management is more appropriately conducted using clinical and electrocardiographic information. With regard to tests of sinus node function it is important to remember two points: first, that a normal test result does not exclude the diagnosis of sinus node disorder and, second, that an abnormal result is not in itself an indication for pacing even in symptomatic patients. Drugs have an important effect on sinus node automaticity, especially in the presence of sinoatrial disease. Both digoxin and betablockers prolong the SNRT and the SACT. Furthermore, almost all class 1 antiarrhythmic agents (lignocaine-quinidine-flecainide group) are known to impair sinus node function and may predispose to abnormal test results. This should be taken into account when interpreting the results of electrophysiological testing.

It would appear that haemodynamic factors should also be taken into account when assessing sinus function by these methods. Nalos et al. (1986) have shown that hypotension induced by rapid atrial pacing may activate autonomic reflexes which tend to shorten the measured indices of sinoatrial function. They show that autonomic blockade (see below) may negate this effect. In another study, an increase in the atrial rate was consistently observed during right ventricular pacing (without retrograde conduction) and was not affected by autonomic blockade. It was suggested that a mechanical effect on the sinus node artery, might explain these findings (Blanc et al., 1981). Systemic hypotension, with its consequent reflexes, could also explain these findings. This effect cannot be excluded because blood pressure was not monitored in this study.

Newer approaches to the investigation of patients with sinus node disorders

Autonomic blockade

Autonomic blockade using propranolol and atropine has been used as an adjunct to sinoatrial function testing. The notion is that autonomic blockade will remove the autonomic influences on the sinus node and reveal the 'true' status of the unmodulated node. The method is time consuming and has not yet made an important clinical contribution to the investigation of sinus node disorders. Because the vagal influence on the sinus node (at rest) exceeds that of the sympathetic system, the use of atropine (0.03 mg/kg i.v.) alone has been recommended (Tonkin and Heddle, 1984). After atropine the heart rate increases (to more than 90 b.p.m.), the sinus node recovery time and sinoatrial conduction time shorten, sinus rate variability decreases and the duration of secondary pauses is minimized. Failure of atropine to produce these effects strongly suggests the presence of important sinoatrial node disease.

Sinus node refractoriness

The point at which sinus node entrance block occurs in response to the test stimulus during extrastimulus testing may be defined as the longest A1A2 interval which results in sinus node reset. This has been regarded as the 'effective refractory period of the sinus node'. The value of this measurement in discriminating between normal and abnormal sinus node function is currently under investigation by several groups. A recent study showed that the ERP of the sinus node was abnormal in all patients with sinus node disease in whom it could be estimated even when the other test results were normal. This method requires further evaluation.

Direct recording of sinus node potentials

Recently, a technique of directly recording potentials from the sinus node has been developed (Fig. 4.7). A standard electrode catheter is used to record signals

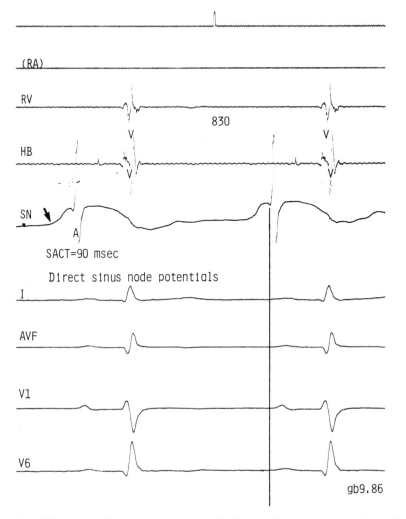

Fig. 4.7 Direct recording of sinus node potentials. Using a bipolar electrode catheter, the junction of the high right atrium and superior vena cava is explored. The electrograms are recorded using a DC amplifier. In the region of the sinus node (SN), low-amplitude, low-frequency deflections are recorded before the onset of the atrial electrogram (A) which itself precedes the onset of the P wave by 25 msec. The time from the onset of the upstroke of the 'preatrial' deflection (arrow) to the onset of the rapid upstroke of the atrial electrogram is 90 msec. This is taken as the sinoatrial conduction time. This interval may be prolonged markedly after rapid pacing in patients with sinoatrial disease.

which are filtered between 0.3 and 50 Hz and highly amplified. A low-frequency, low-amplitude potential just preceding the atrial electrogram has been described as the 'sinus node' electrogram. This method is potentially of considerable interest and clinical value because it may provide insight into the different mechanisms of sinoatrial block, sinus bradycardia and the response of the sinus node to overdrive suppression.

In a recent study, Gomes et al. (1984) investigated the utility of direct sinus node potential recordings in the assessment of sinus node recovery time (SNRT) after overdrive pacing. In 16 patients they compared direct SNRT with indirect SNRT using the conventional method first described by Rosen et al. and Mandel et al. in 1971. They were able to record direct sinus node potentials in each of the 16 patients. The sinoatrial conduction time was measured by the direct method. They noted that the SNRT by the direct method was consistently shorter than by the indirect method and that this was primarily accounted for by prolongation of the sinoatrial conduction time of the first postpacing sinus beat, a phenomenon previously unknown in humans. The site of conduction delay could not be determined in their study. In patients with clinical evidence of sinoatrial disease this effect was more pronounced. The increase in the sinoatrial conduction time was determined by the basic drive cycle length. Thus the shorter the cycle length, the greater the prolongation. It seems, therefore, that the indirect estimation of SNRT includes changes in sinoatrial conduction. A change in the position of the sinus pacemaker site was also documented by an altered morphology in the sinoatrial electrogram corroborated by changes in the surface P wave morphology.

These results have important implications for the interpretation of clinical electrophysiological tests of sinoatrial function. Our present understanding is that sinus node automaticity is depressed in patients with sinus node disorders but this is based on prolongation of the indirect SNRT. The direct estimation suggests that this prolongation may be the result of a marked increase in the sinoatrial conduction time rather than depression of automaticity. The mechanism of this increase is not known.

Several laboratories have reported results of this method but, despite the fairly simple modifications to standard equipment which are required to detect and record these potentials, there have been relatively few publications since the method was first described in 1980 (Hariman et al., 1980). That the direct method has not gained widespread acceptance is somewhat surprising. Technical difficulties may prevent an adequate recording in a high proportion of patients and reproducibility of the method is not known. Nevertheless, technological improvements should make the method more amenable to general use.

Mathematical modelling

A completely different approach has been adopted by Tonkin and Heddle (1984). They have shown that the recovery of the sinus rate after atrial stimulation behaves in an exponential manner, and have devised a mathematical model simulating this response. Using this model they have explored the possibility of separating pacing-induced changes in automaticity, thus enabling computation of the sinoatrial conduction time corrected for these changes (Fig. 4.8). Results to date suggest that the method may be much more sensitive than conventional testing.

As a result of their observations, Tonkin and Heddle (1984) make the following recommendations:

1. Observation of the entire poststimulation sequence.
2. Assessment of sinus node recovery at various pacing rates.

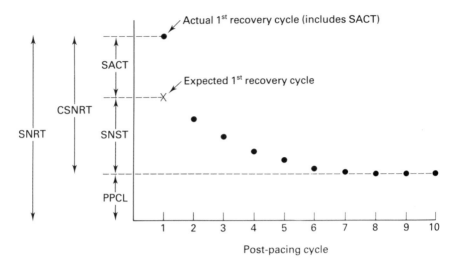

Fig. 4.8 Modelling of sinus node recovery. After a period of atrial pacing, sinus node recovery occurs gradually in an approximately exponential manner (Tonkin and Heddle, 1984). The classic sinus node recovery time (SNRT) includes the prepacing cycle length (PPCL), the sinoatrial conduction time (SACT) and the sinus node suppression time (SNST). The SNST may be estimated by backward extrapolation of the curve of sinus node recovery. CSNRT = corrected sinus node recovery time.

3. Routine evaluation of the effect of atropine on sinus node recovery.
4. Careful evaluation of the direct method of recording sinus node potentials (see above).
5. Determination of subsidiary pacemaker function within the limits of current techniques (see Chapter 5).

The aetiology of the sinoatrial disorders is not fully understood. As a footnote to this chapter we include a hypothesis advanced by Watt (1985), who has suggested that an increased sensitivity to adenosine would account for the clinical findings. Adenosine and adenosine triphosphate have vagal effects and inherent purinergic effects (see Chapter 12). This latter effect seems to predominate in the sinus node because the bradycardias induced by these agents cannot be reversed by atropine. Adenosine can also shorten atrial refractoriness, which, in conjunction with sinus bradycardia, may predispose to atrial fibrillation. Furthermore, suppression of secondary pacemakers can also be accounted for by purinergic activity. This hypothesis has potentially important consequences for both investigation and treatment of these disorders and further studies are required.

References and further reading

Asseman P, Berzin B, Desry D, Vilarem D, Durand P, Delamotte C, Sarkis EH, Lekieffre J, Thery C. (1983) Persistent sinus node electrograms during abnormally prolonged postpacing atrial pauses in sick sinus syndrome in humans: sinoatrial block vs overdrive suppression. *Circulation* **68**, 33

Bashour TT. (1985) Classification of sinus node dysfunction. *American Heart Journal* **110**, 1251

Blanc JJ, Gestin E, Guillerm D, Boschat D, Penther P. (1981) Response of normal and abnormal sinus node to right ventricular stimulation. *American Journal of Cardiology* **48**, 429

Breithardt G, Seipel L. (1978) Comparative study of two methods of estimating sinoatrial conduction time in man. *American Journal of Cardiology* **42**, 965

Crook B, Kitson D, McComisk M, Jewitt D. (1977) Indirect measurement of sinoatrial conduction time in patients with sinoatrial disease and in controls. *British Heart Journal* **39**, 771

Dighton DH. (1974) Sinus bradycardia. Autonomic influences and clinical assessment. *British Heart Journal* **36**, 791

Dhingra R, Amat-y-Leon F, Wyndham C, Deedwania PC, Wu D, Denes P, Rosen KM. (1977) Clinical significance of prolonged sinoatrial conduction time. *Circulation* **55**, 8

Gang E, Reiffel JA, Livelli FD, Bigger JT. (1983) Sinus node recovery time following the spontaneous termination of supraventricular tachycardia and following atrial overdrive pacing: a comparison. *American Heart Journal* **105**, 210

Hatori M, Toyama J, Ito A, Sawada AK, Ito T, Tsuzuki J, Ishikawa S, Kato R, Sotohata I, Yasui S. (1983) Comparative evaluation of depressed automaticity in sick sinus syndrome by Holter monitoring and overdrive suppression test. *American Heart Journal* **105**, 587

Gomes JA, Kang PS, El-Sherif N. (1982) The sinus node electrogram in patients with and without sick sinus syndrome: techniques and correlation between directly measured and indirectly estimated sinoatrial conduction time. *Circulation* **60**, 864

Gomes JA, Hariman RI, Chowdry IA. (1984) New application of direct sinus node recordings in man: assessment of sinus node recovery time. *Circulation* **70**, 663

Gomes JA, Hariman RJ, Kang PS, Chowdry IH. (1985) Sustained symptomatic sinus node re-entrant tachycardia: incidence, clinical significance and the effects of antiarrhythmic agents. *Journal of the American College of Cardiology* **5**, 45

Hariman RF, Krongrad E, Boxer RA, Weiss HB, Steeg CN, Hoffman BF. (1980) Method for recording electrical activity of the sinoatrial node and automatic atrial foci during cardiac catheterization in man. *American Journal of Cardiology* **45**, 775

Josephson ME, Seides S. (1979) *Clinical Cardiac Electrophysiology*, p. 64. Lea & Febiger, Philadelphia, Pa

Kang, PS, Gomes JA, El-Sherif N. (1982) Differential effects of functional autonomic blockade on the variables of sinus node automaticity in sick sinus syndrome. *American Journal of Cardiology* **49**, 273

Kerin NZ, Louridas G, Edlestein, J, Levy MN. (1983) Interactions among the critical factors affecting sinus node function: the quantitative effects of the duration and frequency of atrial pacing and of vagal and sympathetic stimulation upon overdrive suppression of the sinus node. *American Heart Journal* **105**, 215

Kerr CR, Strauss H. (1983) The measurement of sinus node refractoriness in man. *Circulation* **68**, 1231

Kirkorian G, Touboul P, Atallah G, Moleur P, Zuloaga C. (1984) Premature atrial stimulation during regular atrial pacing: a new approach to the study of the sinus node. *American Journal of Cardiology* **54**, 109

Mandel W, Hayakawa H, Danzig R, Marcus HS. (1971) Evaluation of sinoatrial node function in man by overdrive suppression. *Circulation* **44**, 59

Nalos PC, Deng Z, Rosenthal ME, Gang ES, Oseran DS, Mandel WJ, Peter T. (1986) Hemodynamic effects on sinus node recovery time: effects of autonomic blockade. *Journal of the American College of Cardiology* **7**, 1079

Narula OS, Shantha M, Vasquez M, Towne WD, Linhart JW. (1978) A new method for measurement of sinoatrial conduction time. *Circulation* **58**, 706

Narula OS. (1979) Key references; sick sinus syndrome. *Circulation* **60**, 1422

Reiffel JA, Gang E, Gliklick J, Weiss MB, Davis JC, Paton N, Bigger JT. (1980) The human sinus node electrogram: a transvenous catheter technique and a comparison of directly measured and indirectly estimated sinoatrial conduction time in adults. *Circulation* **62**, 1324

Reiffel JA, Gang E, Gliklick J, Bigger JT. (1981) Clinical and electrophysiologic characteristics of sinoatrial entrance block evaluated by direct sinus node electrography: prevalence, relation to antegrade sinoatrial conduction time, and relevance to sinus node disease. *American Heart Journal* **102**, 1011

Reiffel JA, Gang A, Bigger JT, Livelli F, Rolniztky L, Cramer M. (1982) Sinus node recovery time related to paced cycle length in normals and in patients with sinoatrial dysfunction. *American Heart Journal* **104**, 746

Rosen KM, Loeb HS, Sinno MZ, Rahimtoola SH, Gunnar RM. (1971) Cardiac conduction in patients with symptomatic sinus node disease. *Circulation* **42**, 836

Satoh S, Kantsuka H, Kyono H, Suzuki H, Suzuki T, Watanabe J, Nishioka O, Ino-Oka E. (1984) A new indirect method for measurement of sinoatrial conduction time and sinus node return cycle. *Japanese Heart Journal* **26**, 335

Schweitzer P, Mark H. (1984) The values and limitations of deductive analysis and electrophysiological testing in patients with sinoatrial arrhythmias. *Pacing and Clinical Electrophysiology* **7**, 403

Shaw DB, Hocknell JM. (1983) Natural history of sinoatrial disorders. *Clinical Progress in Pacing and Electrophysiology* **1**, 335

Strauss HC, Saroff AL, Bigger Jt, Giardina EGV. (1974) Premature atrial stimulation as a key to the understanding of sinoatrial conduction in man. *Circulation* **47**, 86

Tonkin AF, Heddle WF. (1984) Electrophysiological testing of sinus node function. *Pacing and Clinical Electrophysiology* **7**, 735

Vera Z, Mason DT. (1981) Detection of sinus node dysfunction: consideration of clinical application of testing methods. *American Heart Journal* **102**, 308

Watt AH. (1985) Sick-sinus syndrome: an adenosine-mediated disease. *Lancet* i, 786

5

Atrioventricular Conduction Delays and Block

Delay and block can occur at any level of the conduction system from the atrial myocardium to the ventricular myocardium. Intracardiac studies can provide information about the site of delay or block, and atrial pacing can be used to stress the conduction system to reveal latent conduction disorders. Early applications of the electrophysiological technique were mainly in patients with AV conduction disorders but the emphasis has changed greatly and there are now relatively few indications for this type of study. The information gained from the early studies is, however, important and serves to provide a foundation for the understanding of AV conduction disorders and an appreciation of their electrocardiographic appearances. Furthermore, in patients with unexplained symptoms suggestive of cardiac arrhythmias (such as syncope or collapse – see Chapter 10) useful clinical information may be provided by this type of study.

Intra-atrial delay

Intra-atrial conduction delay is manifest on the surface ECG by prolongation of the P wave and changes in the normal P wave morphology. The main indication for electrophysiological study in patients with isolated intra-atrial conduction defects is to assess the commonly associated atrial tachycardias (see Chapter 8). Occasionally, high degrees of interatrial block (between right and left atria), such as second degree (including Wenckebach conduction) or complete interatrial block, are observed but are relatively uncommon.

Atrioventricular nodal delay

Atrioventricular nodal delay is the most common cause of prolongation of the PR interval. At intracardiac study, the AH interval is prolonged to a variable degree.

The terminology used to describe second degree AV conduction block and delay is confusing. 'Type I AV block' and 'type II AV block' are terms used to describe ECG appearances and do not refer to the site of block. Thus, type I AV block, otherwise referred to as 'Wenckebach-type block', is characterized by a gradual increase in the PR interval prior to the dropped beat, whereas in type II block no such change is evident. Although the former type is usually intranodal and the latter type is usually infranodal, either type of block may (theoretically) occur within or below the node. Typical type I second degree (Wenckebach pattern) AV block is almost always a result of progressive increases in intranodal conduction time (AH intervals) (Fig. 5.1). However, this is not invariable. So-called atypical type I second degree AV block refers to the absence

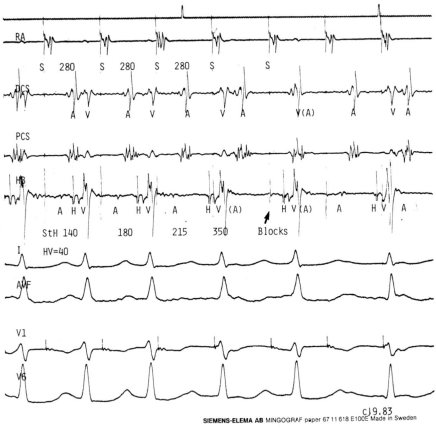

Fig. 5.1 Atrial pacing (S1S2) at a cycle length of 280 msec inducing AH Wenckebach conduction block. The AH interval gradually increases until there is conduction block (blocked stimulus arrowed), manifest by failure of activation of the His bundle (H). Because the atrial electrogram, A, is obscured by the next ventricular electrogram in cycles towards the end of the sequence ('A' is in parentheses), the stimulus to H (StH) interval is given (there is no intra-atrial delay during the sequence). At very short Wenckebach points the His potential may be delayed such that it appears well into the next cycle, as in this recording (the last StH interval of 350 msec exceeds the pacing cycle length). Paper speed 100 mm/sec. DCS and PCS = distal and proximal coronary sinus; HB = His bundle region; RA = right atrium.

of discernible incremental AH prolongation before the blocked impulse but the presence of a shorter PR interval of the first conducted beat after the blocked beat. This pattern is, in fact, common. Agents which decrease AV nodal refractoriness tend to abolish this conduction pattern. First degree and type I second degree AH delay may not be pathological. Type II AV nodal block is rare and has never been adequately demonstrated. Close inspection of the recordings in these instances almost always reveals PR prolongation prior to the dropped beat or PR shortening of the first conducted beat after the dropped beat; that is, type I block. Higher grades of second degree block (sustained 2:1 or 3:1 ratio) within the AV node itself are uncommon. Sustained 2:1 AV block may intermittently progress to higher degrees or regress to lesser degrees (e.g. type I) of block. Clearly, 2:1, 3:1 and higher forms of second degree AV block cannot be classified as either type I or type II by virtue of the definitions of these terms.

The need to implant a permanent pacemaker in patients with these conduction abnormalities is based on clinical grounds. Diagnostic intracardiac studies are unnecessary because the surface ECG is generally sufficient for decision making. Occasionally, type I delay occurs in association with bundle branch block. In this setting the level of type I delay may be within the AV node or the His bundle, and intracardiac recordings may be necessary to localize the site. Whether this is of any therapeutic benefit, however, is dubious. Complete AV nodal block is discussed below.

Intraventricular conduction delays

Delay and block within the distal conduction system are of greater clinical significance than those within the AV node because of the graver prognosis associated with these disorders. All degrees of distal block are encountered in clinical practice, and often the decision to undertake long-term pacing is simple being based on clinical and symptomatic grounds alone. There are, however, several types of distal block which have been regarded as portending total failure of the conduction system and consequent collapse. The continued interest in electrophysiological investigation of distal conduction blocks is therefore primarily to discover information which may be of prognostic value. In clinical practice, the most important of the distal conduction defects (other than complete AV block) is chronic bundle branch block because it is very common and may progress to higher degrees of block.

Prolongation of the HV interval indicates delay in the His bundle itself or in all of the distal fascicles, or both. This is so because the HV interval is determined by the shortest conduction time from the His bundle to the ventricles in any fascicle. HV prolongation rarely exceeds 110 msec and may not be sufficient to give the appearance of first degree AV block on the surface ECG (Fig. 5.2). Type I second degree block within the His–Purkinje system is unusual and is diagnosed by recording progressive beat-by-beat increases in the HV interval prior to infra-His block. Type II distal block is more common than type II AV nodal block. These higher degrees of conduction delays are almost always associated with bundle branch block and indicate severe damage to the distal conduction system. It is widely agreed that long-term pacing is advisable in these patients even in the absence of symptoms because the disease is progressive. Delay or block can also occur within the His bundle itself. Intracardiac recordings may, rarely, demonstrate a 'split His potential' during continued conduction. Occasionally, disappearance of the second spike occurs when the impulse is blocked within the His bundle. The incidence of this phenomenon (intra-His block) is not known but, for clinical purposes, it is treated as second degree distal block.

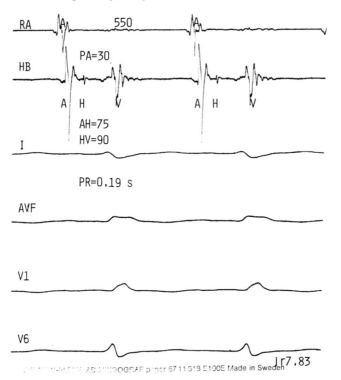

RA   550

HB   PA=30

A H   V   A H   V

AH=75
HV=90

I

PR=0.19 s

AVF

V1

V6

Jr7.83

Fig. 5.2 Prolongation of the HV interval. These recordings were taken after aortic valve replacement during which this 56-year-old man developed right bundle branch block. The HV interval is markedly prolonged at 90 msec and the AH interval is 75 msec. The PR interval, however, is within normal limits. Paper speed 100 mm/sec. HB = His bundle; RA = right atrium.

Prognostic importance of HV prolongation

Patients with idiopathic bundle branch block and symptoms suggestive of intermittent high degree AV block are candidates for long-term pacing even if no definite evidence of AV block has been documented. Intracardiac recording and atrial stimulation studies sometimes expose a distal site of block (see below) but it should be noted that other arrhythmias (e.g. ventricular tachycardia) may be responsible for symptoms in patients with intraventricular conduction delay. In the absence of a positive result, however, pacing may be the most expeditious course. The ultimate decision must be based on individual clinical features. In asymptomatic patients with bundle branch block or bifascicular block the decision is more difficult.

The concept that the HV interval reflects the shortest conduction time from the His bundle to the ventricle has been used as a means of assessing the state of the conducting fascicles in patients with bundle branch block. Thus, HV prolongation in patients with right bundle branch block implies significant damage to the left bundle branch system and a possible risk of progression to complete AV block, with potentially dangerous consequences. It is not certain whether HV prolongation (say >70 msec) can be used to predict which patients with pre-existing bundle branch block are at risk. Several studies conducted over the last decade have not yielded a conclusive answer. Some have concluded that the risk of progression is greater if the HV interval is prolonged, while others have not. Some have shown that mortality in the long HV group was higher compared to a control group but it has not been clear that this was related to progression to complete AV block. Gross prolongation of the HV interval to >100 msec does seem to be predictive of progression to complete AV block but such long values are not common. An interesting finding of several studies is the unexpectedly low incidence of progression to complete block. Even if all these studies are taken into account, it is still not clear that pacemaker implantation reduces the risk of death in symptomatic or asymptomatic patients with a prolonged HV interval and bifascicular block. It must be concluded that prolongation of the HV interval *per se* is not helpful in the assessment of these patients.

Pacing-induced distal block

Block distal to the His bundle may be exposed by atrial pacing but this is very rare in patients with normal atrioventricular conduction (it may be functional in patients with enhanced AV nodal conduction – see Chapter 6, or after atropine administration – see Chapter 12) or in asymptomatic patients with bundle branch block and a normal HV interval. In symptomatic patients, especially those with HV prolongation, infra-His block may be induced by incremental atrial pacing. Extrastimulus testing may also induce distal delay (Fig. 5.3) or block (Fig. 5.4). The sensitivity and specificity of each method of inducing block with regard to predicting late-onset high degree block is not known. Factors such as atrial effective refractoriness and the functional refractoriness of the AV node may limit the ability to expose this propensity to block. The clinical utility of these responses is, however, still unclear and it may be argued that symptomatic patients deserve pacing in any case. To restate the problem, it is clinically inappropriate and probably unethical to deny pacing on the basis of inability to induce distal block in a particular symptomatic patient.

It has been suggested that there is functional longitudinal dissociation of conduction pathways within the His bundle. Localized proximal His bundle lesions could therefore result in an ECG pattern of bundle branch block. This possibility is further suggested by the observation that some examples of bundle branch block can be 'normalized' by selective pacing of the distal (but not proximal) His bundle. The reproducibility of this phenomenon has not be tested and the prognostic importance of this finding is not known.

Drug-induced distal block

Antiarrhythmic drugs with local anaesthetic properties (membrane-stabilizing agents) slow the speed of conduction in excitable myocardial cells. This effect is more pronounced in the presence of pre-existing disease. The concept that these drugs may be used to unmask latent severe conduction defects has been investigated using several different drugs of this type (see Chapter 12).

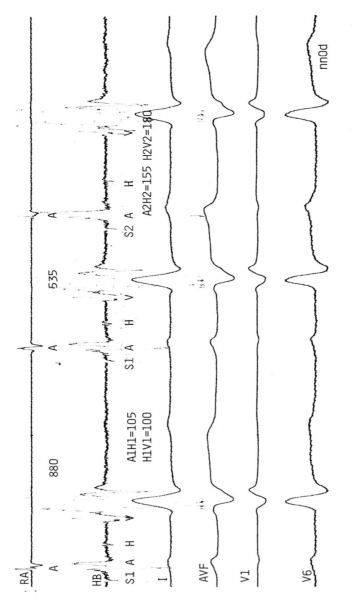
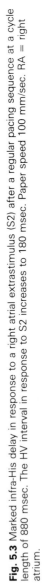

Fig. 5.3 Marked infra-His delay in response to a right atrial extrastimulus (S2) after a regular pacing sequence at a cycle length of 880 msec. The HV interval in response to S2 increases to 180 msec. Paper speed 100 mm/sec. RA = right atrium.

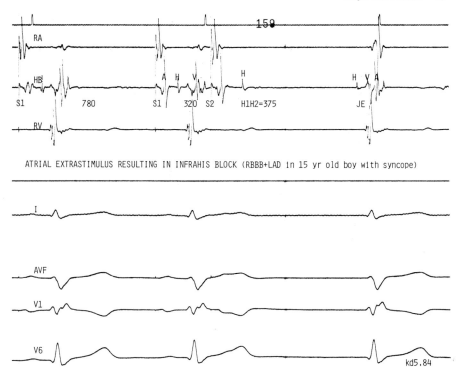

ATRIAL EXTRASTIMULUS RESULTING IN INFRAHIS BLOCK (RBBB+LAD in 15 yr old boy with syncope)

Fig. 5.4 Infra-His block induced by atrial premature stimulation. This 15-year-old had suffered two syncopal episodes. His sister had died suddenly at the age of 14 years. The surface ECG demonstrated left axis deviation and right bundle branch block. After a regular pacing sequence (A1A2) at a cycle length of 780 msec an atrial extrastimulus (S2) coupled at 320 msec results in block below the His bundle. These findings were interpreted as indicative of important distal conduction system disease and a pacemaker was implanted. Paper speed 100 mm/sec. HB = His bundle; RA = right atrium; RV = right ventricle.

Procainamide intravenously may result in conversion of bundle branch block to complete AV block or merely prolong the HV interval. The response is presumably determined by several factors, including the amount of drug given and the degree and location of underlying conduction system disease. A positive response has been defined as:

1. An increase of the HV interval to over 100 msec or doubling of the initial value.
   and
2. Provocation of higher degrees of distal His–Purkinje block.

These effects appear to be predictive of later spontaneous progression to complete block. They have been interpreted as indicating 'critical' distal disease worthy of long-term prophylactic pacing. Similar studies using ajmaline or disopyramide have shown a similar effect. Although these types of studies may be useful in certain patients with undiagnosed symptoms, their predictive value is unknown and further information is required before they can be recommended as routine

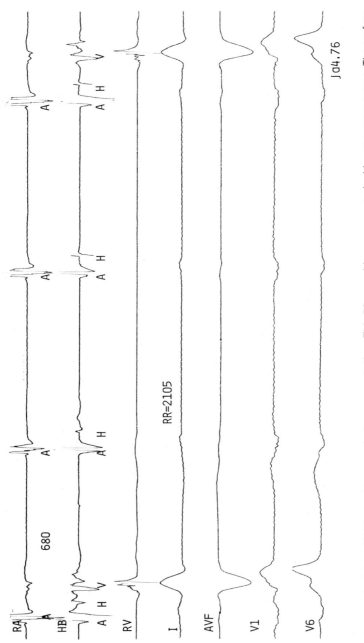

Fig. 5.5 Complete AV block with a ventricular escape rhythm. This 78-year-old man presented with recurrent syncope. The surface ECG showed complete AV block with wide bizarre QRS complexes at a rate of 25–30 b.p.m. Intracardiac recordings show that atrial impulses conduct only to the His bundle. The escape rhythm arises in the distal conduction system. Paper speed 100 mm/sec. HB = His bundle region; RA = right atrium; RV = right ventricle.

procedures in the assessment of patients with asymptomatic AV conduction disorders.

Complete atrioventricular block and escape rhythms

Complete or third degree AV block may be caused by block within the AV node, within the His bundle itself or distal to the His bundle. Electrophysiological investigations have provided much information about these arrhythmias and the associated escape rhythms. By recording the His potential the level of block may be localized to above or below (or, rarely, within) the His bundle. The associated escape rhythm may arise from above or within the His bundle or from the fascicles. Both the level of block and the nature of the escape rhythm are of prognostic importance. The electrocardiographic appearances of complete AV block are determined by the degree of block, the level of block and the nature of the associated escape rhythms.

Complete block distal to the His bundle

Chronic complete AV block caused by idiopathic conduction system disease or anterior myocardial infarction is most commonly a result of block below the bundle of His (Fig. 5.5). The associated escape rhythm arises in the distal conduction system and tends to be slower and behave less predictably than higher levels of escape rhythm. Thus, the surface ECG shows complete AV dissociation with a slow escape rate and wide bizarre QRS complexes. The prognosis of this type of block is generally poor because the disease is progressive and the behaviour of the escape rhythm is unpredictable. Patients with third degree complete infra-His block are therefore candidates for long-term pacing even in the absence of symptoms. The diagnosis can be made from the surface ECG with a high degree of accuracy, and electrophysiological studies are not usually contributory in the management of these patients except in the choice of pacing system (see below).

Complete block proximal to the His bundle

The commonest causes of this type of block are vagotonic influences (e.g. intermittent AV block in fit athletes), inferior myocardial infarction (in which the block is usually transient and not associated with a risk of permanent damage), congenitally complete AV block (Fig. 5.6), myocarditis and drug-related causes. The escape rhythms usually arise from the proximal His bundle or lower AV node and tend to be faster than those of lower escape foci distal to the bifurcation of the His bundle. The ECG appearances are therefore complete AV dissociation with a narrow QRS complex escape rhythm. Intracardiac recordings show that the non-conducted impulses are blocked proximal to the site of the His bundle recording (absence of a His potential after each atrial electrogram) and, in a large proportion of cases, the escape rhythm arises proximal to this site (the QRS complexes are preceded by a His spike). These sites of block and escape are, however, not invariable even in the congenital form. The HV interval of the escape beats is usually normal.

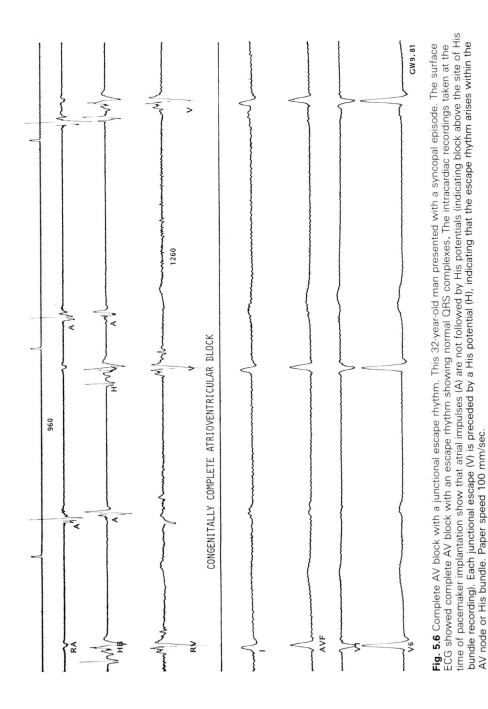

Fig. 5.6 Complete AV block with a junctional escape rhythm. This 32-year-old man presented with a syncopal episode. The surface ECG showed complete AV block with an escape rhythm showing normal QRS complexes. The intracardiac recordings taken at the time of pacemaker implantation show that atrial impulses (A) are not followed by His potentials (indicating block above the site of His bundle recording). Each junctional escape (V) is preceded by a His potential (H), indicating that the escape rhythm arises within the AV node or His bundle. Paper speed 100 mm/sec.

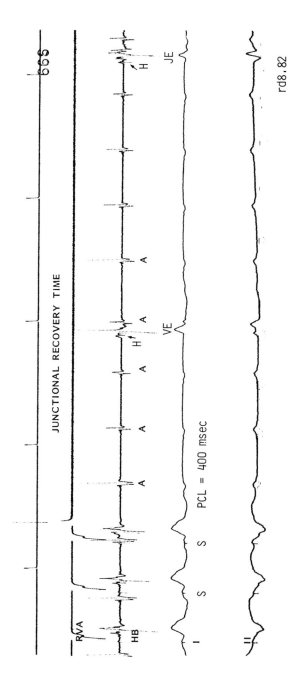

Fig. 5.7 Estimation of junctional recovery time in a patient with complete AV block following His bundle ablation. After right ventricular pacing for 30 seconds at 150 b.p.m., the pacemaker is switched off and an escape beat is recorded 1.66 seconds later. That this is not a junctional escape beat is confirmed by the fact that the His potential (arrowed) is inscribed after the onset of the QRS which is a ventricular escape beat (VE). This QRS shape is different to that seen during conducted rhythm preablation. Ths next complex is a junctional escape (JE) beat. The junctional origin of the beat is confirmed by recording a His potential (arrowed) before the QRS. The QRS complex itself is narrow and of a morphology identical to that seen before ablation. (Note that the latter pause is longer at 2.2 seconds.) Paper speed 50 mm/sec.

Although symptomatic congenitally complete AV block is an undoubted indication for long-term pacing, it should be understood that the first symptom may be collapse and death. Despite extensive investigation, however, there are still no clear guidelines for permament pacing in asymptomatic subjects.

It has been suggested that the site of block in congenital forms is predictive of the risk of syncope but prospective studies have failed to confirm this suggestion. An escape rate of less than 50 b.p.m. is found more commonly in patients who suffer syncope. Formal assessment of the reliability of the escape rhythm by measurement of the junctional recovery time (Fig. 5.7) is another possible approach to the problem. This is achieved by right ventricular pacing at various rates for 15–60 seconds and observing the time taken for the escape rhythm to reappear. Studies have not indicated a clear relationship between the recovery time and the occurrence of later symptoms.

In summary, it appears that electrophysiological studies do not make an important contribution to the management of patients with documented complete AV block because the decision to pace can usually be made on clinical grounds and because the information gained from these studies has not, as yet, been shown to be of prognostic value. Nevertheless, there are occasional patients with unexplained symptoms in whom studies of this type may help to clarify an otherwise difficult decision.

Further reading

Akhtar MM. (1985) Clinical application of electrophysiological studies in the mangement of patients requiring pacemaker therapy. In: *Modern Cardiac Pacing*, p.3. Ed. by S Barold. Futura: Mount Kisco, NY

Alpert B. (1983) Role of electrophysiology study in pacemaker implantation for bradyarrhythmias. *Clinical Progress in Pacing and Electrophysiology* 1, 109

Altschuler H, Fisher JD, Furman S. (1979) Significance of isolated HV prolongation in symptomatic patients without documented heart block. *American Heart Journal* 97, 19

Benson DW, Spach M, Edwards S, Sterba R, Serwer G, Armstrong B, Anderson P. (1982) Heart block in children. Evaluation of subsidiary ventricular pacemaker recovery times and ECG tape recordings. *Pediatric Cardiology* 2, 39

Camm AJ, Levy A, Spurrell RAJ. (1977) Junctional recovery and conduction times in complete congenital atrioventricular block. *British Heart Journal* 39, 933 (abstract)

Castellanos A, Iyengar R, Agha A, Castillo CA. (1972) Wenckebach phenomena within the atria. *British Heart Journal* 34, 1121

Chiale PA, Przybylski J, Laino RA, Halpern S, Nau GJ, Sanchez RA, Lazzari JO, Elizari MV, Rosenbaum MB. (1982) Usefulness of the ajmaline test in patients with left bundle branch block. *American Journal of Cardiology* 49, 21

Denes P, Dhingra RC, Wu D, Chuquimia R, Amat-y-Leon F, Wyndham C, Rosen KM. (1975) HV intervals in patients with bifascicular block (right bundle branch block and left anterior hemiblock). Clinical, electrocardiographic and electrophysiologic correlations. *American Journal of Cardiology* 35, 23

Dhingra R, Winslow E, Pouget M, Rahimtoola SH, Rosen KM. (1973) The effect of isoproterenol on atrioventricular and intraventricular conduction. *American Journal of Cardiology* 32, 629

Dhingra RC, Denes P, Wu D, Chuquimia R, Amat-y-Leon F, Wyndham C, Rosen KM. (1974) Syncope in patients with chronic bifascicular block. Significance, causative mechanisms, and clinical implications. *Annals of Internal Medicine* **81**, 302

Dhingra RC, Denes P, Wu D, Chuquimia R, Amat-y-Leon F, Wyndham C, Rosen KM. (1975) Chronic right bundle branch block and left posterior hemiblock. Clinical, electrophysiologic and prognostic observations. *American Journal of Cardiology* **36**, 867

Dhingra RC, Denes P, Wu D, Wyndham CR, Amat-y-Leon F, Towne WD, Rosen KM. (1976) Prospective observations in patients with chronic bundle branch block and marked HV prolongation. *Circulation* **53**, 600

Dhingra RC, Wyndham CRC, Bauernfeind R, Denes P, Wu D, Swiryn S, Rosen KM. (1979a) Significance of chronic bifascicular block without apparent organic heart disease. *Circulation* **60**, 33

Dhingra RC, Wyndham C, Bauernfeind R, Swiryn S, Deedwania PC, Smith T, Denes P, Rosen KM. (1979b) Significance of block distal to the HI's bundle induced by atrial pacing in patients with chronic bifascicular block. *Circulation* **60**, 1455

Dhingra RC, Wyndham C, Bauernfeind R, Swiryn S, Deedwania PC, Smith T, Denes P, Rosen KM. (1979b) Significance of block distal to the His bundle induced by atrial pacing in patients with chronic bifascicular block. *Circulation* **60**, 1455

Dhingra RC, Wyndham C, Deedwania PC, Bauernfeind R, Swiryn S, Best D, Rosen KM. (1980) Effect of age on atrioventricular conduction in patients with chronic bifascicular block. *American Journal of Cardiology* **45**, 749

Dhingra RC, Palileo E, Strasberg B, Swiryn S, Bauernfeind RA, Wyndham CRC, Rosen KM. (1981) Significance of HV interval in 517 patients with chronic bifascicular block. *Circulation* **64**, 1265

El-Sherif N, Amat-y-Leon F, Schonfield C, Scherlag BJ, Rosen K, Lazzara R, Wyndham C. (1978) Normalization of bundle branch block patterns by distal His bundle pacing. Clinical and experimental evidence of longitudinal dissociation in the pathologic His bundle. *Circulation* **57**, 473

Esscher EB. (1981) Congenital complete heart block in adolescence and adult life. A follow-up study. *European Heart Journal* **2**, 281

Fisher JD, Kulbertus H, Narula O. (1978) Panel discussion: prognostic value of the HV interval. *Pacing and Clinical Electrophysiology* **1**, 132

Jordan J, Yamaguchi I, Mandel WJ, McCullen AE. (1977) Comparative effects of overdrive on sinus and subsidiary pacemaker function. *American Heart Journal* **93**, 367

Karpawich PP, Gillette P, Garson A, Hesslien P, Porter C, McNamara D. (1981) Congenital complete atrioventricular block: clinical and electrophysiologic precursors of need for pacemaker insertion. *American Journal of Cardiology* **48**, 1098

Kastor JA, Goldreyer BN, Moore EN, Shelburne JC, Manchester JH. (1975) Intraventricular conduction in man studied with an endocardial electrode catheter mapping technique. *Circulation* **51**, 786

Lane GK, Kenelly BM. (1978) Ventricular overdrive suppression of idioventricular pacemakers in patients with complete heart block. *Cardiovascular Research* **12**, 712

Lichstein E, Ribas-Meneclier C, Naik D, Chadda KD, Gupta PK, Smith H. (1976) The natural history of trifascicular disease following permanent pacemaker implantation. *Circulation* **54**, 780

Lie KI, Durrer D. (1979) Conduction disorders in acute myocardial infarction. In: *Cardiac Arrhythmias: Electrophysiology, Diagnosis and Treatment*, p. 140. Ed. by OS Narula. Williams & Wilkins: Baltimore, Md

McAnulty JH, Rahimtoola SH, Murphy E, DeMots H, Ritzmann L, Kanarek PE, Kauffman S. (1982) Natural history of 'high-risk' bundle branch block. *New England Journal of Medicine* **307**, 137

McKenna WJ, Rowland E, Davies J, Krikler DM. (1980) Failure to predict development of atrioventricular block with electrophysiological testing supplemented by ajmaline.

Pacing and Clinical Electrophysiology 3, 666

Mangiardi LM, Bonamini R, Conte M, Gaiti F, Orzan F, Presbitero P, Brusca A. (1982) Bedside evaluation of atrioventricular block with narrow QRS complexes: usefulness of carotid sinus message and atropine administration. *American Journal of Cardiology* 49, 1136

Narula OS, Cohen LS, Samet P, Lister JW, Scherlag BJ, Hildner FJ. (1970) Localization of AV conduction defects in man by recording of the His bundle electrogram. *American Journal of Cardiology* 25, 228

Narula OS. (1977) Longitudinal dissociation in the His bundle. Bundle branch block due to asynchronous conduction within the His bundle in man. *Circulation* 56, 996

Narula OS, Narula JT. (1977) Junctional pacemakers in man. Response to overdrive suppression with and without parasympathetic blockade. *Circulation* 57, 880

Narula OS. (1979) Atrioventricular block. In: *Cardiac Arrhythmias: Electrophysiology, Diagnosis and Treatment*, p. 85. Ed. by OS Narula. Williams & Wilkins: Baltimore, Md

Puech P, Wainwright RJ. (1980) Clinical electrophysiology of atrioventricular block. *Cardiology Clinics* 1, 209

Rosen KM, Dhingra R, Loab HS, Rahimtoola SH. (1973) Chronic heart block in adults. Clinical and electrophysiological observations. *Archives of Internal Medicine* 131, 663

Rosenbaum MB, Elizari MV, Lazzari JO. (1970) *The Hemiblocks*. Tampa Tracings: Tampa, Fla

Scheinman MM, Peters RW, Modin G, Brennan M, Mies C, O'Young J. (1977) Prognostic value of infranodal conduction time in patients with chronic bundle branch block. *Circulation* 56, 240

Scheinman MM, Peters RW, Sauve MJ, Desai J, Abbott JA, Cogan J, Wohl B, Williams K. (1982) Value of the HQ interval in patients with bundle branch block and the role of prophylactic permanent pacing. *American Journal of Cardiology* 50, 1316

Scheinman MM, Hughes RW, Morady F, Sauve MJ, Malone P, Modin G. (1983) Electrophysiologic studies in patients with bundle branch block. *Pacing and Clinical Electrophysiology* 6, 1157

Schuilenberg RM, Durrer D. (1970) Observations on atrioventricular conduction in patients with bilateral bundle branch block. *Circulation* 41, 967

Spear JF, Moore EN. (1971) Electrophysiologic studies on Mobitz type II second degree heart block. *Circulation* 44, 1087

Spurrell RAJ, Krikler DM, Sowton E. (1972a) Study of right bundle branch block in association with either left anterior hemiblock or left posterior hemiblock using His bundle electrograms. *British Heart Journal* 34, 800

Spurrell RAJ, Krikler DM, Sowton E. (1972b) Study of intraventricular conduction times in patients with left bundle branch block and left axis deviation and in patients with left bundle branch block and normal QRS axis using His bundle electrograms. *British Heart Journal* 34, 1244

Surawicz B. (1979) Prognosis of patients with chronic bifascicular block. *Circulation* 60, 40

Thomsen PEB, Sterndorff B, Gotzsche H. (1976) Intraventricular trifascicular block verified by His bundle electrocardiography. *American Heart Journal* 92, 497

Tonkin AM, Heddle WF, Tornos P. (1978) Intermittent atrioventricular block: procainamide administration as a provocative test. *Australian and New Zealand Journal of Medicine* 8, 594

Vera Z, Mason DT, Fletcher RD, Awan NA, Massumi RA. (1976) Prolonged His–Q interval in chronic bifascicular block. Relation to impending complete heart block. *Circulation* 53, 46

Ward DE, Jones S, Camm AJ. (1985) Long-term endocardial pacing in congenital heart disease. *Clinical Progress in Electrophysiology and Pacing* 3, 133

Wolff GS, Tamer D, Garcia OL, Ferrer P, Pickoff A, Sung RJ. (1980) His–Purkinje conduction findings after cardiac surgery in children. *Circulation* **62**, 615

Wu D, Denes P, Dhingra R, Rosen KM. (1974) Bundle branch block. Demonstration of the incomplete nature of some 'complete' bundle branch and fascicular blocks by the extrastimulus technique. *American Journal of Cardiology* **33**, 583

Zipes D. (1979) Second degree atrioventricular block. *Circulation* **60**, 465

Part III

Investigation of Tachycardias

6

Pre-excitation

The term 'pre-excitation' was coined by Ohnell (1944) to describe the QRS abnormalities found in patients with the typical Wolff–Parkinson–White (WPW) syndrome. Three major types of pre-excitation are recognized (Fig. 6.1):

1. Anomalous atrioventricular conduction over a pathway connecting the atrial to the ventricular myocardium. This pathway is responsible for the features of the WPW syndrome.
2. Anomalous nodoventricular and His ventricular pathway conduction, the anatomical substrate for which is believed to be fibres discovered by Mahaim (1947). The clinical significance of this form of pre-exitation is not established.
3. Apparent anomalous conduction in atrionodal or atrio-His pathways causing pre-excitation of the AV node or His bundle. The syndrome of a short PR interval associated with a normal QRS complex and paroxysmal tachycardias is thought to reflect this type of pre-excitation.

The terminology of pre-excitation has been confused and misunderstood. In this chapter we have adopted the nomenclature proposed by Anderson et al. (1975), on behalf of the European Study Group for pre-excitation. Thus the terms 'Kent' bundle, 'James' fibre and 'Mahaim' fibre are avoided. The pathways discovered by Kent are accessory nodal structures of a distinctly different morphology from the usual type of anomalous AV connection (Anderson and Becker, 1981).

Anomalous atrioventricular conduction (Wolff–Parkinson–White syndrome)

The anatomical abnormality responsible for abnormal atrioventricular conduction in the WPW syndrome is an anomalous connection capable of conducting atrial impulses to the ventricular mass. This causes an activation wavefront which is separate from that resulting from conduction over the normal AV nodal–His bundle pathway. The eccentric wavefront spreads slowly in the ventricular myocardium, causing slurring of the upstroke of the QRS complex and thus producing the characteristic delta wave appearance. (Fig. 6.2) The abnormal QRS is therefore a result of fusion of two independent wavefronts. The degree of slurring of the QRS depends on the relative contribution to ventricular activation of the normal and anomalous pathways. The QRS abnormality is found in about 1 in 500 people and is associated with symptomatic tachycardias (see Chapter 9) in a small proportion of these. However, these anomalous pathways do not always conduct in the anterograde (AV) direction. Thus, they may be present without causing any QRS abnormality and are then described as

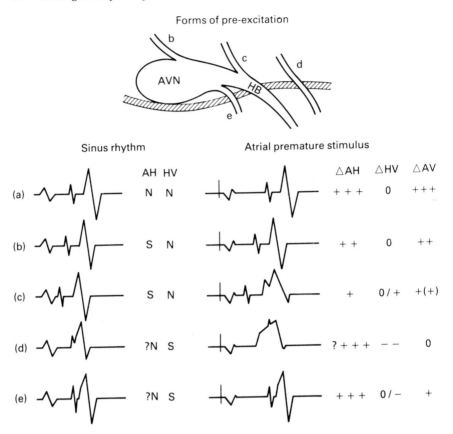

Fig. 6.1 Various types of junctional and ventricular pre-excitation and a schematic representation of the AV conduction pattern in response to atrial premature stimulation. The pathways shown in the upper diagram are: (a) normal pathway; (b) atrionodal pathway; (c) atrio-His pathway; (d) atrioventricular anomalous pathway; and (e) nodoventricular pathway.

Lower diagrams. In the left column, AHV conduction intervals are indicated on the stylized recording during sinus rhythm. The columns labelled 'AH' and 'HV' indicate normal (N) or short (S) intervals. The column labelled 'Atrial premature stimulus' indicates the usual AV conduction response (of the abnormal pathway in combination with the normal AV nodal pathway) to progressively premature atrial stimulation. The columns labelled ΔAH and ΔHV indicate the direction of change in AH and HV intervals in response during extrastimulation. Thus, during sinus rhythm the AH and HV intervals are normal (N) and the AH interval increases considerably with atrial premature stimulation (APS). (*a*) Normal AV conduction. (*b*) An atrionodal pathway shows a short AH interval during sinus rhythm with an attenuated AH increase and no HV change during APS. (*c*) An atrio-His pathway may result in a very short AH interval with a normal HV interval and an attenuated AH increase during APS. The HV interval may also show a slight increase. (*d*) A direct AV anomalous pathway may obscure the His potential but AV nodal intervals during sinus rhythm and responses to APS are unaffected by such a pathway. However, because the ventricles are pre-excited the HV interval is short or negative. This is exaggerated by APS. (*e*) Nodoventricular conduction may also obscure the His potential. When it is apparent (see Fig. 6.14), the interval is normal and the HV interval short. During APS this effect is exaggerated to a variable degree which is determined by the physiology of the nodoventricular pathway and the AV node. Fasciculoventricular pathways (not illustrated) cause a short HV interval which remains constant during APS.

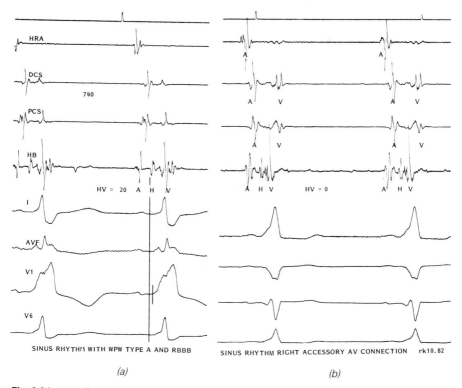

Fig. 6.2 Intracardiac recordings during sinus rhythm and ventricular pre-excitation. (*a*) Recordings in a patient with typical left ventricular pre-excitation and associated right bundle branch block. The QRS complex shows a positive delta wave in leads I, VI and V6. The HV interval is shortened to 20 msec, indicating pre-excitation. The typical right bundle branch block is manifest by deep S waves in I and V6. (*b*) Recordings in a patient with a right accessory AV connection showing an HV interval of zero. Paper speed 100 mm/sec. DCS = distal coronary sinus; HB = His bundle region; PCS = proximal coronary sinus; RA = right atrium.

'concealed anomalous pathways'. These pathways may also give rise to tachycardias if they are capable of conducting in the retrograde (VA) direction. Some pathways conduct only in the anterograde direction and are not able to sustain orthodromic tachycardia. The mechanism of these directional properties is not clear. De la Fuente et al. (1971) investigated undirectional conduction across a narrow isthmus of tissue connecting a large mass of ventricular cells with a sheet of atrium. They concluded that the limited atrial wavefront may not be sufficient to excite the ventricles whereas the conditions in the reverse direction would allow conduction, so-called impedance mismatch.

Electrophysiological features of ventricular pre-excitation

The electrophysiological characteristics of anomalous atrioventricular pathways may be discussed under four categories;

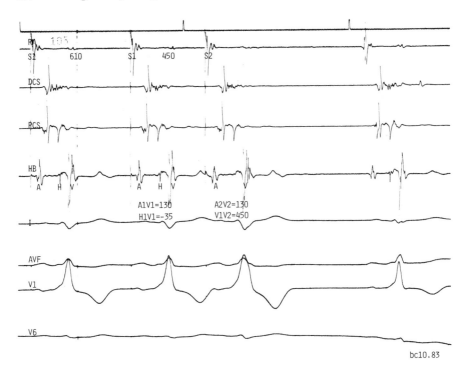

bc10.83

Fig. 6.3 Atrial pacing in a patient with a left free wall anomalous pathway. During regular basic pacing at a cycle length of 610 msec (S1S1) there is evidence of left ventricular pre-excitation (positive delta in V1 and a negative HV interval of −35 msec). An atrial premature stimulus coupled at 450 msec (S2) results in normal prolongation of the AH interval such that the His potential is obscured by the QRS complex. The AV interval remains unchanged at 130 msec because there is no additional delay in the anomalous pathway in response to the premature stimulus (compare with Fig. 6.5). Paper speed 100 mm/sec. A, H and V = atrial, His bundle and ventricular electrograms; DCS and PCS = distal and proximal coronary sinus; His = His bundle; RA = right atrium.

1. Anterograde conduction patterns.
2. Atrial fibrillation and ventricular pre-excitation.
3. Retrograde conduction patterns.
4. Associated junctional tachycardias.

The last of these will be discussed together with other forms of junctional tachycardias (see Chapter 9). When undertaking electrophysiological investigation of anomalous AV or VA conduction it is important to bear in mind the possibility of traumatic block in the pathway induced by catheter manipulation. If an anomalous pathway is strongly suspected but cannot be demonstrated at study, traumatic block may be considered.

Anterograde conduction studies

Intracardiac recordings during ventricular pre-excitation show a short AV

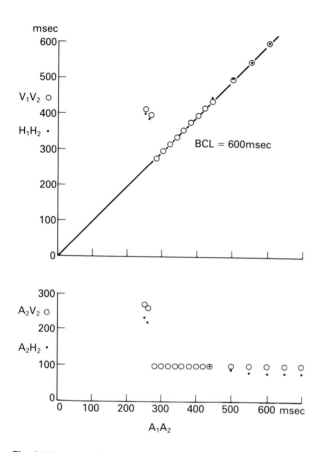

Fig. 6.4 Anterograde conduction curve in a patient with ventricular pre-excitation due to a direct AV anomalous pathway. As the A1A2 interval is decreased, the A2V2 interval remains constant and the V1V2 interval equals the A1A2 interval until block occurs in the anomalous pathway when normal conduction is revealed (Fig. 6.5). The AH interval is prolonged normally and the His potential becomes obscured by the QRS as the A1A2 interval is decreased. BCL = basic cycle length.

interval. The His potential may be obscured by the ventricular electrogram if the AV interval is very short. The His spike may be recorded before the QRS, simultaneous with the onset of the QRS or after the QRS complex depending on the degree of ventricular pre-excitation (Fig. 6.2). During incremental atrial pacing the AV interval, which is determined by conduction over the anomalous pathway, does not increase (compare with AV nodal responses) because these pathways do not possess decremental conduction properties (see Chapters 3 and 12). Similarly, the response to atrial extrastimulation shows no increase in the AV interval. The AV node responds normally and the AH interval gradually lengthens in response to increasingly premature stimulation and the His spike ultimately becomes obscured by the QRS complex (Fig. 6.3). The coupling interval at which anomalous pathway conduction (ventricular pre-excitation) disappears is called the anterograde effective refractory period (ERP) of the

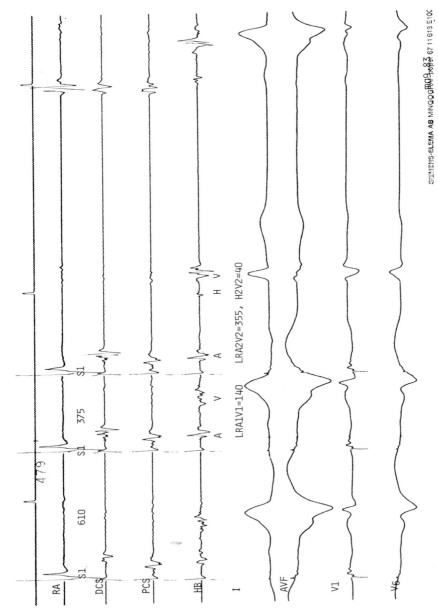

Fig. 6.5 Atrial pacing in a patient with a posteroseptal anomalous pathway. During regular pacing of the right atrium at a cycle length of 610 msec (S1S1) there is ventricular pre-excitation with a negative delta wave in AVF. A premature stimulus (S2) coupled at 375 msec blocks in the anomalous pathway with disappearance of pre-excitation and conducts through the AV node with a normal QRS shape and a normal HV interval. Paper speed 100 mm/sec. LRA = low right atrium on His recording.

anomalous pathway. The typical anterograde conduction pattern is shown in Fig. 6.4. The ERP of the anomalous pathway shortens if the basic driving rate is increased.

If the ERP of the AV node is less than that of the anomalous pathway normal conduction will be revealed with an associated sudden increase in the AV interval (Figs. 6.4 and 6.5). Occasionally this sudden increase in the AV conduction time is associated with the onset of tachycardias (see Chapters 7 and 9) or single atrial echo beats as a result of 're-entry' of the impulse to the atria over the anomalous pathway. These phenomena are in part dependent on the position of the atrial stimulation site in relation to the anomalous pathway and the AV node. For example, remote stimulation from the high right atrium may result in activation of the AV node and a left AV anomalous pathway at approximately the same time, resulting in moderate pre-excitation, whereas stimulation close to the left-sided pathway (with an electrode positioned in the coronary sinus) will allow early activation of the anomalous pathway and later activation of the AV node resulting in a greater degree of pre-excitation. This effect is of importance in the initiation of echo beats and AV re-entrant tachycardias because stimulation near the anomalous pathway will result in earlier activation and thus earlier recovery permitting retrograde conduction and atrial reactivation. Anterograde conduction studies are important in the assessment of tachycardias associated with the WPW syndrome. The relationship of the anomalous and normal pathways is analogous to that of two AV nodal pathways (dual AV nodal pathways – see Chapter 3).

The exact location of an anomalous pathway may be ascertained using several methods, of which the simplest is atrial mapping during sustained AV re-entrant tachycardias (see Chapter 9). Atrial pacing at a constant rate at various sites around the AV ring will result in differing degrees of pre-excitation for the reasons referred to above. However, not all atrial sites are easily accessible. The coronary sinus is in close relationship with the left atrioventricular junction and provides a natural conduit for the mapping electrode. Mapping of the right AV ring is much more difficult and requires skill in manipulation of the catheter and appreciation of radiological cardiac anatomy. A special curved rotatable catheter has been devised for this purpose. Alternatively, in selected patients, a fine bore catheter may be introduced down the right coronary artery for more precise localization of the anomalous pathway (e.g. prior to endocardial ablation from the right atrium). Mapping may also be performed during retrograde conduction studies (see later in this chapter).

Anomalous pathway potentials During anterograde and retrograde conduction studies and re-entrant atrioventricular tachycardia some investigators (Jackman et al., 1983) have observed high frequency deflections between the atrial and ventricular electrograms close to the area of the anomalous pathway (Fig. 6.6). These deflections are usually less than 1 mV in amplitude. They bear a constant relationship to the onset of the QRS complex during atrial fibrillation with varying degrees of pre-excitation, thus excluding the normal atrioventricular conduction system as the source of the signals. During atrial pacing at increasing rates the interval between the atrial electrogram and the anomalous potential and between this and the ventricular activation remains constant, a feature consistent

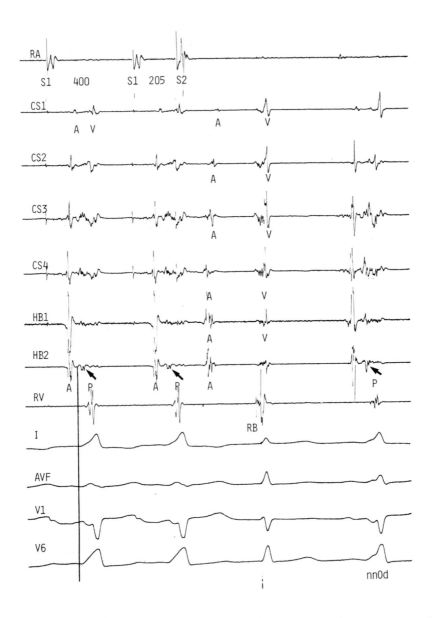

Fig. 6.6 Anomalous pathway potentials. Atrial extrastimulation in a patient with right ventricular pre-excitation due to direct atrioventricular anomalous pathway. During regular pacing (S1S2) at a cycle length of 400 msec, an early potential (labelled P and arrowed), recorded from the His bundle catheter (HB2), occurs immediately prior to the delta wave. This potential is not present when the atrial extrastimulus (S2) blocks in the anomalous pathway and conducts normally. When sinus rhythm resumes, the potential returns, This potential may reflect anomalous pathway activation or ventricular activation in the area immediately adjacent to the anomalous pathway. During AV re-entrant tachycardia, earliest atrial activation was recorded on the same catheter (HB2). Paper speed 100 mm/sec. A = atrial electrograms; CS 1–4 = 'unipolar' coronary sinus recordings; RA = right atrium; RV = right ventricle.

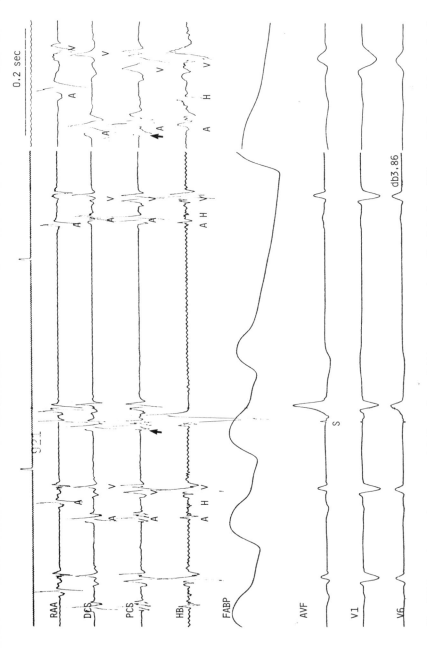

Fig. 6.7 Anomalous pathway potential. Recordings of AV re-entrant tachycardia of the long RP' type. Earliest atrial activation is in the region of the proximal coronary sinus (PCS). The atrial electrogram, A, in this channel is preceded by a distinct sharp deflection (arrowed) which is seen more clearly in the right panel recorded at 250 mm/sec. This deflection was localized to a small region and disappeared when the catheter was moved. It disappeared when sinus rhythm resumed. It was present intermittently during ventricular pacing with retrograde conduction. It is suggested that this potential reflects depolarization of the anomalous pathway itself although rigorous electrophysiological 'proof' was not obtained.

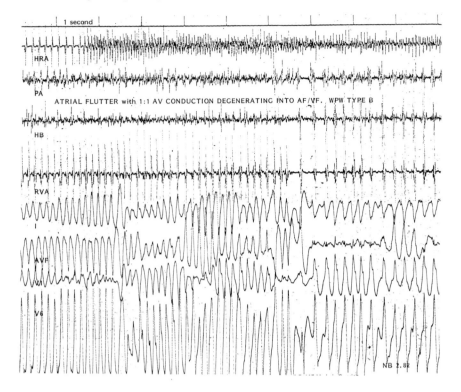

Fig. 6.8 (*a*) Atrial fibrillation in the WPW syndrome. These recordings were taken at electrophysiological study of a 6-year-old boy. Atrial flutter was initiated by rapid atrial pacing. There is a 1:1 response to flutter which then degenerates to atrial fibrillation. The ventricular arrhythmia is rapid and shows axis changes similar to those seen in 'torsade de pointes'. In effect, there is total cardiac fibrillation. Cardioversion was needed to restore sinus rhythm. (*b*) Rapid atrial fibrillation in the WPW syndrome. Atrial fibrillation was induced at electrophysiological study using rapid atrial pacing. The QRS complexes are broad and show variable pre-excitation. The minimum RR interval between successive pre-excited QRS complexes is 220 msec. This value suggests that this patient may be at risk from ventricular fibrillation. Paper speed 25 mm/sec. CSD = distal coronary sinus; CSP = proximal coronary sinus; HB = His bundle region; HRA = high right atrium; PA = pulmonary artery; RA = right atrium.

with non-decremental conduction. It has also been possible to pace the anomalous pathway resulting in simultaneous retrograde conduction to the atria and anterograde conduction to the ventricles. Conduction times from the anomalous pathway to the atria and ventricles are identical to those noted during atrial or ventricular pacing and are consistent with the known properties of these pathways. These potentials may also be recorded during AVRT (Fig. 6.7). Fragmented atrial electrograms are unlikely to explain these potentials because they always precede atrial activation during retrograde conduction and VA block occurs after inscription of the potential.

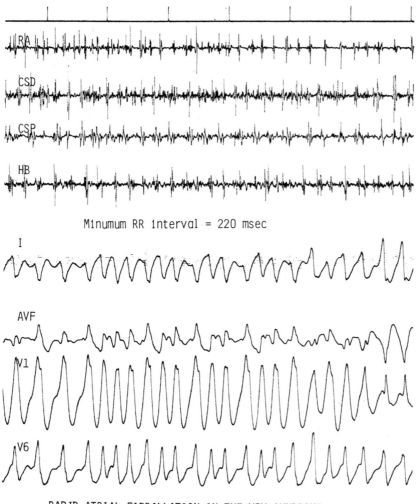

Minumum RR interval = 220 msec

RAPID ATRIAL FIBRILLATION IN THE WPW SYNDROME

Fig. 6.8 (*b*)

These recordings have provided insight into the physiological behaviour and pharmacological responses of direct AV anomalous pathways. Further studies have suggested that such pathways may traverse the AV groove in an oblique rather than an orthogonal manner. Precise localization of the pathway by this method may enhance the success rate of transvenous ablation techniques (see Chapter 15). The potentials may be recorded using a specially constructed 'orthogonal' catheter in which a series of ring electrodes, each quadripolar, is arranged along the catheter. Winters and Gomes (1986) have recorded the potential using standard catheters with a 5 mm interelectrode distance.

Table 6.1 TECHNIQUES FOR INDUCTION OF ATRIAL FIBRILLATION

Rapid atrial pacing
Atrial extrastimulation (S1S2; S1S2S3; S1S2S3S4)
Ultra high frequency stimulation (cycle length <60 msec)
AC current (50 or 60 Hz at 2 × diastolic threshold)

Atrial fibrillation in the WPW syndrome

About one-third of patients with the WPW syndrome have a propensity to develop paroxysmal atrial fibrillation (see also Chapter 8). The reason for this high incidence is not entirely understood but an important factor is the degeneration of atrioventricular re-entrant tachycardias to atrial fibrillation, often with an intervening period of transient atrial flutter. Other contributory factors include associated sinoatrial disorder, multiple anomalous pathways and frequent atrial echo beats. Ventricular premature beats which conduct retrogradely over the anomalous pathway and activate the atria during the vulnerable period may initiate atrial fibrillation. Occasionally, atrial fibrillation may lead to ventricular fibrillation (Fig. 6.8a).

The ventricular rate during atrial fibrillation is determined by many complex factors, of which the ERP of the anomalous pathway is most amenable to reproducible measurement. If the ERP of the anomalous pathway is short, rapid ventricular rates during atrial fibrillation may result from a high frequency of conduction over the anomalous pathway. The minimal RR interval during atrial fibrillation is also determined by several factors other than the anterograde ERP of the anomalous pathway. These include:

1. The ERP of the ventricular myocardium.
2. The ERP of the AV node.
3. Concealed retrograde conduction into the anomalous pathway.
4. Concealed anterograde penetration of the anomalous pathway.

The autonomic status of the patient (posture, respiration, etc.) may affect any of these electrophysiological variables and influence the ventricular response to atrial fibrillation. Whether or not exercise studies during atrial fibrillation provide additional prognostic information is not clear.

During the electrophysiological assessment of patients with ventricular pre-excitation it is important to attempt to initiate atrial fibrillation (Table 6.1) especially in those patients with a history of collapse or syncope. A minimal RR interval (the shortest interval between the onset of delta waves of successive pre-excited QRS complexes) of 250 msec or less during atrial fibrillation with conduction over the anomalous pathway appears to be associated with a higher risk of developing dangerous ventricular arrhythmias (Fig. 6.8b). Minimal RR intervals of 200 msec or less are associated with sustained and rapid ventricular rates which are particularly dangerous.

Induction of atrial fibrillation at electrophysiological study is also useful in revealing the presence of additional anomalous atrioventricular pathways which have not been revealed during atrial pacing studies. These pathways may be manifest by a change in the pattern or vector of the ventricular pre-excitation (Fig. 6.9).

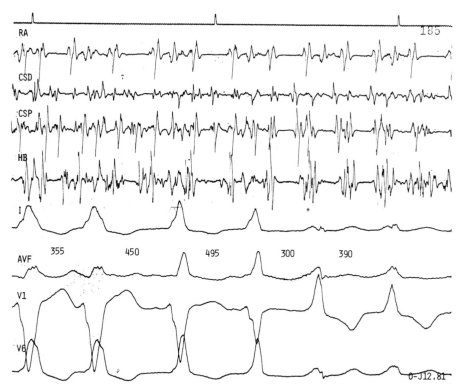

Fig. 6.9 Atrial fibrillation with two forms of ventricular pre-excitation in a patient in whom only right ventricular pre-excitation had been documented on the surface ECG. The left of the recordings show ventricular pre-excitation as a result of conduction over a right atrioventricular pathway (negative delta wave in lead V1). In succeeding beats, the degree of right ventricular pre-excitation decreases and on the fifth beat (*) a different complex (positive delta wave in lead V1) emerges. Further studies confirmed the presence of a left free wall pathway in addition to the right-sided pathway. Atrial fibrillation is useful in eliciting forms of pre-excitation which may not have been documented prior to electrophysiological study. Paper speed 100 mm/sec. CSD = distal coronary sinus; CSP = proximal coronary sinus; HB = His bundle region; RA = right atrium.

Other electrophysiological measurements of anomalous pathway conduction capacity, such as mean RR (of successive pre-excited QRS complexes) during atrial fibrillation, cycle length of second degree block in the anomalous pathway and minimum anomalous pathway ERP (during rapid atrial pacing) are of doubtful prognostic significance.

Concealed conduction in anomalous pathways

The presence of concealed conduction in direct AV anomalous pathways has been the subject of speculation and debate for many years. Klein et al. (1984) have investigated the phenomenon of anterograde concealment using the interpolated blocked atrial stimulus method (see Chapter 3). In this method, an extrastimulus (A2) is delivered at an interval which blocks in the anomalous pathway. This followed by the test stimulus (A3) which is coupled to A2 and adjusted in the usual manner. Retrograde concealment was studied using a similar protocol in the right ventricle. Concealed conduction was defined as an apparent prolongation of the refractory period of the pathway after the non-conducted stimulus. The difference between the true ERP and the apparent ERP of the anomalous pathway may reflect the degree of penetration of the impulse into the anomalous pathway. This difference was found to correlate with the variability of the RR interval during atrial fibrillation (i.e. the greater the degree of concealment, the wider the range of pre-excited RR intervals during atrial fibrillation). Retrograde concealed conduction may be a factor in the production of decremental conduction characteristics in some anomalous pathways. These studies have shown that conduction in anomalous pathways is not necessarily of the 'all-or-none' type. Decremental conduction and Wenckebach type I block have also been documented using the direct method of recording potentials from anomalous pathways (Winters and Gomes, 1986).

Retrograde conduction studies

In the presence of two ventriculoatrial conduction pathways, right ventricular pacing may result in a variety of conduction patterns. These are determined by several factors, including the relative conduction times to the normal and anomalous pathways from the pacing site, the conduction times through these structures and their spatial relationship to each other, and the intra-atrial conduction times. These patterns may be detected by several atrial recording electrodes disposed at suitable sites in the right and left atria. A complete appreciation of the retrograde atrial activation pattern would require many such electrodes but for practical purposes three to five suffice. These are usually positioned in the high right atrium, in the low right atrium (His bundle recording) and in the proximal and distal coronary sinus (Fig. 6.10). These are standard sites and therefore allow comparison within a single study and between one study and another.

During regular ventricular pacing, atrial activation may occur as a result of conduction over the normal and abnormal pathways producing atrial 'fusion'. If the rate is increased, resulting in progressively longer conduction times in the normal pathway, the pattern of fusion will alter accordingly. In some instances there may be complete retrograde block in either the anomalous pathway or the normal pathway resulting in, respectively, a normal retrograde activation pattern or a persistently abnormal pattern with eccentric atrial activation throughout. Most often, there is a contribution to atrial activation from both pathways. This stable state can be disturbed by introducing ventricular premature beats resulting in changes in the activation pattern. These different responses to stimulation are best studied using the ventricular extrastimulus method to construct retrograde conduction curves. Several different patterns may be observed (Fig. 6.11). It is important to appreciate that the typical varieties of anomalous ventriculoatrial connections do not exhibit decremental conduction

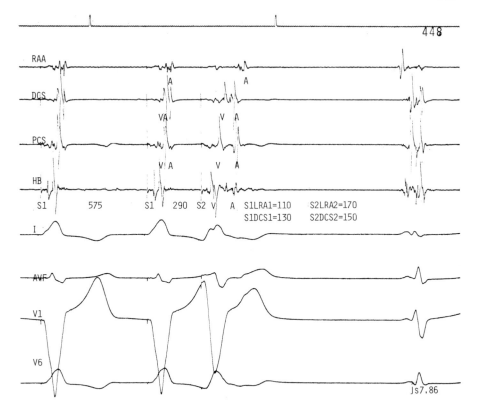

Fig. 6.10 Ventricular pacing in a patient with a left free wall pathway. During regular ventricular pacing at a cycle length of 575 msec (S1S1) there is retrograde conduction over the anomalous pathway and over the normal pathway (retrograde fusion). Earliest activation of the atria is in the low right atrium (LRA) in the region of the His bundle electrode (S1LRA = 110 msec). A ventricular premature stimulus results in a change in the retrograde pattern with earliest activation in the distal coronary sinus (DCS) with S2DCS2 = 150 msec. This reflects slowing or block of conduction in the normal retrograde pathway such that it is pre-empted by anomalous VA conduction. Curves can be constructed to show the various possible patterns of retrograde conduction more clearly (see Fig. 6.11). Paper speed 100 mm/sec. DCS and PCS = distal and proximal coronary sinus; HB = His bundle region; RAA = right atrial appendage.

properties. The retrograde ERP (like the anterograde ERP) of these pathways also decreases with an increase in basic driving rate.

If there is no retrograde conduction over the normal AV nodal pathway, atrial activation is persistently abnormal at all test stimulus intervals (V1V2). If the anomalous pathway is remote from the AV node, the atria are activated eccentrically (Fig. 6.11). If retrograde conduction over the normal pathway is present but conduction time is long compared to that in the anomalous pathway, a normal retrograde atrial pattern will be revealed only if the retrograde ERP of the anomalous pathway is longer than that of the normal retrograde pathway. The

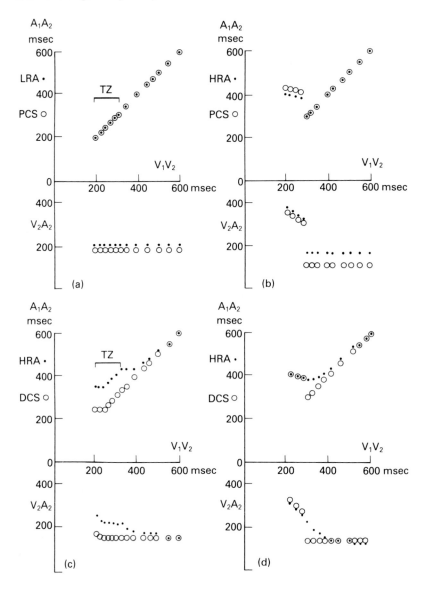

Fig. 6.11 Patterns of retrograde conduction in patients with anomalous pathways. In each graph the upper section is the interval between successive atrial response to ventricular extrastimulation (V2) and the lower section is the corresponding VA conduction interval. These intervals are shown for the high (HRA) or low (LRA) right atrium (dots) and the distal (DCS) or proximal (PCS) coronary sinus (open circles). (*a*) Retrograde conduction of the septal pathway at all coupling intervals (V1V2) of the premature beat. Re-entrant atrioventricular tachycardias (AVRT) were initiated during the zone of VA block in the normal pathway. (*b*) A sudden transition from anomalous to normal pathway conduction at short coupling intervals. There is a corresponding change in the atrial activation sequence. No AVRT was induced. (*c*) Retrograde

converse will exist if the ERPs and conduction times have the opposite relationship; eccentric activation will be recorded at V1V2 intervals which are shorter than the ERP of the normal pathway. An entire spectrum of patterns is possible, and one pattern may convert to another with a change in the basic driving rate which may induce variations in the conduction time and refractoriness in both normal and anomalous pathways.

Retrograde studies are, like anterograde studies, important in the initiation of AV re-entrant tachycardias. Thus if the ERP of the normal pathway is greater than that of the anomalous pathway, conduction to the atria may be followed by anterograde conduction to the ventricles and a ventricular echo beat may result. If the conditions are favourable, continued re-entrant excitation will cause sustained AV re-entrant tachycardia (see Chapter 9).

From the clinical point of view, the purpose of these detailed studies is to reveal anomalous retrograde conduction, make some assessment of pathway location and attempt to initiate tachycardias.

Associated junctional tachycardias Associated junctional tachycardias fall into three categories:

1. Atrioventricular re-entrant tachycardia with anterograde conduction over the normal pathway and retrograde conduction over the anomalous pathway (orthodromic tachycardia). Such a tachycardia shows normal QRS complexes. If conduction proceeds in the reverse direction the QRS complexes show full pre-excitation (antidromic tachycardia).
2. Atrioventricular re-entrant tachycardia involving two anomalous pathways completely excluding the normal AV node–His bundle pathway.
3. Intra-AV nodal re-entrant tachycardia.

These are discussed in Chapter 9.

Anomalous nodoventricular conduction

Anomalous pathways taking their origin from the AV nodal region and the His bundle itself and inserting the ventricular myocardium are described as nodoventricular and His–ventricular pathways respectively (Fig. 6.12). They were discovered by Mahaim and are sometimes eponymously referred to as 'Mahaim pathways'. The clinical significance of these pathways has been debated for many years, the central issue being the role of these pathways in the generation of tachycardias.

---

fusion with a changing atrial pattern as V1V2 is reduced. When conduction over the normal pathway is sufficiently slowed, atrial activation is dominated entirely by retrograde anomalous pathway conduction (unchanging HRA, DCS relationship). In this example, tachycardias could be initiated in this zone (TZ), indicating block rather than delay in the normal VA pathway. (*d*) Atrial fusion at longer coupling intervals with the right atrium activated as a result of normal VA conduction and the left atrium (DCS) activated by the anomalous pathway. When the anomalous pathway becomes refractory, left atrial activation is delayed. No AVRT was induced.

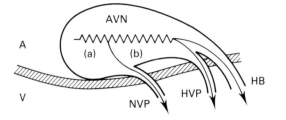

Fig. 6.12 Diagram of a nodoventricular pathway (NVP) and a His–ventricular pathway (HVP). The nodoventricular pathway may arise between zones of AV nodal delay (a) and (b) such that the HV interval is short or negative, and the HV relationship changes during extrastimulation or incremental atrial pacing. In contrast, atrial pacing and extrastimulation does not effect the HV interval associated with HVP conduction, which results in a fixed HV interval (which is short but not negative). The relationship of a nodoventricular pathway to the delaying area of the AV node (AVN) is an important factor influencing the AV conduction pattern during premature atrial stimulation. If the pathway arises distal to the delaying zone (so-called fasciculoventricular pathway) premature stimulation will result in equivalent AH and HV delay with no change in the degree of pre-excitation as the coupling interval of the test beat is reduced. With a very proximal origin, the AV interval lengthens to a small degree while the AH interval lengthens normally, causing increased pre-excitation. AV nodal delay proximal and distal to the anomalous pathway results in increasing pre-excitation with AH delay exceeding AV delay (see Fig, 6.14). HB = His bundle.

The characteristic surface ECG appearances during sinus rhythm due to these pathways are:

1. A variable PR interval.
2. Variable and usually minimal slurring of the upstroke of the QRS.
3. A QRS duration of up to 0.14 second with a left bundle branch block pattern (Fig. 6.13).
4. A small R wave in lead V1.

Often, the ECG is normal during sinus rhythm, with the emergence of the distinctive QRS complex only during tachycardia.

The electrophysiological characterization of these pathways is complex. Conduction in the anomalous pathway itself appears to be of the non-decremental type. During atrial pacing at a fixed rate the degree of ventricular pre-excitation is determined by the relative conduction times in the anomalous and normal pathways. Increasing delay in the AV node will result in a greater degree of pre-excitation (Fig. 6.14). The exact response is, however, also determined by the site of origin of the anomalous pathway relative to the AV nodal delaying area. Thus, if the pathway arises from the His bundle (distal to the AV nodal delaying zone), increasing the atrial rate will merely prolong the PR interval whilst preserving the QRS morphology. In contrast, if the anomalous pathway arises from the AV node itself, with proximal and distal areas of decremental conduction, the response will be more complex. Increasing delay distal to the origin of the anomalous pathway will result in a progressive increase in the degree of pre-excitation without a change in the PR interval whilst proximal delay will increase the PR interval as described above.

These responses may be well characterized by intracardiac studies. The

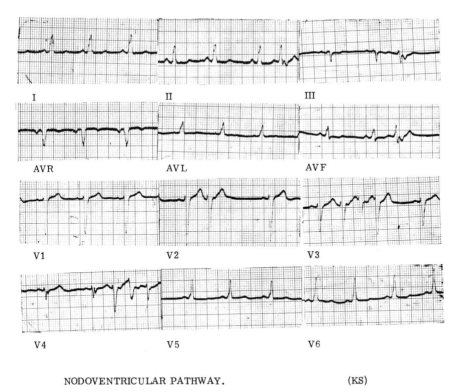

I   II   III

AVR   AVL   AVF

V1   V2   V3

V4   V5   V6

NODOVENTRICULAR PATHWAY.   (KS)

Fig. 6.13 Surface electrocardiogram showing anomalous nodoventricular conduction in a 30-year-old woman with frequent attacks of regular palpitations. During regular sinus rhythm the QRS complexes are slightly widened with a slurred initial positive wave clearly seen in leads I, II, AVF, V5 and V6. The QRS complexes also show variable pre-excitation during brief runs of tachycardia (lead V3) and premature beats (leads III and AVF). The LBBB morphology of the QRS complexes is typical of nodoventricular pre-excitation.

extrastimulus method is particularly useful in this respect. When the anomalous pathway arises from the AV node itself, with proximal and distal areas of delay (see Fig. 6.12), the AH interval increases as a result of delay throughout the entire AV node as the A1A2 interval is shortened. The nodoventricular pathway is activated during conduction through the delaying area of the AV node, with subsequent activation of the myocardium as indicated by the onset of the pre-excited QRS complex. Thus, increasing AV nodal delay distal to the origin of the nodoventricular pathway results in progressive delay of the His potential relative to the onset of the QRS and the HV interval shortens (see Fig. 6.14). The AV interval, determined by conduction over the AV node proximal to the origin of the anomalous pathway and over the pathway itself, increases as A1A2 is decreased. This response is quite different from that seen with typical direct AV anomalous connections (see Fig. 6.1).

In many patients with nodoventricular pathways, dual AV nodal pathways can be demonstrated. Occasionally, a sudden increase in the AV interval is associated

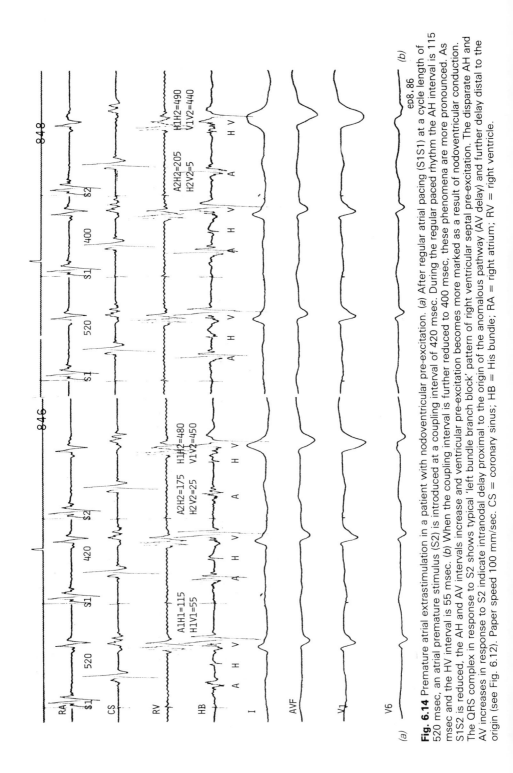

Fig. 6.14 Premature atrial extrastimulation in a patient with nodoventricular pre-excitation. (*a*) After regular atrial pacing (S1S1) at a cycle length of 520 msec, an atrial premature stimulus (S2) is introduced at a coupling interval of 420 msec. During the regular paced rhythm the AH interval is 115 msec and the HV interval is 55 msec. (*b*) When the coupling interval is further reduced to 400 msec, these phenomena are more pronounced. As S1S2 is reduced, the AH and AV intervals increase and ventricular pre-excitation becomes more marked as a result of nodoventricular conduction. The QRS complex in response to S2 shows typical 'left bundle branch block' pattern of right ventricular septal pre-excitation. The disparate AH and AV increases in response to S2 indicate intranodal delay proximal to the origin of the anomalous pathway (AV delay) and further delay distal to the origin (see Fig. 6.12). Paper speed 100 mm/sec. CS = coronary sinus; HB = His bundle; RA = right atrium; RV = right ventricle.

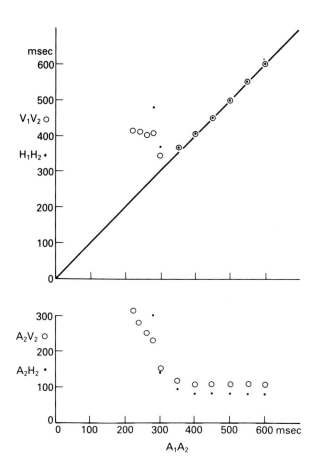

Fig. 6.15 Anterograde conduction curve in the presence of anomalous nodoventricular conduction in a 16-year-old girl with Ebstein's anomaly. During regular atrial pacing there is no evidence of pre-excitation. As the coupling interval of the test beat (A1A2) is decreased the AH interval and AV interval are prolonged as indicated by deviation from the line of identity. With early coupling intervals of A2, pre-excitation emerges (the AH interval prolongs more than the AV interval) with consequent shortening of the interval. Atrial echo beats occurred at the three shortest coupling intervals of A2.

with either disappearance or emergence of anomalous nodoventricular conduction, implying close association of the pathway with one of two AV nodal pathways (Figs. 6.15 and 6.16). This event may be associated with the appearance of atrial echo beats or sustained tachycardia, leading to the suggestion that AV nodal re-entrant excitation is the mechanism of tachycardia in these patients. The wide 'LBBB' type QRS complex during tachycardia has been interpreted as reflecting incidental ('bystander') anterograde nodoventricular conduction rather than participation of the anomalous pathway in the anterograde limb of the re-entrant circuit. This is discussed further in Chapter 9.

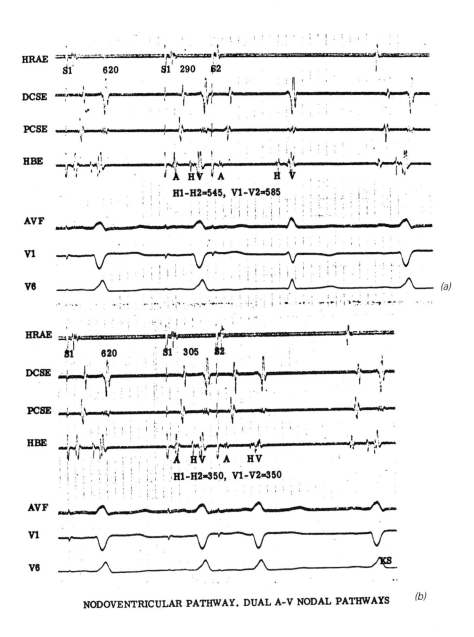

NODOVENTRICULAR PATHWAY. DUAL A-V NODAL PATHWAYS   *(b)*

Fig. 6.16 Recordings during atrial extrastimulus testing in a patient with anomalous nodoventricular conduction. During regular atrial pacing (S1S1 = 620 msec) there is ventricular pre-excitation with HV = zero. An atrial premature stimulus (S1S2 = 305 msec) conducts with the same degree of pre-excitation (*b*) and the His potential does not change its relationship with the QRS (cf. Fig 6.14). In (*a*) the test beat is delivered earlier (S1S2 = 290 msec) and conducts with a sudden jump in both the AH interval and the AV interval. The QRS complex is normalized and the HV interval is prolonged to 40 msec). At faster rates of pacing the same

There is no good information about the retrograde conduction properties of these anomalous pathways. During ventricular pacing and during re-entrant tachycardia the atria are activated in the normal retrograde manner consistent with spread of activation from the AV node rather than directly from the abnormal pathway itself. A subtle change in retrograde atrial activation during tachycardia or ventricular pacing may be explained by predominant activation of the right atrionodal junction.

Associated junctional tachycardias include AV nodal re-entry and macrore-entry involving the anomalous pathway in the anterograde limb (really a 'subjunctional' or even a ventricular tachycardia).

The short PR interval/normal QRS complex syndrome

The syndrome was originally described by Clerc, Levy and Cristesco in 1938 but was rediscovered by Lown, Ganong and Levine who published their findings in 1952 and whose names are eponymously linked to the syndrome (Lown–Ganong–Levine; LGL). The syndrome has been a constant source of perplexity and is still not clearly understood. Whereas there is pathological evidence for both types of anomalous pathway described above, there is no corresponding pathologically or anatomically accepted basis for this syndrome. Both James (1961) and Brechenmacher (1975) described fibres which connect the atrial myocardium to the AV node or His bundle. However, the structures described in these reports differed and in neither report were there adequate electrophysiological correlations. The histological demonstration of the existence of these pathways does not provide any information about their function during life.

The LGL syndrome is defined as the association of:

1. Paroxysmal tachycardias in otherwise healthy people.
2. A normal QRS complex.
3. A paroxysmal tachycardias in otherwise healthy people.

Because the original descriptions were rather vague ('paroxysmal palpitations') it is felt that the modern definition should restrict the associated tachycardias to atrial and junctional tachycardias.

Several explanations for this collection of observations have been advanced. These include a hypoplastic AV node, supernormal conduction, anatomical variation of the normal AV node, an intranodal 'fast' pathway bypassing the normal delaying zone of the AV node or an extranodal bypass tract inserting at variable points along the main AV nodal structure (so-called James pathways).

---

phenomenon was observed with occasional atrial echo beats. Sustained tachycardias (with similar QRS complexes and HV of zero) could be induced only by ventricular pacing and extrastimulation. These findings are interpreted as reflecting an anomalous nodoventricular pathway in association with the faster of dual AV nodal pathways. The associated tachycardias are intranodal re-entrant in type. Paper speed 100 mm/sec. DCSE and PCSE = distal and proximal coronary sinus electrograms; HBE = His bundle electrogram; HRAE = high right atrial electrogram.

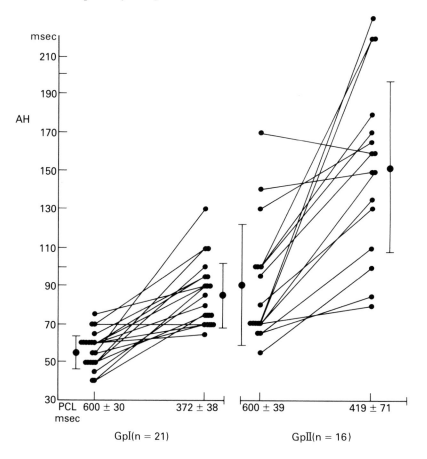

Fig. 6.17 The AH interval response to changes in pacing rate in a group of patients with junctional tachycardias associated with the Lown–Ganong–Levine syndrome (group I) and a group with similar tachycardias not associate with the syndrome (group II). The mean slower pacing cycle length (left columns in each graph) is approximatley 100 b.p.m., and the mean faster rate (right column) is approximately 150 b.p.m. The mean AH interval at the slower pacing rate (mean indicated by large dot with bars denoting 1 s.d.) is significantly shorter in group I than in group II. The increase in AH is also much less in group I compared to group II. This attenuated increase in AH interval is a characteristic of AV conduction in the LGL syndrome.

The electrophysiological correlates of the short PR interval have been well studied. The important features are:

1. A short AH interval during sinus rhythm.
2. An attenuated AH increase during atrial stimulation (Fig. 6.17).
3. A high Wenckebach rate during atrial pacing.
4. A short AH effective refractory period.
5. A short AH functional refractory period.

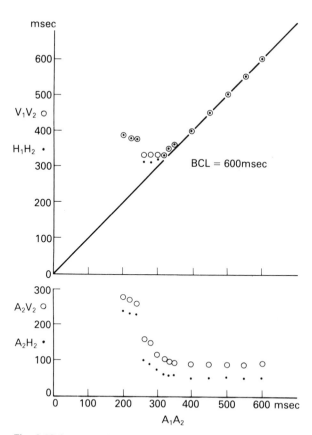

Fig. 6.18 Anterograde conduction curve demonstrating dual AH pathways in a patient with the Lown–Ganong–Levine syndrome. The AH interval during sinus rhythm is 50 msec and the HV interval is 45 msec. The effective refractory period (ERP) of the AV node (equal to that of the slow pathway) is short at 220 msec at a basic pacing cycle length (BCL) of 600 msec. The ERP of the fast pathway is 275 msec. Early coupling intervals of A2 which conduct in the fast pathway result in HV prolongation. Block in the fast pathway allows slow pathway conduction to be revealed with a sudden increase in the AH and HH intervals with a normal HV interval.

Associated features include:

1. Prolongation of the HV interval and bundle branch delay at short coupling intervals of A2 (see Fig. 3.7).
2. The presence of gap phenomena (see Fig. 3.9).
3. Occasional presence of dual AH pathways (Fig. 6.18).

Because many of these phenomena are a result of rapid conduction through the AV node to the His bundle, they may be referred to as manifestations of 'junctional pre-excitation'.

The AH interval in these patients is not only abnormally short but also shows an attenuated increase in response to incremental atrial stimulation (see Fig. 3.3). Extrastimulus testing shows a similar phenomenon. The normal AH increase as the A1A2 interval is decreased is absent or attenuated. It has been suggested that a more attenuated AH increase is evidence for a more distal insertion of the bypass tract. However, since the bypass tract theory is unproven, this argument is specious.

Dual 'AH' pathways, analogous to dual intranodal pathways, (so-called because their anatomical basis is unknown) are found in about 50 per cent of these patients during extrastimulus testing. This has been interpreted as reflecting block in the extranodal bypass tract with continued conduction in the normal AV node. The ERP of the fast pathway in these patients may be normal or short. Interestingly, the ERP of the slow pathway and the maximum AH conduction time via the slow pathway are very short compared to the normal single AV nodal pathway, an unexpected finding if the bypass theory is correct. The attenuated slow pathway properties (compared to normal AV nodal conduction) may account for the faster AV nodal tachycardias in the LGL syndrome.

The FRP of the fast pathway is also short and may be exceeded by the RRP or ERP of the His–Purkinje system when HV prolongation or bundle branch delay or block may occur until proximal AH delay lengthens the H1H2 interval to a value above the RRP of the distal conduction system. This is in effect a type of gap (see Chapter 3). Sometimes proximal delay with relief of distal delay or block is caused by a shift from slow to fast pathway conduction. Occasionally, tachycardias are initiated by such a shift. Although some of these tachycardias are analogous to intranodal re-entrant tachycardias, others involve an anomalous AV connection in the retrograde limb (see Chapter 9).

Atrial flutter or fibrillation are commonly associated with this syndrome and may result in rapid ventricular rates because the normal filtering properties of the AV junction are attenutated. Rarely, ventricular fibrillation can occur in response to atrial fibrillation.

References and further reading

Anderson RH, Becker AE, Brechenmacher C, Davies MJ, Rose L. (1975) Ventricular preexcitation: a proposed nomenclature for its substrates. *European Heart Journal* **3**, 27

Anderson RH, Becker AE. (1981) Stanley Kent and accessory atrioventricular connections. *Journal of Thoracic and Cardiovascular Surgery* **81**, 649

Anderson RH, Becker A, Tranum-Jensen J, Janse MJ. (1981) Anatomico-electrophysiological correlations in the conduction system: a review. *British Heart Journal* **45**, 67

Bardy GH, Fedor JM, German LD, Packer DL, Gallagher JJ. (1984) Surface electrocardiographic clues suggesting presence of a nodofascicular Mahaim fiber. *Journal of the American College of Cardiology* **3**, 1161

Bauernfeind RA, Ayres BF, Wyndham CRC, Dhingra R, Swiryn S, Strasberg B, Rosen KM. (1980) Cycle length in atrioventricular reentrant paroxysmal tachycardia with observations on the Lown–Ganong–Levine syndrome. *American Journal of Cardiology* **45**, 1148

Bauernfeind RA, Wyndham CR, Swiryn SP, Palileo E, Strasberg B, Lam W, Westveer D, Rosen KM. (1981) Paroxysmal atrial fibrillation in the Wolff–Parkinson–White syndrome. *American Journal of Cardiology* **47**, 562

Bauernfeind RA, Swiryn S, Strasberg B, Palileo E, Wyndham C, Duffy CE, Rosen KM. (1982) Analysis of anterograde and retrograde fast pathway properties in patients with dual atrioventricular nodal pathways. Observations regarding the pathophysiology of the Lown–Ganong–Levine syndrome. *American Journal of Cardiology* **49**, 283

Befeler B, Castellanos A, Aranda J, Guiterrez R, Lazzara R. (1976) Intermittent bundle branch block in patients with accessory atrio–His or atrio–AV nodal pathways. *British Heart Journal* **38**, 173

Benditt DG, Epstein ML, Arentzen CE, Kriett JM, Klein GJ. (1982) Enhanced atrioventricular conduction in patients without preexcitation syndrome: relation to heart rate in paroxysmal reciprocating tachycardia. *Circulation* **65**, 1474

Benditt DG, Klein GJ, Kriett JM, Dunnigan A, Benson DW. (1984) Enhanced atrioventricular nodal conduction in man: electrophysiologic effects of pharmacologic autonomic blockade. *Circulation* **69**, 1088

Benditt DG, Klein GJ, Kriett KM, Dunnigan A, Benson DW. (1984) Enhanced atrioventricular nodal conduction in man: electrophysiologic effects of pharmacologic autonomic blockade. *Circulation* **69**, 1088

Boineau JP, Moore EN. (1970) Evidence for propagation of activation across an accessory atrioventricular connection in types A and B preexcitation. *Circulation* **41**, 375

Brechenmacher C. (1975) Atrio–His bundle tracts. *British Heart Journal* **37**, 853

Camm AJ, Ward DE, Spurrell RAJ. (1977) Manifestations of junctional preexcitation in the Lown–Ganong–Levine syndrome. In: *Advances in the Management of Arrhythmias*, p. 319. Ed. by D Kelly. Telectronics: Sydney

Campbell RWF, Smith RA, Gallagher JJ, Pritchett ELC, Wallace AG. (1977) Atrial fibrillation in the preexcitation syndrome. *American Journal of Cardiology* **40**, 514

Castellanos A, Chapunoff E, Castillo C, Maytin O, Lemberg L. (1970) His bundle electrograms in two cases of Wolff–Parkinson–White (preexcitation) syndrome. *Circulation* **41**, 399

Castellanos A, Castillo CA, Agha AB, Befeler B, Myerburg RJ. (1973) Functional properties of accessory AV pathways during premature atrial stimulation. *British Heart Journal* **35**, 578

Clerc A, Levy R, Cristesco C. (1938) A propos du racourcissement permanent du l'espace PR de l'electrocardiogramme sans deformation du complexe ventriculaire. *Archives des Maladies du Coeur* **31**, 569

Coumel P, Waynberger M, Garnier JC, Slama R, Bouvrain Y. (1971) Syndrome de preexcitation ventriculaire associant P-R court et onde delta, sans elargissement de QRS. (A propos de 3 cas de syndrome de W–P–W a complexes de fin.) *Archives des Maladies du Coeur* **64**, 1234

Critelli G, Grassi G, Perticone F, Coltorti F, Monda V, Condorelli M. (1983) Transesophageal pacing for prognostic evaluation of preexcitation syndrome and assessment of protective therapy. *American Journal of Cardiology* **51**, 513

De la Fuente D, Sasyniuk B, Moe GK. (1971) Conduction through a narrow isthmus in isolated canine atrial tissue. A model of the Wolff–Parkinson–White syndrome. *Circulation* **44**, 803

Denes P, Wyndham CR, Amat-y-Leon F, Wu D, Dhingra R, Miller RH, Rosen KM. (1977) Atrial pacing at multiple sites in the Wolff–Parkinson–White syndrome. *British Heart Journal* **39**, 506

Denes P, Wu D, Amat-y-Leon F, Dhingra R, Bauernfeind R, Kehoe R, Rosen KM. (1978) Determinants of atrioventricular reentrant paroxysmal tachycardia in patients with the Wolff–Parkinson–White syndrome. *Circulation* **58**, 415

Dreifus LS, Haiat R, Watanabe Y, Arriaga J, Reitman N. (1971) Ventricular fibrillation. A possible mechanism of sudden death in patients with Wolff–Parkinson–White syndrome. *Circulation* **43**, 520

Dreifus LS, Wellens HJ, Watanabe Y, Kibiris D, Truex R. (1976) Sinus bradycardia and atrial fibrillation associated with the Wolff–Parkinson–White syndrome. *American Journal of Cardiology* **38**, 149

Durrer D, Wellens HJJ. (1970) Pre-excitation revisted. *American Journal of Cardiology* 25, 690

Durrer D, Wellens HJJ. (1974) The Wolff–Parkinson–White syndrome anno 1973. *European Journal of Cardiology* 1, 347

Frank R, Phan-Thuc H, Blanc P, Allali I, Goutte R, Vedel J, Fontaine G, Grosgogeat Y. (1980) La response nodal attenuee *Archives des Maladies du Coeur* 73, 1007

Furlanello F, Vergara G, Bettini R, Disertori M, Inama G, Guarnerio M, Visona L. (1984) Progress in the study of Wolff–Parkinson–White syndrome of the athletes. The transesophageal atrial pacing during bicycle exercise. *Journal of Sports Cardiology* 1, 102

Gallagher JJ, Pritchett ELC, Sealy WC, Kasell J, Wallace AG. (1978) The preexcitation syndromes. *Progress in Cardiovascular Diseases* 20, 285

German LD, Gallagher JJ, Broughton A, Guarnieri T, Trantham J. (1983) Effects of exercise and isoproterenol during atrial fibrillation in patients with Wolff–Parkinson–White syndrome. *American Journal of Cardiology* 51, 1203

Gomes JA, Dhatt MS, Rubenson DS, Damato AN. (1979a) Electrophysiologic evidence for selective retrograde utilization of a specialized conducting system in atrioventricular nodal reentrant tachycardia. *American Journal of Cardiology* 43, 687

Gomes JA, Dhatt MS, Damato AN, Akhtar M, Holder CA. (1979b) Incidence, determinants and significance of fixed retrograde conduction in the region of the atrioventricular node. Evidence for retrograde atrioventricular nodal bypass tracts. *American Journal of Cardiology* 44, 1089

Gulamhusein S, Ko P, Carruthers SG, Klein GJ. (1982) Acceleration of the ventricular response during atrial fibrillation in the Wolff–Parkinson–White syndrome after verapamil. *Circulation* 65, 348

Hammill SC, Pritchett ELC, Klein GJ, Smith WM, Gallagher JJ. (1980) Accessory pathways that conduct only in the antegrade direction. *Circulation* 62, 1335

Harper RW, Whitford E, Middlebrook K, Federman S, Pitt A. (1982) Effects of verapamil on the electrophysiologic properties of the accessory pathway in patients with the Wolff–Parkinson–White syndrome. *American Journal of Cardiology* 50, 1323

Huang SK, Rosenberg MJ, Denes P. (1984) Short PR interval and narrow QRS complex associated with pheochromocytoma: electrophysiologic observations. *Journal of the American College of Cardiology* 3, 872

Jackman WM, Prystowsky EN, Naccarelli GV, Fineberg NS, Rahilly T, Heger JJ, Zipes DP. (1983a) Reevalulation of enhanced atrioventricular nodal conduction: evidence to suggest a continuum of normal atrioventricular nodal physiology. *Circulation* 67, 441

Jackman WM, Friday KJ, Scherlag BJ, Dehning MM, Schechter E, Reynolds DW, Olsen EG, Berbari EJ, Harrison LA, Lazzara R. (1983b) Direct endocardial recording from an accessory atrioventricular pathway: localization of the site of block, effect of antiarrhythmic drugs, and attempt at nonsurgical ablation. *Circulation* 68, 906

James TN. (1961). The morphology of the human atrioventricular node with remarks pertinent to its electrophysiology. *American Heart Journal* 62, 756

Josephson ME, Seides SF, Damato AN. (1976) Wolff–Parkinson–White syndrome with 1:2 atrioventricular conduction. *American Journal of Cardiology* 37, 1094

Klein GJ, Bashore TM, Sellers TD, Pritchett ELC, Smith WM, Gallagher JJ. (1979) Ventricular fibrillation in the Wolff–Parkinson–White syndrome. *New England Journal of Medicine* 310, 1080

Klein GJ, Gulamhusein SS. (1983) Intermittent preexcitation in the Wolff–Parkinson–White syndrome. *American Journal of Cardiology* 52, 292

Klein GJ, Yee, R, Sharma AD. (1984) Concealed conduction in accessory atrioventricular pathways: an important determinant of the expression of arrhythmias in patients with the Wolff–Parkinson–White syndrome. *Circulation* 70, 402

Lin FC, Yeh SJ, Wu D. (1985) Double atrial responses to a single ventricular impulse due to simultaneous conduction via two retrograde pathways. *Journal of the American College of Cardiology* 5, 168

Lloyd EA, Hauer RN, Zipes DP, Heger JJ, Prystowsky EN. (1983) Syncope and ventricular tachycardia in patients with ventricular preexcitation. *American Journal of Cardiology* 52, 79

Lown B, Ganong W, Levine SA. (1952) The syndrome of short PR interval, normal QRS complex and paroxysmal rapid heart action. *Circulation* 5, 693

Mandel WJ, Danzig R, Hayakawa H. (1971) Lown–Ganong–Levine syndrome. A study using His bundle electrograms. *Circulation* 44, 696

Mandel W, Yamaguchi I, Laks MM. (1978) Syndromes of accelerated conduction. *Advances in Cardiology* 22, 80

Mahaim I. (1947) Kent's fibres and the AV paraspecific conduction through the upper connections of the bundle of His–Tawara. *American Heart Journal* 33, 651

Milstein S, Sharma AD, Klein GJ. (1986) Electrophysiologic profile of asymptomatic Wolff–Parkinson–White pattern. *American Journal of Cardiology* 57, 1097

Morady F, Sledge C, Shen E, Sung RJ, Gonzales R, Scheinman MM. (1983) Electrophysiologic testing in the management of patients with the Wolff–Parkinson–White syndrome and atrial fibrillation. *American Journal of Cardiology* 51, 1623

Narula OS. (1973) Wolff–Parkinson–White syndrome. A review. *Circulation* 47, 872

Narula OS. (1974) Retrograde pre-excitation. Comparison of antegrade and retrograde conduction intervals in man. *Circulation* 50, 1129

O'Callaghan WC, Colavita PG, Kay N, Ellenbogen KA, Gilbert MR, German LD. (1986) Characterization of retrograde conduction by direct endocardial recording from an accessory atrioventricular pathway. *Journal of the American College of Cardiology* 7, 167

Ohnell RF. (1944) Preexcitation, a cardiac abnormality. *Acta Medica Scandinavica* 1, 152

Pritchett ELC, Benditt DG, Smith WM, Gallagher JJ. (1978a) Effect of catheter position on the initiation of atrial echoes with atrial pacing and premature stimulation in patients with accessory pathways. *American Journal of Cardiology* 42, 738

Pritchett ELC, Gallagher JJ, Scheinman MM, Smith WM. (1978b) Determinants of the antegrade echo zone in patients with the Wolff–Parkinson–White syndrome. *Circulation* 57, 671

Prystowsky EN, Pritchett ELC, Gallagher JJ. (1984) Concealed conduction preventing anterograde preexcitation in Wolff–Parkinson–White syndrome. *American Journal of Cardiology* 53, 960

Prystowsky EN, Pritchett ELc, Gallagher JJ. (1984) Concealed conduction preventing anterograde preexcitation in Wolff–Parkinson–White syndrome. *American Journal of Cardiology* 53, 960

Przybylski J, Chiale PA, Halpern S, Nau GJ, Elizari MV, Rosenbaum MB. (1980) Unmasking of ventricular preexcitation by vagal stimulation or isoproterenol infusion. *Circulation* 61, 1030

Rosenbaum FF, Hecht HH, Wilson FN, Johnston FD. (1945) The potential variation of the thorax and the esophagus in anomalous atrioventricular excitation (Wolff–Parkinson–White syndrome). *American Heart Journal* 29, 281

Rowland E, Curry P, Fox K, Krikler D. (1981) Relation between atrioventricular pathways and ventricular response during atrial fibrillation and flutter. *British Heart Journal* 45, 83

Seipel L, Breithardt G, Both A. (1976) Atrioventricular (AV) and ventriculoatrial (VA) conduction patterns in patients with short PR interval and normal QRS complex. In: *Cardiac Pacing*, p. 152. Ed. by B Luderitz. Springer Verlag: Berlin

Sharma AD, Klein GJ, Guiraudon GM, Milstein S. (1985) Atrial fibrillation in patients with the Wolff–Parkinson–White syndrome: incidence after surgical ablation of the accessory pathway. *Circulation* 72, 161

Shen EN, Sung RJ. (1982) Initiation of atrial fibrillation by spontaneous ventricular premature beats in concealed Wolff–Parkinson–White syndrome. *American Heart Journal* **105**, 911

Sherf L, Heufeld HN. (1978) *The Preexcitation Syndromes: facts and theories.* Yorke Medical Books: New York

Spurrell RAJ, Krikler DM, Sowton E. (1975) Problems concerning assessment of anatomical site of accessory pathway in Wolff–Parkinson–White syndrome. *British Heart Journal* **37**, 127

Sung RJ, Castellanos A, Mallon S, Gelband H, Mendoza S, Myerburg RJ. (1977) Mode of initiation of reciprocating tachycardia during programmed ventricular pacing in the Wolff–Parkinson–White syndrome. *American Journal of Cardiology* **40**, 24

Svenson RH, Miller HC, Gallagher JJ, Wallace AG. (1975) Electrophysiological evaluation of the Wolff–Parkinson–White syndrome. Problems in assessing antegrade and retrograde conduction over the accessory pathway. *Circulation* **52**, 552

Svinarich JT, Tai DY, Mickelson J, Keung EC, Sung RJ. (1985) Electrophysiologic demonstration of concealed conduction in anomalous atrioventricular bypass tracts. *Journal of the American College of Cardiology* **5**, 898

Tonkin AM, Miller HC, Svenson RH, Wallace AG, Gallagher JJ. (1975a) Refractory periods of the accessory pathway in the Wolff–Parkinson–White syndrome. *Circulation* **52**, 563

Tonkin AM, Gallagher JJ, Wallace AG, Sealy WC. (1975b) Anterograde block in accessory pathways with retrograde conduction in reciprocating tachycardia. *European Heart Journal* **3**, 143

Touboul P, Tessier Y, Magrina J, Clement C, Delahaye JP. (1972) His bundle recording and electrical stimulation of atria in patients with Wolff–Parkinson–White syndrome type A. *British Heart Journal* **34**, 623

Ward DE, Camm AJ. (1979) Patterns of atrial activation during right ventricular pacing in patients with concealed left sided Kent pathways. *British Heart Journal* **42**, 192

Ward DE, Camm AJ, Spurrell RAJ. (1979) Ventricular preexcitation due to anomalous nodoventricular pathways: report of 3 patients. *European Heart Journal* **9**, 111

Ward DE, Bexton RS, Camm AJ. (1983) Characteristics of atrio–His conduction in the short PR interval, normal QRS complex syndrome. Evidence for enhanced slow pathway conduction. *European Heart Journal* **4**, 882

Ward DE. (1984) Ventricular preexcitation. *European Heart Journal* **5**, supp. A, 119

Wellens HJJ, Durrer D. (1974a) Patterns of ventriculoatrial conduction in the Wolff–Parkinson–White syndrome. *Circulation* **49**, 22

Wellens HJJ, Durrer D. (1984b) Effect of procaine-amide, quinidine, and ajmaline on the Wolff–Parkinson–White syndrome. *Circulation* **50**, 114

Wellens HJ, Durrer D. (1974c) Wolff–Parkinson–White syndrome and atrial fibrillation. Relation between refractory period of accessory pathway and ventricular rate during atrial fibrillation. *American Journal of Cardiology* **34**, 777

Wellens HJJ. (1975) Contribution of cardiac pacing to our understanding of the Wolff–Parkinson–White syndrome. *British Heart Journal* **37**, 231

Weiner I. (1983) Syndromes of Lown–Ganong–Levine and enhanced atrioventricular conduction. *American Journal of Cardiology* **52**, 637

Winters SL, Gomes JA. (1986) Intracardiac electrode catheter recordings of atrioventricular bypass tracts in Wolff–Parkinson–White syndrome: techniques, electrophysiologic characteristics and demonstration of concealed and decremental propagation. *Journal of the American College of Cardiology* **7**, 1392

Wolff L, Parkinson J, White PD. (1930) Bundle branch block with short PR interval in healthy young people prone to paroxysmal tachycardia. *American Heart Journal* **5**, 685

Yee R, Klein GJ. (1984) Syncope in the Wolff–Parkinson–White syndrome: incidence and electrophysiological correlates. *Pacing and Clinical Electrophysiology* **7**, 381

7

Mechanisms of Tachycardia

There are two basic mechanisms of tachycardias in man: 'abnormal automaticity' and 're-entrant excitation'. Several other mechanisms of experimental arrhythmias such as 'triggered automaticity' and 'reflection' have not yet been shown to be clinically important. The most thoroughly investigated mechanism and the only one for which the evidence of clinical significance is substantial is re-entrant excitation or circus movement.

Normal automaticity

Normally automatic cells, such as those of the sinus and AV nodes, slowly lose membrane polarization (by slow inward movement of sodium) during diastole until a critical potential is reached when the cell rapidly depolarizes. The gradual

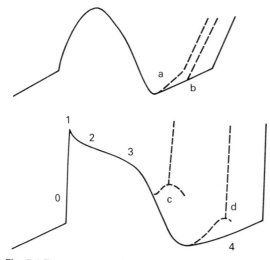

Fig. 7.1 There are several mechanisms of increased automaticity. (*above*) Two ways in which normally automatic cells may increase their discharge frequency: (a) an increase in the slope of spontaneous diastolic depolarization, and (b) negative shift in the threshold potential. (*below*) Early (c) and late (d) afterdepolarizations occurring in abnormal cells. The numbers indicate the phases of the action potential: phase 0 is the initial rapid upstroke due to a sudden increase in sodium permeability; phase 1 may be due to the diminishing influx of sodium; phase 2 is the plateau phase due to a slow inward calcium current; phase 3 is the repolarization phase due to potassium leakage from the cell; phase 4 represents spontaneous diastolic depolarization which may have a variety of ionic bases, depending on the tissue in which it is occurring.

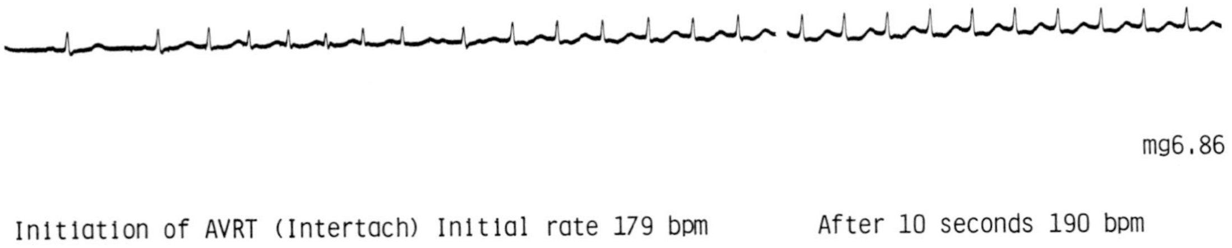

Initiation of AVRT (Intertach)   Initial rate 179 bpm   After 10 seconds 190 bpm

Fig. 7.2 'Warm-up' phenomenon. Initiation of AV re-entrant tachycardia using an implanted antitachycardia device (Intertach). The initial rate of tachycardia is 179 b.p.m. but after 10 seconds the rate has increased to 190 b.p.m. The warm-up phenomenon is not useful in distinguishing automatic from re-entrant tachycardias.

loss of diastolic potential is called 'phase 4 depolarization' and the membrane potential at which the cell fires is the 'threshold potential'. There are several possible mechanisms (Fig. 7.1) by which a normally automatic cell may increase its firing rate, including increased slope of phase 4, lowering (more negative) of the threshold voltage and shortening of the action potential. The rate of discharge of a normal automatic focus is decreased by depolarization from another, faster, pacemaker. This is referred to as 'overdrive suppression'.

Abnormal automaticity

In the presence of disease or metabolic disturbance other cells which are not normally automatic may generate propagated impulses which, if repetitive, cause tachycardias. Unlike normal cells, these cells are partially depolarized (i.e. the membrane potential is reduced). This mechanism may be responsible for some atrial tachycardias and some types of ventricular arrhythmia in acute ischaemia. A clinical diagnosis of abnormal automaticity has been made on the basis of responses to electrical stimulation. Abnormal automaticity in cells is not initiated or terminated by electrical stimuli. It has been assumed that inability to terminate a clinical tachycardia by electrical stimulation is an indication of an automatic rather than a re-entrant mechanism. Furthermore, unlike normal automaticity, overdrive suppression (slowing of the rate of the rhythm after a period of pacing at a faster rate) of abnormal automaticity is unusual. Failure of external cardioversion has also been suggested as indicative of abnormal automaticity. These criteria are, however, not sound, and it is still not clear whether abnormal automaticity of the type well characterized in cells is a mechanism of clinical tachycardias.

The main clinical electrophysiological characteristics of these tachycardias are a tendency to 'warming up' – that is, a gradual increase in rate – after initiation (Fig. 7.2) and their inability to be initiated or terminated by premature stimulation. However, all kinds of exceptions to these concepts have been observed.

Re-entrant excitation

Re-entrant excitation was first observed in animal experiments in the late nineteenth and early twentieth centuries (see Chapter 8, section on atrial flutter). Of the more notable investigators associated with its characterization were Mayer (1906), Garrey (1914), Mines (1914), Kinoshita (1911), Lewis (1918) and Schmitt and Erlanger (1928). It was not until the advent of clinical electrophysiological techniques, however, that this mechanism of tachycardia production was demonstrated to be clinically important.

Other terms that have been used to describe the phenomenon are 'circus movement', 'reciprocation' and 're-entry'. For re-entrant excitation to occur (Fig. 7.3) several conditions must be satisfied:

1. Two or more anatomically distinct or functionally separate pathways which are in electrical continuity.
2. Transient or permanent one-way block in one of these pathways.

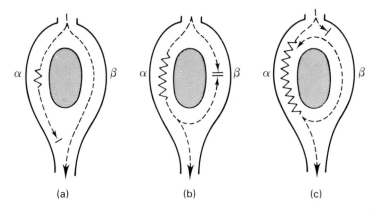

Fig. 7.3 Re-entrant excitation around an anatomical or fixed obstacle (shaded). During the normal rhythm the impulse penetrates both the slow (alpha) and the fast (beta) pathways (a). A premature beat (b) results in block in the fast pathway and conducts in the slower pathway, but cannot return in the fast pathway because of residual tissue refractoriness. An earlier impulse (c) which encounters more delay in the slow pathway finds the fast pathway recovered and can return to initiate continuous re-entrant excitation.

3. The induction of sufficiently slow conduction in the other pathway to allow previously excited tissue to recover excitability. The impulse may then re-enter the area of slowed conduction. Without slowed conduction the initiation and maintenance of circus movement cannot occur (cf. triggered automaticity, later in this chapter).
4. Sustained re-entrant excitation is possible only if the tachycardia cycle length always exceeds the longest refractory period of any part of the circuit.

Pathways

The concept of two pathways is an oversimplification but is useful in understanding the mechanism of circus movement and re-entrant excitation. These pathways provide the 'limbs' of the tachycardia circuit and are connected to form a circuit around a central obstruction which is electrically insulated from the pathways. In some instances the limbs of the circuit are readily identifiable, the most typical example being the anomalous and normal pathways in the tachycardia circuit of the Wolff–Parkinson–White (WPW) syndrome (Fig. 7.4) (see Chapters 6 and 9). This is, however, a simplification because the atrial and the ventricular myocardium are also essential parts of the circuit. Another example is the circuit comprising the 'slow' and 'fast' pathways of intra-AV nodal tachycardia. There is no known anatomical basis for these pathways but their functional reality is not in dispute. The essential element of the two-pathway concept is the notion that one of them contains an area of slowed conduction (see below). Hence in the WPW syndrome, the area of slowed conduction is the AV node. In intranodal re-entrant tachycardia (of the usual type) the limbs are the 'fast' anterograde and 'slow' retrograde pathways. In other parts of the heart giving rise to arrhythmias (e.g. the borders of a myocardial infarct as a substrate for ventricular tachycardia) the two pathways are not so easily characterized by

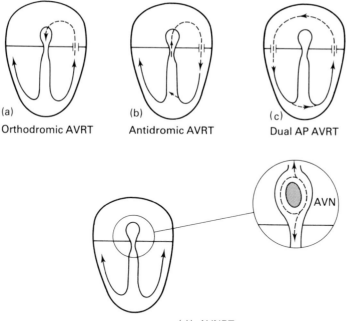

(a) Orthodromic AVRT (b) Antidromic AVRT (c) Dual AP AVRT

(d) AVNRT

Fig. 7.4 (a–c) possible tachycardia circuits in the presence of anomalous AV pathways: (a) the usual form of atrioventicular re-entry (orthodromic) in which the tachycardia impulse circulates towards the ventricle over the normal AV node and His bundle, and returns to the atrium over the anomalous pathway; (b) the reverse of this circulation (antidromic tachycardia), which is unusual; (c) a rare form of atrioventricular re-entry involving anomalous pathways in both anterograde and retrograde limbs of the circuit. (d) AV nodal re-entry in which circulation is confined to the AV node or the perinodal region.

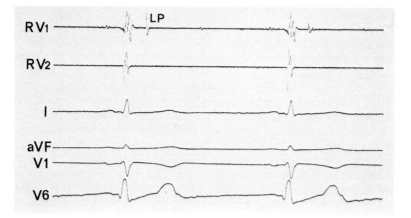

Fig. 7.5 A discrete late potential (LP) during sinus rhythm from the right ventricular outflow tract in a patient with ventricular tachycardia showing 'left bundlle branch block' pattern and right axis deviation (not shown). Paper speed 100 mm/sec. RV1 = distal right ventricular outflow; RV2 = proximal right ventricular outflow (quadripolar catheter).

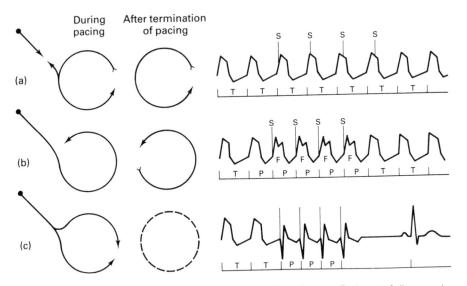

Fig. 7.6 Schematic diagram showing the mechanism of entrainment. Each set of diagrams is accompanied by a stylized ECG tracing (as for ventricular tachycardia). (a) During tachycardia, pacing at a slow rate or remote from the circuit results in failure to penetrate the circuit. Thus the tachycardia continues undisturbed. (b) Pacing at a slightly faster rate or closer to the circuit results in invasion of the circuit by the paced impulse. This impulse drives, or 'entrains', the circuit such that the tachycardia is accelerated to the rate of pacing. The tachycardia complexes are the result of fusion between the tachycardia activation and the pacing activation patterns. When pacing is switched off, tachycardia continues but note that the first cycle after switch-off is at the same rate as the pacing rate. This occurs because the last pacing impulse circulates to produce the first postpacing tachycardia complex, which is not fused with a paced wavefront. (c) Pacing at a still faster rate progressively invades both limbs of the circuit preventing continuation of tachycardia. In this case pacing results in an activation pattern which is not fused with the spontaneous tachycardia. When pacing is discontinued, tachycardia is no longer present. F = fusion beat; P = pace cycle length; S = pacing stimulus; T = tachycardia cycle length.

clinical electrophysiological techniques. However, endocardial electrogram mapping may reveal delayed potentials which probably reflect slowed activation (Fig. 7.5).

Re-entrant excitation and slow conduction pathways important to the continuation of a tachycardia can be identified by pacing techniques even if the circuit itself cannot be precisely defined. The concept, introduced by Waldo et al. (1977), is called 'entrainment' and is now accepted as an important marker for re-entry in the human heart (Fig. 7.6). Entrainment was studied initially in patients with atrial flutter after open heart surgery. During atrial pacing at increasing rates during atrial flutter (see Chapter 8), the morphology of the atrial electrograms and surface flutter waves alters, indicating progressive fusion and a change in the atrial activation pattern consistent with entrainment (Waldo et al., 1977). Entrainment is further evidence for the presence of a re-entrant pathway which is invaded and 'driven' by the stimulation. The entrainment phenomenon has now been shown in almost all arrhythmias known to be of the re-entrant type, including atrioventricular re-entry (Fig. 7.7), AV nodal re-entry

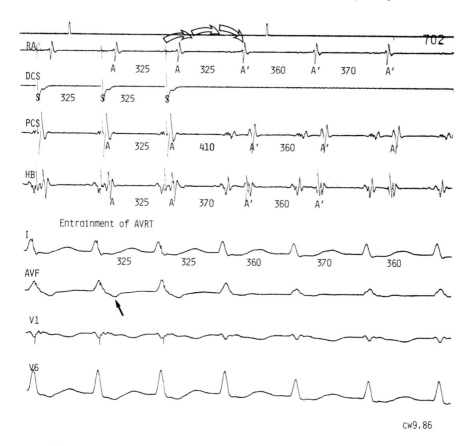

702

A 325 A 325 A′ 360 A′ 370 A′

DCS
S 325 S 325 S

PCS
A 325 A 410 A′ 360 A′ A

HB
A 325 A′ 370 A′ 360 A′

Entrainment of AVRT

I
325 325 360 370 360

AVF

V1

V6

CW9.86

Fig. 7.7 Transient entrainment of atrioventricular re-entrant tachycardia involving a right anterolateral anomalous pathway. Left atrial pacing (SS) at a cycle length of 325 msec results in atrial fusion between the wavefront originating from the pacing site and the retrograde activation of the atria via the anomalous pathway. The fused P wave on the surface ECG is clearly visible (arrowed). Tachycardia continues at a cycle length of 360–370 msec when pacing is turned off. The morphology of the anteromedial right atrial (RA) electrograms during pacing is identical to those seen during tachycardia, suggesting retrograde rather than anterograde or fused activation of this region. In the same site, the first postpacing cycle is the same duration as the pacing cycle but the fused P wave is absent following the last entrained QRS, also of the same cycle length, because it results entirely from retograde atrial activation (A). The open arrows indicate that this site was activated retrogradely by the preceding stimulus. At other atrial sites, the first postpacing cycle is longer than the paced cycle length because these sites were activated anterogradely (from the pacing site) during pacing. These phenomena indicate that the tachycardia circuit is driven and 'entrained' by the left atrial pacing and that the arrhythmia is re-entrant in type. Paper speed 100 mm/sec. A′ = retrograde atrial electrogram; DCS and PCS = distal and proximal coronary sinus; HB = His bundle region; RA = right atrium.

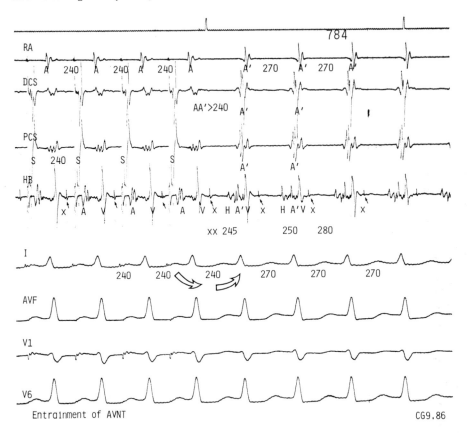

Entrainment of AVNT   CG9.86

Fig. 7.8 Recordings showing transient entrainment of AV nodal re-entrant tachycardia in a patient with the Lown–Ganong–Levine syndrome (see Chapters 6 and 9). Atrial pacing (in the proximal coronary sinus at a cycle length of 240 msec) was initiated during tachycardia at a cycle length of 270 msec. Termination of pacing reveals tachycardia. The tachycardia was entrained as shown by the fact that the first postpacing QRS cycle (open arrows) is the same duration as that during pacing. The His potential would also show this were it not concealed by the low right atrial electrogram during atrial pacing. The atrial return cycles all exceed the paced cycle length because, during pacing, all were the result of anterograde conduction from the pacing site, whereas the last paced atrial beat activates the atria retrogradely (A'). The atrial activation sequence (A') during tachycardia begins in the low right atrium adjacent to the AV node and precedes tha ventricular electrograms. This is typical of AV nodal re-entrant·tachycardia. The deflection labelled 'x' (arrowed) is present after each ventricular electrogram. Its cause is not clear. The XX intervals during tachycardia bear no relationship to the preceding or following VV interval. It is unlikely, therefore, to reflect activation of a site which is 'on-circuit' (e.g. the anterograde slow AV nodal pathway). Paper speed 100 mm/sec. DCS and PCS = distal and proximal coronary sinus; HB = His bundle region; RA = right atrial appendage.

(Fig. 7.8), long RP′ tachycardia and ventricular tachycardia (Fig. 7.9). Demonstration of entrainment implies a re-entrant mechanism.

The criteria for entrainment are as follows (it is not necessary to satisfy all of these criteria to demonstrate entrainment):

1. Progressively increasing fusion as the pacing rate is increased (in discrete

increments rather than like a 'ramp') above the tachycardia rate. At each pacing rate, the degree of fusion should remain constant and unvarying but as the rate is increased the degree of fusion increases. This reflects the increased contribution to activation from the pacing site. For example, in ventricular tachycardia, pacing at the same site and rate during sinus rhythm should produce unfused QRS complexes of a distinctly different morphology (Fig. 7.9).

2. The last entrained beat is not fused and its coupling interval is identical to the pacing cycle length. This phenomenon occurs because the last paced impulse enters and completes the circuit, producing a tachycardia complex. Fusion does not occur because pacing has ceased.
3. Tachycardia returns to the original rate on cessation of pacing after the first return cycle described in criterion 2.
4. The occurrence of localized block for one beat followed by activation of the area from a different direction with a shorter conduction time (e.g. reversal of the circuit in AVRT).

Inability to fulfil any of these criteria does not mean that entrainment is not possible. The site of pacing is critically important in the demonstration of the criteria. Thus, entrainment of orthodromic atrioventricular re-entrant tachycardia (AVRT) can be demonstrated during atrial pacing (see Fig. 7.7) but not ventricular pacing, and entrainment of the antidromic form of tachycardia can be shown during ventricular but not atrial pacing (Okumura et al., 1985). Although entrainment may occur in these situations, because the criteria cannot be demonstrated, the entrainment is said to be 'concealed'. These examples illustrate the principle that the criteria for entrainment can be demonstrated only when the site of pacing is proximal to an area of slow conduction (pacing the atrium in the case of orthodromic AVRT, and pacing the ventricle in the case of antidromic AVRT, the area of slowed conduction being the AV node). During pacing distal to the area of conduction delay, the paced antidromic (against the direction of tachycardia) wavefront will enter the area of slow conduction and the paced orthodromic (in the same direct as tachycardia) impulse will conduct in the faster limb, in the direction of the tachycardia circuit. The paced antidromic wavefront blocks in the area of slowed conduction and prevents orthodromic conduction of the wavefront from the previous paced beat. Thus, progressive fusion between the paced antidromic wavefront and the tachycardia orthodromic wavefront is not possible.

In ventricular tachycardia, it is frequently possible to demonstrate progressive fusion but without a return cycle at the paced rate. Failure to observe a third criterion (the first non-fused tachycardia beat after pacing occurs at the same cycle length as pacing) does not mean that the tachycardia is not entrained. (One reason for such failure is too few recording sites.) It may be difficult to demonstrate any of the criteria for entrainment if pacing is close to the site of origin of ventricular tachycardia. The demonstration of 'concealed' entrainment (no criteria demonstrable) of ventricular tachycardia would seem to be difficult, if not impossible, without detailed information about the re-entrant loop itself. This would require multiple electrode recordings.

Another phenomenon related to entrainment is 'resetting' of tachycardia by a single premature stimulus (Fig. 7.10). This response has been observed in a

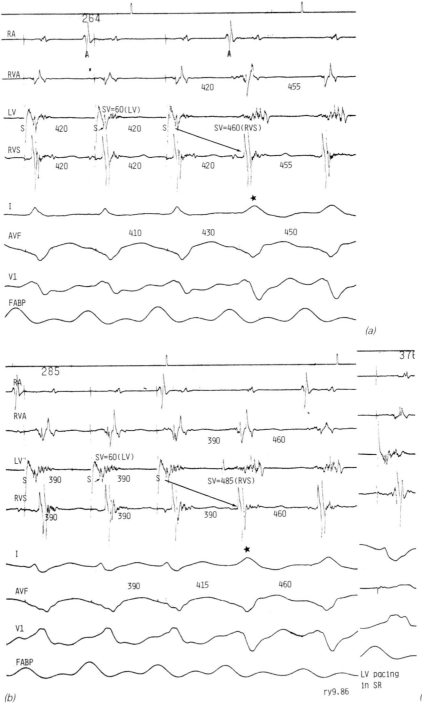

(a)

(b)

ry9.86

(c)

LV pacing
in SR

variety of re-entrant tachycardias and is thought to reflect advancement of the circulating impulse in the circuit. If so, it is equivalent to entrainment by a single beat rather than a train of beats. It should be noted, however, that similar responses can be observed in automatic rhythms, presumably as a result of rephasing phase 4 depolarizing currents. Resetting, therefore, is supportive rather than confirmatory evidence for re-entrant excitation.

These refinements to the concept of entrainment may be especially useful in the identification of areas of slowed conduction (see Fig. 7.9) needed to maintain re-entrant excitation, especially in relation to the mechanisms of ventricular tachycardia (MacLean et al., 1981; Anderson et al., 1984; Waldo et al., 1984; Mann et al., 1985; Okumura et al., 1987).

In another form of re-entry, described in experimental preparations and in animals, a central obstacle or a fixed path length is not necessary. In this model, first studied in detail in rabbit atrial myocardium by Allessie and colleagues (1977), the wavefront circulates around a central refractory zone which is maintained by electrotonic influences and 'blind loops' colliding in the central area. In this form of re-entry the length of the pathway is equal to the length of the circulating wave and no fully excitable gap is present. The time taken for the impulse to circulate (assuming the circuit tissue has homogeneous properties) is therefore proportional to the refractory period of the tissue. Thus, if either the conduction velocity (V) or the refractory period (RP) increases, this will lead to an increase in the wavelength (wavelength $= V \times RP$) and therefore the circuit size will tend to increase. In this model the wavelength (rather than the refractory period of conduction velocity) appears to be the most important determinant (in

---

Fig. 7.9 Entrainment of ventricular tachycardia. (*a*) The left of the recording shows termination of left ventricular (LV) pacing (S) at a cycle length of 420 msec. The site of pacing was close to the tachycardia source in the septum. Note the fractionated electrograms, starting before and extending throughout the QRS complex, at the LV recording site. During tachycardia at different rates the QRS complexes showed fixed fusion (unvarying QRS complexes at a given stable pacing rate). The first unfused QRS complex (★) occurs at a longer cycle length than the paced rate, possibly due to fusion of the onset of the previous paced complex. Examination of the RV septal (RVS) recordings, however, shows that the first postpacing electrogram occurs at the same cycle length as pacing (420 msec). This site is therefore entrained. The morphology of the electrogram during pacing at this site is identical to that seen during tachycardia, giving further evidence that activation of the site during pacing is identical to that during tachycardia (i.e. orthodromically from the tachycardia origin). The morphology of the LV site during tachycardia is different from that during pacing and the return cycle is in excess of the pacing cycle length, indicating orthodromic activation with respect to the pacing site. The stimulus–RV septal interval is 460 msec whereas the stimulus–LV interval is 60 msec. The RV apical site also appears to be entrained but the electrogram shape is varying. The stimulus–RVA time is 480 msec. Pacing at the LV site during sinus rhythm at various rates of tachycardia produced distinctly different QRS complexes (*c*). (*b*) Similar phenomena are observed during pacing at 390 msec. The last unfused complex is entrained but the stimulus–RV septal interval is now prolonged to 485 msec but the stimulus–LV interval is unchanged at 60 msec. Thus, as the pacing rate is increased there is increasing delay across an area of slow conduction. It is not possible to conclude that this area is part of the re-entrant loop because localized conduction block at this site followed by termination of tachycardia as the pacing rate was increased did not occur (Okumura et al., 1986). The stimulus–RVA interval was also unchanged at 480 msec. Entrainment could not be demonstrated (according to the usual criteria) during right ventricular pacing. Paper speed 100 mm/sec. FABP = femoral artery blood pressure; RA = right atrium; RVA = right ventricular apex.

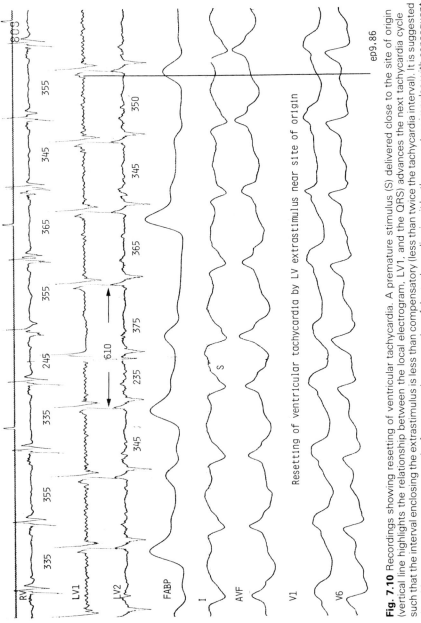

Fig. 7.10 Recordings showing resetting of ventricular tachycardia. A premature stimulus (S) delivered close to the site of origin (vertical line highlights the relationship between the local electrogram, LV1, and the QRS) advances the next tachycardia cycle such that the interval enclosing the extrastimulus is less than compensatory (less than twice the tachycardia interval). It is suggested that this response occurs as a result of anterograde penetration of the tachycardia circuit by the premature impulse with consequent earlier re-entrant excitation and emergence of the next beat. This tachycardia could also be entrained. Paper speed 100 mm/sec. LV1 and LV2 = left ventricular electrograms; RV = right ventricular electrogram.

experimental dog preparations) of the type of arrhythmia induced (Allessie, 1986, personal communication). Very short wavelengths are associated with atrial fibrillation, longer wavelengths with atrial flutter, and even longer wavelengths in transient repetitive atrial responses.

The features of the classical and leading circle mechanisms are compared and contrasted in Fig. 7.11 and Table 7.2. These concepts of re-entry are also discussed in the section on atrial flutter because this arrhythmia has provided an insight into both mechanisms (see Chapter 8).

Unidirectional block

A depolarizing wavefront approaching 'two' pathways will activate both unless one pathway is refractory or incapable of propagating an impulse travelling in a particular direction. If both limbs of the potential re-entry circuit are activated in this way, circus movement cannot take place. Thus the wavefront must encounter block in either one or the other limb of the circuit. This may be functional (i.e. determined by local physiological conditions at the time) or permanent. Functional block can be induced by premature impulses (or an increase in rate of impulses) which arrive at both limbs at a time when only one has recovered. This is the typical mode of initiation of junctional tachycardias associated with the WPW syndrome or dual anterograde AV nodal pathways (see Chapter 9). Thus, functional block may be determined by differences in the refractory periods of the limbs of the circuit.

The mechanisms of permanent unidirectional block are thought to be related to various asymmetries (one end of the pathway compared to the other), including fibre geometry and conduction properties. An example of permanent unidirectional block in one limb is so-called concealed anomalous pathways. In this setting, initiation of tachycardia by a premature atrial beat is dependent not on unidirectional block (because it is already present) but on slowed conduction in the other limb.

Slowed conduction

Re-entry occurs when the 'distal' end of the blocked pathway is excited and conducts the impulse to its starting point. If this has recovered, circulating impulse conduction will continue. Slowed conduction allows recovery of proximal tissue in readiness for reactivation. This principle is illustrated most clearly in paroxysmal junctional tachycardias (see Chapter 9). Anterograde block (in either an anomalous or a slow AV nodal pathway) allows emergence of slow conduction, which is manifest during extrastimulus testing, by a sudden increase in the AV interval. This event alone is sometimes sufficient to initiate tachycardia but often further increases in AV conduction time are required before tachycardia is started (this explains why tachycardia is not always induced coincident with a sudden 'jump' in the AV interval). Similar 'critical' delays at the initiation of a tachycardia have been observed in relation to re-entrant ventricular tachycardia (Chapter 10) although the site of slowed conduction is more difficult to demonstrate.

It has been shown experimentally that the velocity of impulse propagation in

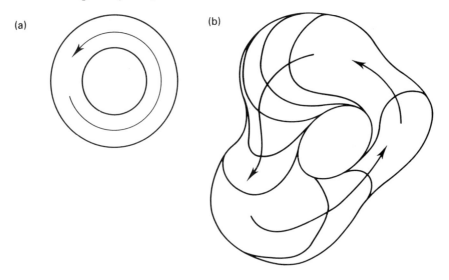

Fig. 7.11 Types of re-entrant excitation. (*a*) Re-entrant excitation around an anatomical or fixed obstacle. This is the classic type of re-entry first described by Mines (1913). (*b*) The concept of re-entry around an area of functionally refractory tissue, as described by Allessie and colleagues (1977). The typical features of these mechanisms are summarized in Table 7.2.

Table 7.1 VARIETIES AND CLASSIFICATION OF TACHYCARDIAS

Supraventicular	Atrial	Sinus node re-entry Atrial automatic tachcardia * Intra-atrial re-entrant tachycardia Atrial flutter Atrial fibrillation *
	Junctional	Intra–AV nodal re-entry Long RP' tachycardia Orthodromic atrioventricular tachycardia Antidromic atrioventricular tachycardia Dual bypass atrioventricular tachycardia Junctional ectopic tachycardia *
Ventricular	Subjunctional	Nodoventricular pathway Macrore-entry Bundle branch re-entry
	Ventricular	Ventricular re-entry Ventricular automaticity * Torsade de pointes * Ventricular fibrillation *

* Possibly automatic mechanisms.

Table 7.2 COMPARISON OF TYPES OF RE-ENTRY

	Classic re-entry	Leading circle re-entry
Circulation time	Dependent on tissue conduction velocity	Dependent on tissue refractoriness
Excitable gap	Present	May be absent
Circuit length	Fixed	Variable
Circuit variation	Little	Substantial

myocardium is related to the orientation of the muscle fibres with respect to the propagating wavefront (Spach and Dolber, 1985). Thus, conduction in the direction of the fibres is faster than that in a direction perpendicular to the fibres. This phenomenon is a property of 'anisotropic' muscle. Furthermore, conduction in a transverse direction may be associated with fractionation of the electrograms. It is conceivable that such anisotropic properties may, in certain circumstances, provide a basis for the slowed conduction necessary for re-entry (see below).

Continued re-entrant excitation

Stable continuous re-excitation of the re-entrant loop results in a sustained tachycardia. Thus there is activation of tissue throughout the cardiac cycle. This is readily demonstrable in experimental preparations where multiple electrodes can be used. It is shown less easily in the clinical situation because electrograms from fewer sites can be sampled and often it is not possible to record potentials from critical sites (e.g. the AV node) with current recording techniques. However, such continuous electrical activity has been recorded during ventricular tachycardia (see Chapter 10), particularly at the time of surgery (Fig. 7.12).

The concept of re-entrant excitation implies the presence of a time interval between the advancing head of the wavefront and the receding tail (defined by refractory tissue). As the refractory tissue recovers, an 'excitable gap' is created. In a fixed anatomical circuit of homogeneous properties (conduction time and refractory period) the gap duration is constant throughout the tachycardia cycle (and whatever its spatial position). In contrast, if the circuit is not homogeneous (for example with respect to refractoriness), the duration of the gap will change cyclically depending on the position of the advancing wavefront. Thus, if the impulse traverses an area of prolonged refractoriness, the duration of the excitable gap is diminished but increases again as it passes through tissue with shorter refractoriness. These corollaries of the re-entry theory are of relevance to the effects of drugs on tachycardias (see Chapter 12) and the use of pacing stimuli (see Chapter 13) to terminate tachycardias.

The interrelationship between the conduction time around the circuit and the maximum refractory period of any part of the circuit determines the stability of tachycardia. Thus, if the conduction time is less than the relative refractory period of any part of the circuit, progressive conduction delay results in slowing and perhaps termination of tachycardia. If the effective refractory period exceeds conduction time the advancing wavefront is extinguished and re-entry ceases.

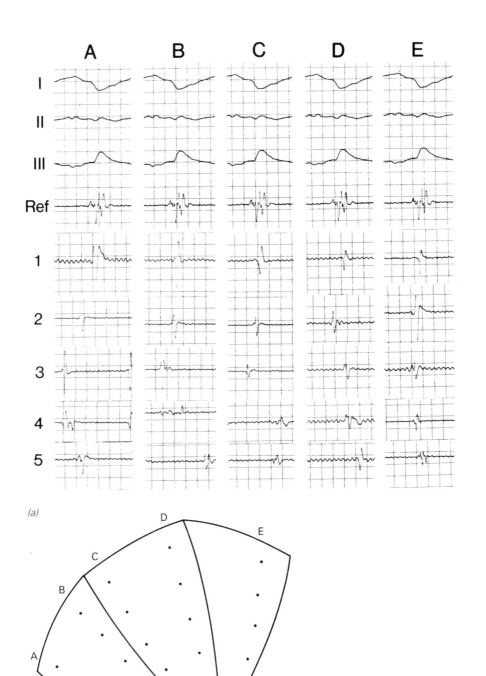

(a)

(b)

The leading circle model does not incorporate an excitable gap, characteristic of the fixed pathway model. Recently, however, Allessie and his group (1986, personal communication) have studied a model (isolated rabbit heart) of ventricular tachycardia (in a thin, uniform, normal layer of muscle) in which the central area of functional block (or delay) was an elongated zone aligned with the muscle fibres. At each end of this zone where the impulse turns (the pivotal point) there is slowed transverse conduction which allows the formation of an excitable gap. It is hypothesized that the slowed conduction is related to anisotropic properties (see above). This 'mixed' type of re-entry, in which an excitable gap is present in a wave which circulates around a central functional obstacle in anisotropic muscle, has been termed 'anisotropic re-entry'. Experimental atrial flutter in dogs exhibits properties that could be explained by such a mechanism (Waldo et al., unpublished observations).

Related phenomena have been studied in detail in experimental myocardial infarction models (Gardner et al., 1984; Wit, 1986, personal communication). During sustained ventricular tachycardia in a uniform layer of epicardial myocardium, an elongated zone of apparent functional block was repeatedly and consistently observed in the direction of fibre orientation. Detailed electrogram mapping of the 'line of block' suggested, however, that this line (of densely packed isochrones) probably reflected markedly slowed conduction across muscle fibres (perpendicular to the direction of the muscle fibres) rather than complete block due to refractoriness. This elongated area of slowed conduction could be explained by anisotropic conduction. These phenomena need further study but are likely to result in considerable revisions of the classic theory.

Triggered activity

This phenomenon, previously discussed only within the context of cellular electrophysiological responses, has recently received considerable attention as a possible mechanism of arrhythmias in man. In cells the basis for these responses is the production of two different types of afterpotential called 'early' and 'delayed' afterdepolarizations.

Early afterdepolarizations are seen on the downstroke of the action potential and may initiate a sequence of repetitive responses. The role of this mechanism

---

Fig. 7.12 (a) Intraoperative mapping of the pattern of endocardial activation during ventricular tachycardia (cycle length 290 msec) in a patient with an anteroseptal myocardial infarction. In each panel surface leads I, II and III are shown together with a reference (Ref) electrogram and local electrograms from the 25 sites which were sampled. Each local electrogram has been mounted using the reference electrogram to align the trace. (b) The opened left ventricular endocardial surface. Columns A and E are contiguous along the lateral free wall. A and B are on the anterior wall, C and D are on the septum and E recorded on the posterolateral wall. Earliest activity is seen in A3 (preceding the onset of the QRS compex); fractionated activity is present in B4 and late activation occurs in C4. These recordings show that, at any point in the cycle, an area of myocardium is depolarized. The mechanism of tachycardia could be a continuous macrore-entrant loop rather than a localized microre-entrant focus. The fractionation may reflect activation of the area of slowed conduction within the loop. Paper speed 100 mm/sec. (*Kindly supplied by Dr E. Rowland*)

in clinical arrhythmias is completely obscure but it is known that factors such as low partial pressure of oxygen, digitalis and high concentrations of catecholamines (which are thought to be clinically important) predispose to its emergence in experimental conditions.

Delayed afterdepolarizations are seen as additional contours after the end of the normal action potential. These delayed potentials may increase in amplitude during rapid stimulation or after a premature stimulus and reach a threshold sufficient to trigger a sustained train of responses. As the stimulation rate is increased, so the coupling interval of the first threshold response is also reduced and the amplitude is increased. This latter relationship is also seen when single stimuli are used. A train of responses can be accelerated by rapid pacing but may also be terminated by rapid pacing and a single stimulus. The afterdepolarizations are suppressed by calcium antagonists, such as verapamil.

These observations have led clinical electrophysiologists to suggest that some human tachycardias behave in a manner predicted by the dynamics of cellular afterdepolarizations. The following criteria have all been suggested as possible criteria for diagnosing triggered activity in the clinical setting:

1. Initiation by timed stimuli.
2. A direct relationship between the coupling interval of the initiating stimulus and the coupling interval of the first response (Fig. 7.13).
3. Overdrive acceleration by rapid pacing.

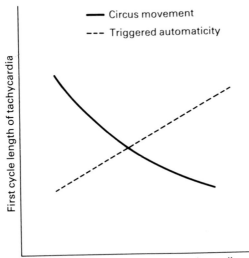

Fig. 7.13 Graphical representation of the relationship between the coupling interval of the initiating stimulus and the first tachycardia cycle length in re-entrant excitation and triggered automaticity. The solid line shows that the shorter the initiating coupling interval, the longer the first cycle length (signifying the critical importance of 'delay' in the initiation of the arrhythmia. The broken line shows a direct relationship between the two intervals. This is consistent with phenomena caused by cellular triggered automaticity but there is little evidence for a clinical counterpart.

4. A direct relationship between the cycle length of an initiating pacing burst and the subsequent tachycardia cycle length.
5. Termination by verapamil where such a response would not be expected (e.g. atrial or ventricular tachycardias but not those involving the AV node).

Triggered responses have been demonstrated in isolated human atrial fibres. Despite the considerable volume of speculative literature on human triggered automaticity, it must be concluded at the present time that there is little evidence for its existence as a clinically important mechanism. Tachycardias initiated by one or two premature stimuli are more likely to be re-entrant than triggered, and for clinical purposes they are best considered as such. If rapid pacing is the only method of initiation, an attempt at clinical demonstration of those cellular features characteristic of triggered activity may be fruitful but so far this evidence has not been forthcoming. Those instances of clinical tachycardias where triggered activity has been mooted have shown some but not all of the features of triggered activity.

Reflection

The definition of this term has been confusing. It has been applied to several *in vitro* responses, including 'microre-entry' in unbranched Purkinje fibres, re-excitation of distal normal fibres by slowly conducting impulses in adjacent depressed fibres and re-excitation of fibres with shorter action potentials by adjacent cells with markedly prolonged action potentials. It has also been used to describe AV nodal re-entry where the fast pathway refractory period is less than that of the slow pathway (i.e. concealed slow pathway conduction leading to re-entry without a sudden jump in the AH interval). The term is best used to describe two types of experimental response:

1. Stimulation of a single fibre at a site proximal to an inexcitable gap (sucrose gap model) can cause excitation of a distal segment across the gap by electronic spread. If conduction across the depressed segment is slow enough to allow recovery of the proximal stimulated segment, electronic spread the impulse in the reverse direction may result in reactivation of the proximal segment (Antzelevitch, et al., 1980). This mechanism has been shown to account for modulation of experimental parasystole. This experimental model accurately predicts modulation of clinical parasystole. Whether or not this type of reflection can cause sustained clinical tachycardias is not clear. The sucrose gap model also predicts many of the features associated with dual AH pathways (see Chapter 3). Conduction across the depressed segment in response to extrastimulation can show decremental features, with or without discontinuous output curves (mimicking dual pathways) and echo responses (Jalife, 1983).
2. If adjacent areas of tissue have markedly disparate electrophysiological properties, this may generate current flow between one area and the other. For example, if one area has normal duration of action potential and the other has markedly prolonged depolarization, a potential gradient will exist at the end of repolarization of the normal area. A similar situation exists when the action potential duration of one area is markedly shortened compared to the other.

Table 7.3 SUMMARY OF ELECTROPHYSIOLOGICAL CHARACTERISTICS OF RE-ENTRANT TACHYCARDIA

	Sinoatrial	Atrial	AV nodal		Atrioventricular		Fasciculoventricular		Ventricular
			Usual	Unusual	Ortho	Anti	Ortho	Anti	
Atrial activation	Norm	Ab	Retro	Retro	Ab	Retro	Retro	Retro	Retro
Atrial dissociation	Poss	NA	Poss	Poss	Imp	Imp	Poss	Poss	Poss
HV time	Norm	Norm	Norm	Norm	Norm	Norm	Norm	Neg	Neg/?
Ventricular activation	Norm	Norm	Norm	Norm	Norm	Pre-ex	Norm	Pre-ex	Ab
Ventricular dissociation	Poss	Poss	Poss	Poss	Imp	Imp	Imp	Imp	NA
Tachycardia initiation and termination: *									
atrium	Poss	Poss	Poss	Poss	Imp	Imp	Imp	Imp	Imp
ventricle	Imp	Imp	Poss	Poss	Imp	Imp	Poss	Poss	Poss

Ab = abnormal; Imp = impossible; NA = not applicable; Neg = negative; Norm = normal; Poss = possible; Pre-ex = pre-excited; Retro = normal retrograde activation.

* For the purposes of this table tachycardia initiation or termination from the atrium (or ventricle) implies that the tachycardia can be affected by a premature beat(s) which does not conduct to the ventricle (or atrium).

These gradients may cause current flow and re-excite adjacent tissue. This mechanism is responsible for some arrhythmias in experimental acute ischaemia but evidence for its existence in clinical arrhythmias is limited. It may account for arrhythmias associated with prolonged repolarization syndromes. This type of reflection has also been called 'the re-excitation theory'. Reflection is a mechanism distinct from triggered activity due to early afterdepolarizations. Thus, there are many basic mechanisms which account for the production of experimental arrhythmias but their exact relevance to clinical tachycardias is far from certain. However, it is clear that circus movement is the mechanism responsible for the majority of recurrent paroxysmal tachycardias (see Table 7.2, p. 141). The clinical electrophysiological characteristics of the re-entrant tachycardias are summarized in Table 7.3 and will be discussed in subsequent chapters.

References and further reading

Allessie MA, Bonke FIM, Schopman FJG. (1973) Circus movement in rabbit atrial muscle as a mechanism of tachycardia. *Circulation Research* **33**, 54

Allessie MA, Bonke FIM, Schopman FJG. (1976) Circus movement in rabbit atrial muscle as a mechanism of tachycardia. II. The role of nonuniform recovery of excitability in the occurrence of unidirectional block, as studied with multiple electrodes. *Circulation Research* **39**, 168

Allessie MA, Bonke FIM, Schopman FJG. (1977) Circus movement in rabbit atrial muscle as a mechanism of tachycardia. III. The 'leading circle' concept: a new model of circus movement in cardiac tissue without the involvement of an anatomical obstacle. *Circulation Research* **41**, 9

Almendral JM, Gottlieb C, Marchlinski FE, Buxton AE, Doherty JU, Josephson ME. (1985) Entrainment of ventricular tachycardia by atrial depolarizations. *American Journal of Cardiology* **56**, 298

Anderson KP, Swerdlow CD, Mason JW. (1984) Entrainment of ventricular tachycardia. *American Journal of Cardiology* **53**, 335

Antzelevitch C, Jalife J, Moe GK. (1980) Characteristics of reflection as a mechanism of reentrant arrhythmias and its relationship to parasystole. *Circulation* **61**, 182

Brugada P, Wellens HJJ. (1984a) The role of triggered activity in clinical ventricular arrhythmias. *Pacing and Clinical Electrophysiology* **7**, 260

Brugada P, Wellens HJJ. (1984b) Entrainment as an electrophysiologic phenomenon. *Journal of the American College of Cardiology* **3**, 451

Castellanos A, Portillo B, Leon-Portillo N, Saoudi N, Zaman L. (1985) Entrainment of circus movement tachycardia utilizing an accessory pathway with long retrograde conduction times during ventricular and atrial pacing. *Journal of the American College of Cardiology* **6**, 1431

Fisher JD. (1981) Entrainment of ventricular tachycardia: all aboard or end of the line. *Pacing and Clinical Electrophysiology* **4**, 467

Frame LH, Hoffman BF. (1984) Mechanisms of tachycardia. In: *Tachycardias*, p. 7. Ed. by B Surawicz, CP Reddy, EN Prystowsky. Martinus Nijhoff: Boston, Mass

Gardner PI, Ursell PC, Pham TD, Fenoglio JJ, Wit AL. (1984) Experimental chronic ventricular tachycardia: anatomic and electrophysiologic substrates. In: *Tachycardias: Mechanisms, Diagnosis and Treatment*, p. 29. Ed. by HJJ Wellens, ME Josephson. Lea & Febiger: Philadelphia, Pa

Garrey WE. (1914) The nature of fibrillary contraction of the heart. Its relation to tissue mass and form. *American Journal of Physiology* **33**, 397

Jalife J. (1983) The sucrose gap preparation as a model of AV nodal transmission: are dual pathways necessary for reciprocation and AV nodal 'echoes'? *Pacing and Clinical Electrophysiology* **6**, 1106

Janse MJ, van Capelle FJL, Freud GE, Durrer D. (1971) Circus movement within the AV node as a basis for supraventricular tachycardia as shown by multiple microelectrode recording in the isolated rabbit heart. *Circulation Research* **28**, 403

Janse M, van Capelle FJL. (1982) Electrotonic interactions across an inexcitable region as a cause of ectopic activity in acute regional myocardial ischemia: a study in intact porcine and canine hearts and computer models. *Circulation Research* **50**, 527

Kinoshita H. (1911) Initiation of entrapped circuit wave in a scyphomedusae, mastigia papua. *Japanese Journal of Zoology* **9**, 209

Lehmann MH, Denker S, Mahmud R, Addas A, Akhtar M. (1985) Linking: a dynamic electrophysiologic phenomenon in macroreentry circuits. *Circulation* **71**, 254

Lewis T. (1918) Observations upon flutter and fibrillation. IV. Atrial flutter: theory of circus movement. *Heart* **8**, 293

MacLean WAH, Plumb VJ, Waldo AL. (1981) Transient entrainment and interruption of ventricular tachycardia. *Pacing and Clinical Electrophysiology* **4**, 358

Macwilliam JA. (1897) Fibrillar contraction of the heart. *Journal of Physiology* **8**, 296

Mann DE, Lawrie GM, Luck JC, Griffin JC, Magro SA, Wyndham CRC. (1985) Importance of pacing site in entrainment of ventricular tachycardia. *Journal of the American College of Cardiology* **5**, 781

Mayer AG. (1906) *Rhythmical Pulsation in Scyphomedusae*, publication no. 47. Carnegie Institute: Washington DC

Mendez C, Moe GK. (1966) Demonstration of a dual AV nodal conduction system in the isolated rabbit heart. *Circulation Research* **19**, 378

Mines GR. (1913) On the dynamic equilibrium in the heart. *Journal of Physiology* **46**, 349

Mines GR. (1914) On circulating excitations in heart muscles and their possible relationship to tachycardias and fibrillation. *Transactions of the Royal Society of Canada* series 3, section IV, **8**, 43

Moe GK, Cohen W, Vick RL. (1963) Experimentally induced paroxysmal AV nodal tachycardia in the dog. A 'case' report. *American Heart Journal* **65**, 87

Okumura K, Henthorn RW, Epstein AE, Plumb VJ, Waldo AL. (1985) Further observations on transient entrainment: importance of pacing site and properties of the components of the reentry circuit. *Circulation* **72**, 1293

Okumura K, Olshansky B, Henthorn RW, Epstein AW, Plumb VJ, Waldo AL. (1987) Demonstration of the presence of slow conduction during sustained ventricular tachycardia in man: use of transient entrainment of the tachycardia. *Circulation* **75**, 369.

Portillo B, Leon-Portillo N, Zaman L, Myerburg RJ, Castellanos A. (1984) Entrainment of atrioventricular nodal reentrant tachycardias during overdrive pacing from the high right atrium and coronary sinus. *American Journal of Cardiology* **53**, 1570

Reddy CP, Surawicz B. (1983) Terminology of tachycardias: historical background and evolution. *Pacing and Clinical Electrophysiology* **6**, 1123

Rosen MR, Feder RF. (1981) Does triggered activity have a role in the genesis of cardiac arrhythmias? *Annals of Internal Medicine* **94**, 794

Schmitt FO, Erlanger J. (1928) Directional differences in the conduction of the impulse through heart muscle and their possible relation to extrasystolic and fibrillary contractions. *American Journal of Physiology* **87**, 326

Spach MS, Dolber PC. (1985) The relation between discontinuous propagation in anisotropic cardiac muscle and the 'vulnerable period' of reentry. In: *Cardiac Electrophysiology and Arrhythmias*, p. 28. Ed. by DP Zipes, J Jalife. Grune & Stratton: Orlando, Fla

Waldo AL, Kaiser GA. (1973) Study of ventricular arrhythmias associated with acute myocardial infarction in the canine heart. *Circulation* **47**, 1222

Waldo AL, MacLean WAH, Karp RB, Kouchoukos NT, James TN. (1977) Entrainment and interruption of atrial flutter with atrial pacing. Studies in man following open heart surgery. *Circulation* **56**, 737

Waldo AL, Plumb V, Arciniegas JG, MacLean WAH, Copper TB, Priest MF, James TN. (1983) Transient entrainment and interruption of the atrioventricular bypass type of paroxysmal atrial tachycardia. A model for understanding and identifying reentrant arrhythmias. *Circulation* **67**, 73

Waldo AL, Henthorn RW, Plumb VJ, MacLean WAH. (1984) Demonstration of the mechanism of transient entrainment of ventricular tachycardia with rapid atrial pacing. *Journal of the American College of Cardiology* **3**, 422

Wallace AG, Daggett WM. (1964) Reexcitation of the atrium. 'The echo phenomenon'. *American Heart Journal* **67**, 661

Wallace AG, Mignone RJ. (1966) Physiologic evidence concerning the reentry hypothesis for ectopic beats. *American Heart Journal* **72**, 60

Watanabe Y, Dreifus LS. (1965) Inhomogeneous conduction in the AV node. A model for reentry. *American Heart Journal* **70**, 505

Wellens HJJ. (1971) *Electrical Stimulation of the Heart in the Study and Treatment of Tachycardias*. University Park Press: Baltimore, Md

Wellens HJJ. (1978) Value and limitations of programmed electrical stimulation of the heart in the study and treatment of tachycardias. *Circulation* **57**, 845

Wit AL, Cranefield PF. (1982) Reentrant excitation as a cause of cardiac arrhythmias. In: *Excitation and Neural Control of the Heart*, p. 113. Ed. by M Levy, M Vassalle. American Physiological Society: Bethesda, Md

Zipes DP, Bailey JC, Elharrar V. (1980) *The Slow Inward Current and Cardiac Arrhythmias*. Martinus Nijhoff: The Hague

8

Atrial Tachycardias

Atrial arrhythmias arise in and are sustained by atrial myocardium. They usually occur in association with organic heart disease (e.g. ischaemic heart disease, valvular disease, congenital heart disease, cardiomyopathy) or metabolic disturbances (e.g. thyrotoxicosis, electrolyte disorder, drug toxicity – particularly digoxin). Sometimes there is an isolated abnormality of the atria (idiopathic dilation). Patients who have delayed atrial depolarization and associated atrial arrhythmias in the absence of any evidence for organic disease may be regarded as having a primary electrical disorder. Atrial tachycardias, especially atrial flutter and fibrillation, are also associated with anomalous AV conduction and atrioventricular tachycardias (Chapters 6 and 9).

As an incidental point, it is appropriate to mention the continuing debate about the importance of so-called 'specialized internodal tracts', as these apparent structures are often referred to in discussions concerning the mechanisms of atrial conduction and atrial arrhythmias. A discussion proposing the existence of these pathways has been presented by James (1963, 1984). Another school of thought, however, has denied the existence of such pathways on the basis that histological evidence for them has not been forthcoming (Anderson and Becker, 1978, 1985; Anderson et al., 1981). If such tracts do exist, it would appear that they are distinctly different from the intraventricular specialized pathways in that they are not readily characterized by standard histological or electrophysiological techniques. It seems likely that the electrophysiological properties of the atria as a whole can be attributed to the anatomical complexity of these chambers (e.g. numerous orifices which act as obstacles to conduction and thick bands of muscle running through thinner sheets of tissue) rather than specialized intra-atrial conduction pathways which have defined morphological characteristics.

Sustained atrial tachycardias may be classified into three groups: (1) atrial fibrillation; (2) atrial flutter; and (3) atrial tachycardia.

Atrial fibrillation

Clinical observations

This is one of the commonest clinical cardiac arrhythmias. It is a functional disturbance of atrial myocardium in which atrial activation is rapid, disorganized and mechanically ineffective. The frequency of atrial depolarization is difficult to ascertain because it is so disorganized. It is often said to be between 350 and 600 per minute but this varies with time and location (Fig. 8.1). The arrhythmia

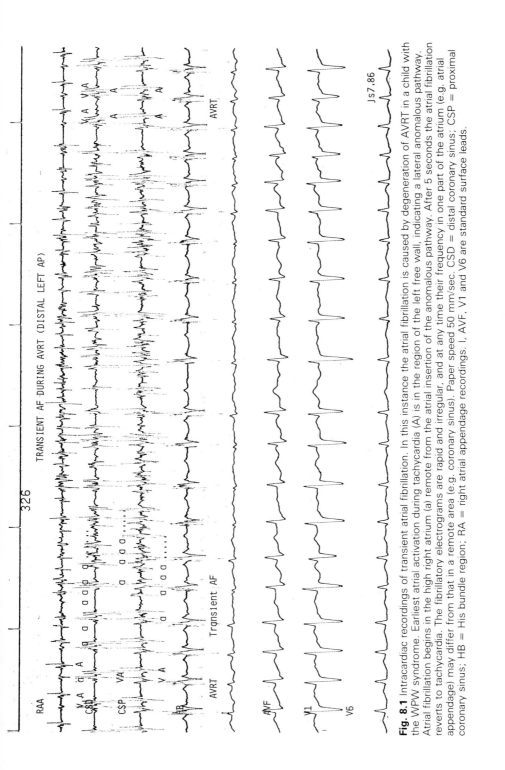

Fig. 8.1 Intracardiac recordings of transient atrial fibrillation. In this instance the atrial fibrillation is caused by degeneration of AVRT in a child with the WPW syndrome. Earliest atrial activation during tachycardia (A) is in the region of the left free wall, indicating a lateral anomalous pathway. Atrial fibrillation begins in the high right atrium (a) remote from the atrial insertion of the anomalous pathway. After 5 seconds the atrial fibrillation reverts to tachycardia. The fibrillatory electrograms are rapid and irregular, and at any time their frequency in one part of the atrium (e.g. atrial appendage) may differ from that in a remote area (e.g. coronary sinus). Paper speed 50 mm/sec. CSD = distal coronary sinus; CSP = proximal coronary sinus; HB = His bundle region; RA = right atrial appendage recordings. I, AVF, V1 and V6 are standard surface leads.

is found most commonly in patients with heart disease, especially if there is atrial enlargement. Atrial fibrillation may be permanent or paroxysmal, the latter often being found in patients with no evidence of structural heart disease. There is a higher incidence of atrial fibrillation in patients with the Wolff–Parkinson–White (WPW) syndrome either because of associated sinoatrial disease (rare) or due to spontaneous degeneration of atrioventricular tachycardias (common) (Fig. 8.1). Almost 30 per cent of patients with paroxysmal supraventricular tachycardia have episodes of atrial fibrillation from the underlying tachycardia (Roark et al., 1986). In patients with anomalous atrioventricular pathways, surgical section of the pathway results in abolition of the atrial fibrillation as well as the re-entrant tachycardia (Sharma et al., 1985). Atrial flutter (see below) often degenerates to fibrillation. The clinical effects of atrial fibrillation are related to loss of effective atrial contraction and normal atrioventricular synchrony and abnormally fast or slow ventricular rates in response to atrial fibrillation.

Atrioventricular conduction during atrial fibrillation is determined by the electrophysiological properties of the AV node. The normal AV node is a complex network of pathways of differing properties which act as a filter to supraventricular impulses. The high frequency of stimulation of the node means that many intranodal pathways will be excited while they are still in a partially refractory state, with consequent slow conduction and gradual extinction of the impulse within the node. This phenomenon is described as concealed conduction (i.e. not manifest directly on the ECG). Repetitive concealed conduction prevents high frequency depolarization of the His bundle and therefore protects the ventricles against rapid rates. Another consequence of the filtering mechanism is an irregular ventricular response. The distribution of responses per unit time is described statistically by a Poisson exponential distribution. Detailed mathematical studies of the ventricular response have shown cyclical variations in the RR interval (Meijler, 1986; Rawles and Rowland, 1986). In the presence of enhanced AV nodal conduction the ventricular rate is faster because the filtering properties of the AV node are attenuated. This is especially evident in patients with the Lown–Ganong–Levine syndrome (see Chapter 6).

Ventricular bigeminy during atrial fibrillation may result in regularization of the ventricular response (Fig. 8.2). This effect is most probably due to concealed retrograde invasion of the AV node. This slowing and regularizing effect may have therapeutic applications to the control of atrial fibrillation. If the minimum interval between successive depolarizations of the His bundle is less than the effective refractory period of the right or left bundle branch, aberrant bundle branch conduction is induced. Because a longer preceding cycle length increases the refractory period of the His–Purkinje system (see Chapter 3), aberration tends to occur when a short cycle follows a long cycle during atrial fibrillation. This is known as the Gouaux–Ashman phenomenon.

In the presence of an anomalous AV pathway of the type found in the WPW syndrome (see Chapter 6) the ventricular response is determined by the properties of the abnormal pathway as well as the normal pathway. Thus, pathways with short anterograde refractory periods may conduct with a high frequency, causing a fast irregular rhythm with broad pre-excited QRS complexes. Such episodes of fast rate are often interspersed with periods of rapid rates with normal AV conduction (Fig. 8.3).

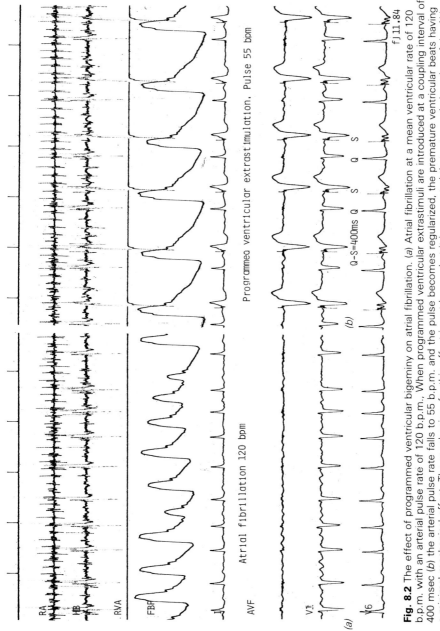

RA

HB

RVA

FBP

II

AVF   Atrial fibrillation 120 bpm   Programmed ventricular extrastimulation, Pulse 55 bpm

V1

V6   Q-S=400ms Q S   Q S

(a)   *(b)*   fJ11.84

Fig. 8.2 The effect of programmed ventricular bigeminy on atrial fibrillation. (*a*) Atrial fibrillation at a mean ventricular rate of 120 b.p.m. with an arterial pulse rate of 120 b.p.m., (*b*) When programmed ventricular extrastimuli are introduced at a coupling interval of 400 msec (*b*) the arterial pulse rate falls to 55 b.p.m. and the pulse becomes regularized, the premature ventricular beats having a minimal mechanical effect. The mechanism for this effect is not known but it is suggested that retrograde invasion of the AV node may rephase nodal tissue and at the same time impair anterograde conduction. Such a mechanism could be useful in controlling the ventricular response to rapid atrial fibrillation. Paper speed 25 mm/sec. FBP = femoral artery blood pressure; HB = His bundle region; RA = right atrium; RVA = right ventricular apex.

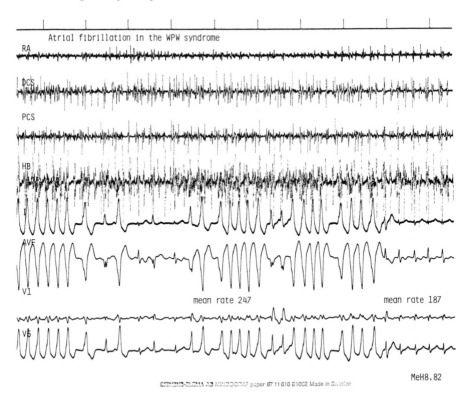

Fig. 8.3 Atrial fibrillation in the WPW syndrome. This recording shows a rapid ventricular response (mean 247 b.p.m) to atrial fibrillation during pre-excited AV conduction. There are also periods of normal AV conduction during which the ventricular rate remains rapid with a mean of 187 b.p.m. Paper speed 25 mm/sec. DCS and PCS = distal and proximal coronary sinus; HB = His bundle region; RA = right atrium.

Electrophysiological observations in patients with paroxysmal atrial fibrillation

The mechanism of atrial fibrillation is probably microre-entry with multiple wavefronts circulating around areas of refractoriness until they are extinguished and new fronts emerge. The autonomic nervous system has important modulating effects on the electrophysiological properties of the atrial myocardium which may predispose to the development of atrial fibrillation. Coumel and colleagues (1979b) have shown that vagal activity may trigger 'lone' atrial fibrillation (Fig. 8.4) and it is known that vagal stimulation in animals shortens atrial refractoriness more in some areas than in others (inhomogeneity of refractoriness), predisposing to re-entry.

The electrophysiological abnormalities of the atria found in patients with paroxysmal atrial fibrillation are variable and are determined largely by the predisposing causes. In patients with heart disease, intra-atrial conduction times may be prolonged correlating with increased P wave duration on the ECG. The

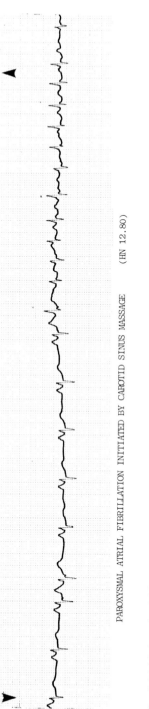

PAROXYSMAL ATRIAL FIBRILLATION INITIATED BY CAROTID SINUS MASSAGE   (HN 12.80)

Fig. 8.4 Initiation of atrial fibrillation by carotid sinus massage. This middle-aged man had suffered from paroxysmal atrial fibrillation for several years, especially at night. Tape-monitored attacks were often preceded by sinus bradycardia. Carotid sinus massage consistently initiated attacks often with preceding atrial ectopic beats. He had been treated with digoxin but noticed a marked deterioration in symptoms and stopped the drug. Paper speed 25 mm/sec.

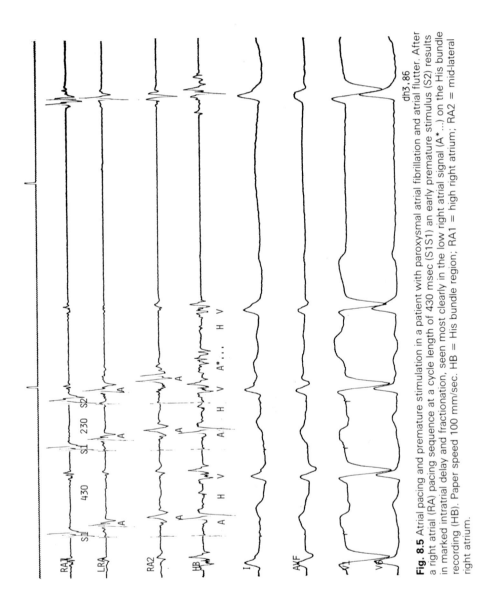

Fig. 8.5 Atrial pacing and premature stimulation in a patient with paroxysmal atrial fibrillation and atrial flutter. After a right atrial (RA) pacing sequence at a cycle length of 430 msec (S1S1) an early premature stimulus (S2) results in marked intratrial delay and fractionation, seen most clearly in the low right atrial signal (A*...) on the His bundle recording (HB). Paper speed 100 mm/sec. HB = His bundle region; RA1 = high right atrium; RA2 = mid-lateral right atrium.

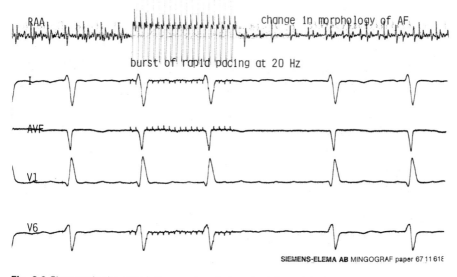

Fig. 8.6 Changes in the morphology and cycle length of the atrial electrograms following a burst of rapid pacing (20 Hz) during apparent atrial fibrillation. Paper speed 50 mm/sec. RAA = right atrial appendage.

atrial ERP has been documented as normal, prolonged or shortened in these patients. Extrastimulus testing at several different sites may reveal marked inhomogeneity of refractoriness. More recently, it has been shown that the normal rate-dependent shortening of the atrial ERP is attenuated or absent in patients with atrial arrhythmias.

In patients with atrial disease, early atrial premature stimulation may induce marked intra-atrial delay (Fig. 8.5), fractionation of electrograms and the initiation of atrial fibrillation. This correlates with the observation that spontaneous episodes are initiated by atrial premature beats. In patients with vagally related paroxysmal atrial fibrillation and without atrial disease, the electrophysiological characteristics of the atria are normal and atrial fibrillation cannot be induced by extrastimulation in the majority. Spontaneous onset is usually preceded by sinus slowing. Because there is no detectable excitable gap in atrial fibrillation, pacing the atria usually has no effect on the rhythm. However, the form of atrial fibrillation may sometimes be changed by atrial pacing (Fig. 8.6).

An interesting phenomenon sometimes observed when atrial fibrillation is induced at study is interatrial dissociation (or even intra-atrial dissociation) in which atrial fibrillation is seen in one part of the atrial mass and atrial flutter in another (Fig. 8.7). Several different varieties have been described (another is right atrial sinus rhythm and left atrial flutter). The coexistence of atrial flutter and atrial fibrillation is a cause of the ECG pattern of so-called flutter–fibrillation (tremulation, 'flutter', etc.). Abnormalities of sinus node function (see Chapter 4)

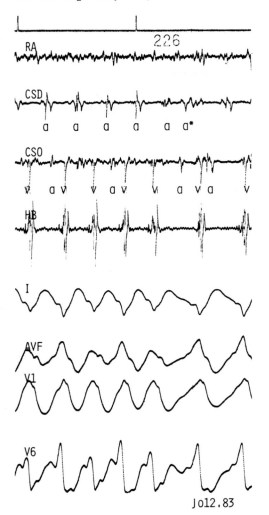

Fig. 8.7 Intracardiac recordings showing interatrial dissociation in a patient with left ventricular free wall pre-excitation (positive delta wave in V1, negative in lead I. The right atrial (RA) recordings show atrial fibrillation whereas the left atrial (recorded from the extreme distal coronary sinus) recordings show atrial tachycardia (a). Occasional fibrillatory activity is seen in the recording of the coronary sinus ostium (CSO) and also in the distal coronary sinus (a*). The ventricular response over the anomalous pathway seems to be determined by the left atrial rhythm rather than by the right atrial rhythm. Paper speed 25 mm/sec. RV = right ventricle.

are found in a small proportion of patients with paroxysmal atrial fibrillation.

Atrial fibrillation can be induced at electrophysiological study in about 1 in 20 patients with normal hearts and without spontaneous atrial fibrillation. The arrhythmia is transient in the majority of these, lasting from several seconds to a few hours. Usually the arrhythmia terminates within a few minutes.

Clinical electrophysiological studies of atrial fibrillation

Electrophysiological studies in patients with established atrial fibrillation are not helpful (excepting other reasons such as the study of associated ventricular tachycardia). In patients with paroxysmal atrial fibrillation the main indications for study are assessment of drug therapy and investigation of associated abnormalities such as pre-excitation.

Most of the information about drug testing in patients with atrial fibrillation comes from patients with ventricular pre-excitation and atrial fibrillation with rapid ventricular rates (see Chapter 6). In general, the aim of the studies is to identify a drug which prevents initiation of atrial fibrillation by premature or burst stimulation (see Chapter 11). Bauernfeind et al. (1982) were able to prevent induction of sustained atrial fibrillation in all patients studied and this seemed to predict long-term suppression on oral treatment. In patients with severely symptomatic recurrent paroxysmal atrial fibrillation not responding to empirical treatment, drug testing using the methods described in Chapter 11 should be considered. In patients with the WPW syndrome the aim of the study is primarily to identify a drug which will prevent a rapid ventricular response by altering the properties of the anomalous pathway.

Rapid rates causing symptoms, despite drug treatment, can be controlled by ablation of the His bundle or the anomalous pathway, whichever is appropriate (see Chapter 14).

Atrial flutter

Clinical observations

Spontaneous atrial flutter is usually found in patients with organic heart disease although, like atrial fibrillation, it may occur in patients with otherwise normal hearts. It may be transient, lasting several seconds or minutes, or may be sustained over weeks, months or years. Atrial flutter is often an unstable tachycardia and may degenerate spontaneously into atrial fibrillation rather than convert to sinus rhythm.

Most usually, atrial flutter conducts to the ventricles in a 2:1 ratio. Not infrequently (especially in those who are not taking AV nodal blocking drugs) this ratio may decrease to 1:1 on exertion (Fig. 8.8). Therapy with AV blocking drugs (digoxin, verapamil, beta blockers) may increase the ratio to 4:1 but more often there is variable conduction with Wenckebach patterns. Higher degrees of stable block are usually in ratios of 4:1, 6:1 or 8:1 but rarely 3:1, 5:1 or 7:1. Wenckebach-type conduction of every other flutter impulse is taken to indicate two levels of block within the AV node. Alternate impulses are always completely blocked at one level while interpolated impulses encounter an area of decremental conduction producing the typical Wenckebach type of pattern. Enhanced AV nodal conduction may cause block below the His bundle. Atrial flutter in the presence of an anomalous AV connection produces an arrhythmia resembling ventricular tachycardia with wide pre-excited complexes at a rate of 300 b.p.m.

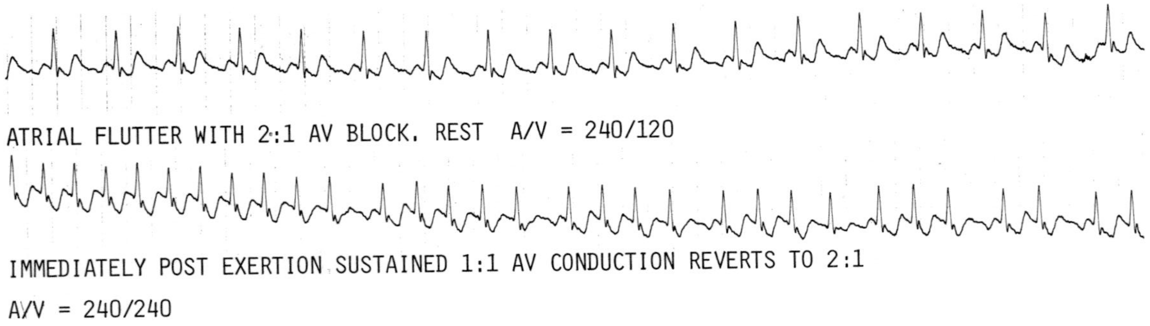

ATRIAL FLUTTER WITH 2:1 AV BLOCK. REST A/V = 240/120

IMMEDIATELY POST EXERTION SUSTAINED 1:1 AV CONDUCTION REVERTS TO 2:1

A/V = 240/240

Fig. 8.8 The effect of exertion on atrial flutter. At rest there is stable atrial flutter with 2:1 AV block (atrial rate 240, ventricular rate 120). After 1 minute of the Bruce protocol treadmill test the ventricular rate suddenly doubled (atrial rate 240, ventricular rate 240) as a result of a change from 2:1 to 1:1 AV conduction. Immediately postexertion, 2:1 AV conduction resumes. The relatively slow flutter rate is due to oral amiodarone treatment. Paper Speed 25 mm/sec.

Electrophysiological observations in patients with atrial flutter

The mechanism of atrial flutter has been debated for many years. The historical aspects of the investigation of this arrhythmia have had an important bearing on the understanding of re-entrant excitation in general. The elegant dog experiments conducted by Thomas Lewis led him to conclude that 'circus movement' (the term was his) was the mechanism responsible. He suggested that the circuit was of large but not fixed dimensions, with the AV wave rings and venous orifices acting as central obstacles. He also suggested that the path length was potentially variable and contrasted this with re-entry in a pathway of fixed dimensions. He proposed that the refractoriness of tissue in the centre of the circulating impulse determined the dimensions of the more peripheral pathways. Increases in the area of central refractoriness would tend to increase the outer path length. Lewis also referred to Garrey's idea that such a mechanism could exist in the absence of a central fixed orifice such as the caval orifices. The studies of Allessie and colleagues with small sheets of rabbit atrium have confirmed many of these hypotheses and led to the formulation of the 'leading circle' concept in which a vortex of excitation circulates around a small refractory area which is maintained by electrotonic influences from the surrounding excited tissue. Boineau et al. (1980) have further refined the model of atrial flutter by studying intact dogs. They have shown macrore-entry in a definable anatomical circuit containing areas of inhomogeneous refractoriness and slowed conduction. Klein et al. (1986) have studied the activation sequence of the common type of atrial flutter at surgery designed to interrupt the arrhythmia. Using the extrastimulus method at preoperative electrophysiological studies, they were able to entrain the flutter cycle. At surgery, earliest activation of the atrial mass was found close to the ostium of the coronary sinus. The left atrium did not seem to be part of the circuit and was activated 'passively'. The area of slow conduction in the circuit was found to be in right atrial tissue bounded by the mouth of the inferior vena cava, the tricuspid annulus and the coronary sinus ostium. Cryoablation (see Chapter 14), in this the narrowest area of the circuit, abolished the flutter. Cosio et al. (1986), using multiple bipolar electrode recordings, demonstrated fragmentation of electrograms, double and triple 'spikes' and continuous electrical activity during atrial flutter (see Chapter 10). The evidence for a re-entrant mechanism of atrial flutter in both clinical and experimental settings is, therefore, considerable and convincing.

Prolonged intra-atrial conduction (PA interval >50 msec) is present in most patients with atrial flutter whether spontaneous or induced at electrophysiological study. This is reflected by an increased P wave duration on the surface ECG. The atrial ERP is normal in the majority but may be prolonged. Atrial flutter can be initiated by rapid atrial stimulation (Fig. 8.9) or extrastimulation. Early premature stimuli may cause marked fractionation of electrograms (see Fig. 8.5) and repetitive atrial responses preceding stable flutter. The cycle length of flutter appears to be closely related to the atrial ERP, suggesting that refractoriness rather than conduction time is the main factor which determines the flutter rate. This is consistent with the experimental evidence.

Using right atrial extrastimulation it is possible to shorten the atrial cycle which follows that containing the extrastimulus, suggesting that the stimulated impulse enters a circuit and conducts anterogradely (in the direction of the circus movement), advancing the next flutter electrogram. Other responses indicating the presence of a circuit with an excitable gap have also been reported. Similar phenomena are seen during rapid atrial pacing.

Atrial flutter may be terminated by rapid atrial pacing in 50–100 per cent of patients. Waldo et al. (1977) studied this phenomenon in great detail, using epicardial electrodes in patients with postoperative atrial flutter. They noted that critical rates (15–25 per cent faster than the flutter rate) and durations (up to 40 seconds) of pacing were essential if it were to succeed in terminating the arrhythmia. They also observed that pacing from the high right atrium failed to terminate flutter of faster rates (340–430 b.p.m.). This type of flutter sometimes converted spontaneously to the slower type (240–340 b.p.m.). On the basis of these observations, Wells et al. (1979) classified the slower form as type I and the faster form as type II flutter. Type I seems to correspond with the classic or 'common' variety of flutter which is characterized by typical sawtooth flutter waves on the ECG, a stable cycle length and the presence of an excitable gap. Type II flutter is similarly stable but faster and not influenced by pacing.

During these studies Waldo et al. (1977) discovered the phenomenon of 'entrainment' during atrial pacing (see Chapter 7). As the rate of atrial pacing is increased, the morphology of the atrial electrograms and surface flutter waves alters, indicating progressive fusion and a change in the atrial activation pattern. The flutter rate is increased to the pacing rate without the termination of flutter. Entrainment is further evidence for the presence of a re-entrant pathway for atrial flutter.

Clinical electrophysiological studies of atrial flutter

The main indications for study are to assess the effect of drugs on the inducibility of the arrhythmia, to terminate an attack by rapid atrial pacing (Chapter 12) and to investigate any associated abnormalities (enhanced AV nodal conduction, anomalous connections, etc.). As with atrial fibrillation, there is little to be gained from these studies if the arrhythmia is established. In some patients, however, rate control using drugs may to be achieved and conversion to atrial fibrillation by rapid atrial pacing may permit drug control. There is little information about the value of drug studies in paroxysmal atrial flutter. Such studies should be considered in patients with severe symptoms uncontrolled by empirical treatment. In severely symptomatic refractory atrial flutter, electrical ablation of the His bundle may be undertaken.

Atrial tachycardias

Atrial tachycardia is defined as an abnormal rhythm arising from atrial myocardium (i.e. excluding the AV junction) somewhat slower (150–250 b.p.m. in adults) than atrial flutter, with a distinct P wave preceding each QRS complex. The morphology of the P wave is determined by the origin of the tachycardia. The mechanism of atrial tachycardia may be re-entrant or automatic. In the former type the episodes are usually paroxysmal whereas the automatic form is

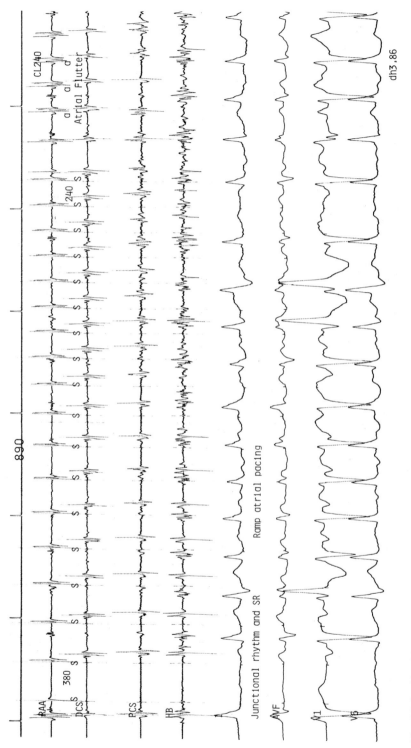

Fig. 8.9 Rapid atrial pacing initiating atrial flutter. In this example the atrial pacing (S) cycle length is gradually decreased over 5 seconds from 380 to 240 msec. After cessation of pacing, stable atrial flutter was induced. Other methods of inducing atrial flutter include atrial premature stimulation and fixed rate pacing at a cycle length near to that of the spontaneous flutter cycle length. Paper speed 100 mm/sec. DCS and PCS = distal and proximal coronary sinus; HB = His bundle region; RAA = right atrial appendage.

often persistent. The main forms of atrial re-entrant tachycardia are: (1) sinoatrial re-entrant tachycardia; and (2) intra-atrial re-entrant tachycardia.

Sinoatrial re-entrant tachycardia

Clinical observations

This type of re-entrant atrial tachycardia is relatively rare and probably is often not recognized for what it is. It is usually found in patients with heart disease although it is also seen in patients where organic disease is absent. The prevalence of the arrhythmia is not known because it is suspected that most cases are asymptomatic. A minority of patients have clinically manifest sinoatrial disease. The tachycardia is characteristically paroxysmal. The diagnosis is suggested by a sudden change in the atrial rate (usually triggered by an atrial premature beat) with either no change in the normal sinus P wave morphology or very minor changes. The rate of tachycardias is in the range of 80–140 b.p.m. The brief runs of sinus tachycardia which often immediately follow termination of paroxysmal junctional tachycardias are probably sinoatrial re-entry.

Electrophysiological observations in patients with sinoatrial re-entrant tachycardia

The tachycardia can be initiated by atrial premature stimulation after a period of atrial pacing or by atrial extrastimulation during sinus rhythm. In relation to the sinoatrial response curve the tachycardia is initiated during zone 4 or the sinoatrial re-entry zone (see Chapter 4). Often a distinct initiation 'window' can be identified. The atrial activation sequence during tachycardia is indistinguishable from that of sinus rhythm (Fig. 8.10). It is necessary to record from several intra-atrial sites to verify this. The tachycardia can also be readily terminated by atrial premature stimulation (Fig. 8.11). Occasionally, other mechanisms of re-entrant tachycardia (AV nodal re-entry, AV re-entry) coexist in the same patient and may interact with sinoatrial re-entry.

At the onset of tachycardia the PR interval is often prolonged because the AV node has not adapted to the sudden rate increase (during physiological sinus tachycardia the autonomic nervous system acts on the AV node to shorten the intranodal conduction time appropriately). The exact site of the re-entrant pathway in sinoatrial re-entrant tachycardia has not been identified. It has been assumed to be near to, or within, the sinus node because of the absence of any change in the atrial activation pattern. Abnormalities of sinoatrial function tests (sinus node recovery time and sinoatrial conduction time) are found in a minority of patients. The criteria for sinoatrial re-entry tachycardia are summarized in Table 8.1.

Clinical electrophysiological studies of sinoatrial re-entrant tachycardia

Studies of sinoatrial re-entrant tachycardia are generally not indicated unless the attacks are disabling and unresponsive to empirical drug treatment. The attacks can be suppressed by beta-blocking drugs although verapamil, amiodarone and

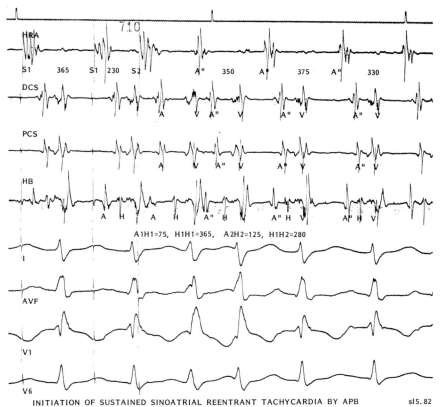

INITIATION OF SUSTAINED SINOATRIAL REENTRANT TACHYCARDIA BY APB   sI5.82

Fig. 8.10 Initiation of sustained sinoatrial re-entrant tachycardia in a 6-year-old boy. Following regular atrial pacing at a cycle length of 365 msec (S1S1) an atrial premature stimulus (S2) was introduced. This resulted in a sustained tachycardia of cycle length 330 msec. The atrial activation sequence during the tachycardia (A″) is identical to that seen during sinus rhythm (see Fig. 8.11). This child also had AV nodal re-entrant tachycardia. Paper speed 100 mm/sec. DCS = distal coronary sinus; HB = His bundle; HRA = high right atrium; PCS = proximal coronary sinus.

Table 8.1 ELECTROPHYSIOLOGICAL CHARACTERISTICS OF SINUS NODE RE-ENTRANT TACHYCARDIA

P wave morphology identical to sinus rhythm P wave

Atrial activation sequence identical to that during sinus rhythm

Tachycardia initiated by atrial premature beats:
1. within critical zone
2. independent of intra-atrial delay
3. independent of atrioventicular delay

Tachycardia termination by atrial premature stimulation or vagal manoeuvres

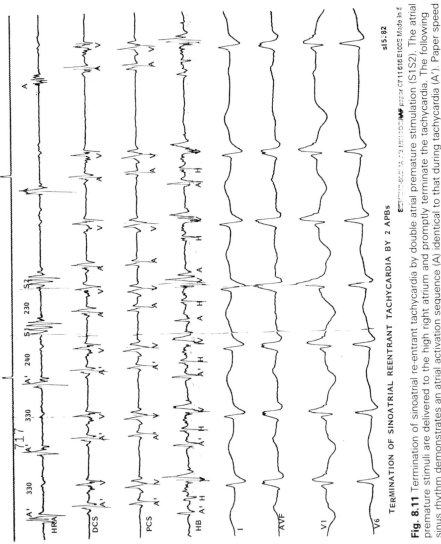

TERMINATION OF SINOATRIAL REENTRANT TACHYCARDIA BY 2 APBs

Fig. 8.11 Termination of sinoatrial re-entrant tachycardia by double atrial premature stimulation (S1S2). The atrial premature stimuli are delivered to the high right atrium and promptly terminate the tachycardia. The following sinus rhythm demonstrates an atrial activation sequence (A) identical to that during tachycardia (A'). Paper speed 100 mm/sec. DCS = distal coronary sinus; HB = His bundle; HRA = high right atrium; PCS = proximal coronary sinus.

quinidine-like agents are also effective. Beta-blocking agents are not always effective.

Intra-atrial re-entrant tachycardia

Clinical observations

Atrial re-entrant tachycardias are associated with organic heart disease in about 50 per cent of patients. A very small proportion of these patients have had previous atrial surgery (closure of atrial septal defect, cardiopulmonary bypass, etc.). The surface ECG during sinus rhythm may be normal or show evidence of abnormal atrial activation. The tachycardias may be chronic and established or occur in paroxysms. The rate of the atrial tachycardia varies from about 140 to 250 b.p.m. At the faster rates there is often variable (Wenckebach type) or fixed second degree AV conduction block, especially if the patient is receiving treatment with AV nodal blocking drugs.

Electrophysiological observations in patients with intra-atrial re-entrant tachycardia (Table 8.2)

Intra-atrial conduction time (PA interval) and the atrial ERP are prolonged in some patients but not in others. Early premature stimuli usually induce intra-atrial conduction delay and the atrial FRP is often prolonged. Associated abnormalities of sinoatrial function are uncommon. The tachycardia can be initiated by early coupled atrial premature stimuli, often within a definable 'initiation zone'. The atrial activation pattern during tachycardia shows early activation at a site remote from the sinus node. Occasionally, earliest atrial activation is in the region of the AV node and it may be difficult to distinguish between one mechanism and the other. The demonstration of second degree AV block during tachycardia favours an atrial origin but this can occur during AV

Table 8.2 ELECTROPHYSIOLOGICAL CHARACTERISTICS OF INTRA-ATRIAL RE-ENTRANT TACHYCARDIA

Abnormal atrial activation sequence *

Normal atrioventricular conduction †

Ventricular dissociation may occur

Provoked by atrial premature beats with critical range of coupling intervals, usually close to the atrial relative refractory period

Termination by atrial premature beats (which may not conduct to the ventricles)

---

* In sinoatrial re-entrant tachycardia normal atrial activation may be seen (see Table 8.1); atrial tachycardia arising from the region of the AV node may produce a normal retrograde atrial activation sequence.

† His–Purkinje block or delay may occur without affecting tachycardia; in the presence of an anterogradely conducting anomalous pathway, ventricular pre-excitation may occur.

nodal re-entrant tachycardia. Termination of the arrhythmia by a ventricular premature stimulus which fails to conduct to the atria excludes atrial re-entry. Atrial re-entrant tachycardia is usually capable of termination by an atrial premature stimulus. Occasionally, it is possible to locate the area of re-entry to a site known to have been incised or damaged at surgery but direct demonstration of a re-entrant pathway by clinical endocardial studies is usually not possible.

Clinical electrophysiological studies of intra-atrial re-entrant tachycardia

Intracardiac studies are not generally required unless the diagnosis is not clear or drug studies are indicated in a patient who has not responded to empirical treatment. There is very little information about the value of drug studies in this setting, but in patients with refractory arrhythmias this approach is worth considering. In patients with disabling symptoms (e.g. caused by associated poor left ventricular function) direct electrical ablation of the atrial focus or His bundle ablation should be considered (see Chapter 15).

Atrial tachycardia due to abnormal automaticity

Clinical observations

In adults, this type of atrial tachycardia is almost always associated with cardiac disease or chronic pulmonary disease. Precipitating factors include myocardial ischaemia, digoxin toxicity and metabolic disturbances. In children the arrhythmia may occur without associated heart disease. The P wave morphology is determined by the site of origin of the tachycardia. Changing P wave morphology from beat to beat has been taken to imply a 'multifocal' origin. It is by no means certain, however, that a multiple re-entry phenomenon could not also account for this observation. The tachycardia may be paroxysmal and repetitive or incessant. It is thought that incessant or frequently repetitive tachycardia may itself cause ventricular dilatation and cardiomyopathy. The mechanism of tachycardia is probably abnormal automaticity.

Electrophysiological observations in patients with automatic atrial tachycardia

These tachycardias have been distinguished from re-entrant atrial tachycardias primarily on the basis that they cannot be initiated or terminated by atrial premature stimulation. Rapid pacing for a short period sometimes suppresses the tachycardia which returns after a latent period that may be directly proportional to the rate or duration of overdrive pacing (Fig. 8.12). The tachycardia can very occasionally be triggered by rapid atrial pacing, an observation which has led to the suggestion that some of these tachycardias may be due to 'triggered automaticity'. Spontaneous onset of tachycardia often shows a gradual increase in rate, referred to as the 'warming up' phenomenon. Although thought to be a feature of abnormal automaticity, it is also seen in re-entrant supraventricular tachycardias. Another feature, said to be characteristic of this type of tachycardia, is the observation that the initiating atrial beat has a P wave morphology (and

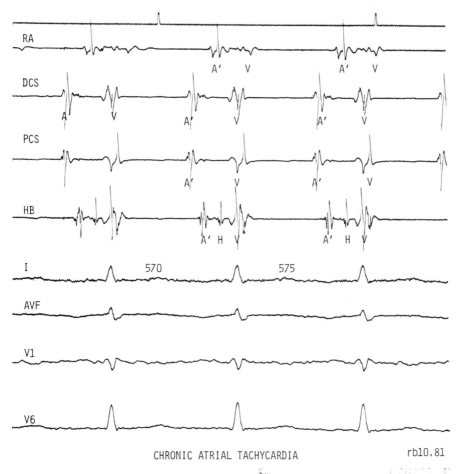

CHRONIC ATRIAL TACHYCARDIA   rb10.81

Fig. 8.12 Chronic atrial tachycardia in a 15-year-old boy complaining of shortness of breath on exertion. The recordings show that atrial activation (A′) begins in the left atrium. The atrial electrograms in the coronary sinus recordings precede the right atrial signal in the low right atrium (His recording) by 65 msec. The arrhythmia could not be terminated by short bursts (less than 10 seconds) of rapid atrial pacing but prolonged periods of rapid pacing (more than 20 seconds) suppressed the tachycardia for a period directly proportional to the rate and duration of pacing. Paper speed 100 mm/sec. DCS = distal coronary sinus; HB = His bundle region; PCS = proximal coronary sinus; RA = right atrium.

atrial endocardial activation pattern) identical to that seen during sustained tachycardia. Clearly, this is not a useful distinguishing feature because many re-entrant junctional tachycardia (especially the long RP′ type – see Chapter 9) begin with an atrial echo beat caused by re-entrant excitation of the circuit which sustains the tachycardia. The atrial ERP is normal, and early premature atrial stimulation does not tend to induce marked intra-atrial delay and repetitive beats as in atrial fibrillation, flutter and re-entrant tachycardia.

Clinical electrophysiological studies of these arrhythmias are not indicated unless a therapeutic procedure (such as atrial or His bundle ablation or continuous overdrive suppression) is being considered.

References and further reading

Allessie MA, Bonke FIM, Schopman FJG. (1977) Circus movement in rabbit atrial muscle as a mechanism of tachycardia. III. The 'leading circle' concept: a new model of circus movement in cardiac tissue without the involvement of an anatomical obstacle. *Circulation Research* **41**, 9

Anderson RH, Becker A. (1978) Anatomy of the conduction tissues revisited. *British Heart Journal* **40** (suppl.), 2

Anderson RH, Becker AE, Tranum-Jensen J, Janse MJ. (1981) Anatomico-electrophysiological correlations in the conduction system: a review. *British Heart Journal* **45**, 67

Anderson RH, Becker A. (1985) Pathways of preferential conduction. *British Heart Journal* **53**, 350

Attuel P, Childers R, Cauchemez B, Poveda J, Mugica J, Coumel P. (1982) Failure in the rate adaptation of the atrial refractory period: its relationship to vulnerability. *International Journal of Cardiology* **2**, 179

Bauernfeind RA, Wyndham CR, Swiryn SP, Palileo E, Strasberg B, Lamb W, Westveer D, Rosen KM. (1981) Paroxysmal atrial fibrillation in the Wolff–Parkinson–White syndrome. *American Journal of Cardiology* **47**, 562

Bauernfeind RA, Swiryn SP, Strasberg B, Palileo E, Scagliotti D, Rosen KM. (1982) Electrophysiologic drug testing in prophylaxis of sporadic paroxysmal atrial fibrillation: technique, application, and efficacy in severely symptomatic preexcitation patients. *American Heart Journal* **103**, 941

Bennett MA, Pentecost BL. (1970) The pattern of onset and spontaneous cessation of atrial fibrillation in man. *Circulation* **41**, 981

Boineau JP, Schuessler RB, Mooney CR, Miller CB, Wylds AC, Hudson RD, Borremans JM, Brockus CW. (1980) Natural and evoked atrial flutter due to circus movement in dogs. Role of abnormal atrial pathways, slow conduction, nonuniform refractory period distribution and premature beats. *American Journal of Cardiology* **45**, 1167

Boineau JP. (1985) Atrial flutter: a synthesis of concepts. *Circulation* **72**, 249

Camm AJ, Ward DE, Spurrell RAJ. (1980) Response of atrial flutter to overdrive atrial pacing and intravenous disopyramide phosphate, singly and in combination. *British Heart Journal* **44**, 240

Childers RW, Arnsdorf MF, De la Fuente DJ, Gambetta M, Svenson R. (1973) Sinus node echoes. Clinical case report and canine studies. *American Journal of Cardiology* **31**, 220

Chung EK. (1971) A reappraisal of atrial dissociation. *American Journal of Cardiology* **28**, 111

Cosio FG, Palacios J, Vidal JM, Cocina EG, Gomez-Sanchez MA, Tamargo L. (1983) Electrophysiologic studies in atrial fibrillation. Slow conduction of premature impulses: a possible manifestation of the background for reentry. *American Journal of Cardiology* **51**, 123

Cosio FG, Arribas F, Palacios J, Tason J, Lopez-Gil M. (1986) Fragmented electrograms and continuous electrical activity in atrial flutter. *American Journal of Cardiology* **57**, 1309

Coumel P, Flammang D, Attuel P, Leclercq JF. (1979a) Sustained intraatrial reentrant tachycardia; electrophysiologic study of 20 cases. *Clinical Cardiology* **2**, 167

Coumel P, Leclercq JF, Attuel P, Lavalle JP, Flammang D. (1979b) Autonomic influences in the genesis of atrial arrhythmias: atrial flutter and fibrillation of vagal origin. In: *Cardiac Arrhythmias: Electrophysiology, Diagnosis and Management*, p. 243. Ed. by OS Narula. Williams & Wilkins: Baltimore, Md

Coumel P, Attuel P, Friocourt P, Couty F, Mugica J. (1984) Arrhythmogenic effect of vagal drive on the atrium. *Pacing and Clinical Electrophysiology* 7, 1380

Curry PVL, Evans TR, Krikler DM. (1977) Paroxysmal reciprocating sinus tachycardia. *European Journal of Cardiology* 6, 199

Disertori M, Inama G, Vergara G, Guarnerio M, del Favero A, Furlanello F. (1983) Evidence of a reentry circuit in the common type of atrial flutter in man. *Circulation* 67, 434

Gillette PC, Garson A. (1977) Electrophysiologic and pharmacologic characteristics of automatic atrial ectopic tachycardia. *Circulation* 56, 571

Goldreyer BN, Gallagher JJ, Damato AN. (1973) The electrophysiologic demonstration of atrial ectopic tachycardia in man. *American Heart Journal* 85, 205

Gomes JA, Hariman RJ, Kang PS, Chowdry IH. (1985) Sustained symptomatic sinoatrial reentrant tachycardia: incidence, clinical significance, electrophysiologic observations and the effects of antiarrhythmic agents. *Journal of the American College of Cardiology* 5, 45

Gouaux JL, Ashman R. (1947) Auricular fibrillation with aberration simulating ventricular paroxysmal tachycardia. *American Heart Journal* 34, 366

Inoue H, Matsuo H, Takayanagi K, Murao S. (1981) Clinical and experimental studies of the effects of atrial extrastimulation and rapid pacing on atrial flutter cycle. *American Journal of Cardiology* 48, 623

James TN. (1963) The connecting pathways between the sinus node and the AV node and between the right and the left atrium in the human heart. *American Heart Journal* 66, 498

James TN. (1984) Sir Thomas Lewis redivivus: from pebbles in a quiet pond to autonomic storms. *British Heart Journal* 52, 1

Kerr CR, Chung DC. (1985) Atrial fibrillation: fact, controversy and future. *Clinical Progress in Electrophysiology and Pacing* 3, 319

Klein GJ, Guiraudon GM, Sharma AD, Milstein S. (1986) Demonstration of macroreentry and feasibility of operative therapy in the common type of atrial flutter. *American Journal of Cardiology* 57, 587

Leier CV, Meacham JA, Schaal SF. (1978) Prolonged atrial conduction. A major predisposing factor for the development of atrial flutter. *Circulation* 57, 213

Lewis T. (1925) Theory of circus movement and its application to atrial flutter. In: *The Mechanism and Graphic Registration of the Heart Beat*, p. 319. Shaw: London

Luck JC, Engel TR. (1979) Dispersion of atrial refractoriness in patients with sinus node dysfunction. *Circulation* 60, 404

Meijler F. (1986) The pulse in atrial fibrillation. *British Heart Journal* 56, 1

Moe GK. (1962) On the multiple wavelet theory of atrial fibrillation. *Archives Internationale de Pharmacodynamie et de Therapie* 140, 183

Narula OS. (1974) Sinus node reentry. A mechanism for supraventricular tachycardia. *Circulation* 50, 1114

Pastelin G, Mendez R, Moe GK. (1978) Participation of atrial specialized conduction pathways in atrial flutter. *Circulation Research* 42, 386

Prystowsky EN, Naccarelli GV, Jackman WM, Rinkenberger RL, Heger JJ, Zipes DP. (1983) Enhanced parasympathetic tone shortens atrial refractoriness in man. *American Journal of Cardiology* 51, 96

Peuch P. (1956) *L'Activite Electrique Auriculaire Normale et Pathologique*, p. 214. Masson: Paris

Rawles JM, Rowland E. (1986) Is the pulse in atrial fibrillation irregularly irregular? *British Heart Journal* 56, 4

Roark SF, McCarthy EA, Lee KL, Pritchett ELC. (1986) Observations on the occurrence of atrial fibrillation in paroxysmal supraventricular tachycardia. *American Journal of Cardiology* **57**, 571

Rosenblueth A, Garcia-Ramos J. (1947) Studies of flutter and fibrillation. II. Influence of artificial obstacles on experimental auricular flutter. *American Heart Journal* **33**, 677

Rytand DA. (1966) The circus movement (entrapped circuit wave) hypothesis and atrial flutter. *Annals of Internal Medicine* **65**, 125

Scheinman MM, Basu D, Hollenberg M. (1974) Electrophysiologic studies in patients with persistent atrial tachycardia. *Circulation* **50**, 266

Sharma AD, Klein GJ, Guiraudon GM, Milstein S. (1985) Atrial fibrillation in patients with Wolff–Parkinson–White syndrome: incidence after surgical ablation of the accessory pathway. *Circulation* **72**, 161

Simpson R, Foster JR, Mulrow JP, Gettes LS. (1983) The electrophysiological substrate of atrial fibrillation. *Pacing and Clinical Electrophysiology* **6**, 1166

Sung RJ, Castellanos A, Malon SM, Bloom MG, Gelband H, Myerberg RJ. (1977) Mechanisms of spontaneous alternation between reciprocating tachycardia and atrial flutter-fibrillation in the Wolff–Parkinson–White syndrome. *Circulation* **56**, 409

Tenczer J, Littmann L, Molnar F, Kekes E. (1980) Atrial reentry in chronic repetitive supraventricular tachycardia. *American Heart Journal* **99**, 349

Waldo AL, MacLean WAH, Karp RB, Kouchoukos NT, James TN. (1977) Entrainment and interruption of atrial flutter with atrial pacing. Studies in man following open heart surgery. *Circulation* **56**, 737

Waldo AL. (1983) Some observations concerning atrial flutter in man. *Pacing and Clinical Electrophysiology* **6**, 1181

Waldo AL. (1984) Atrial flutter. Recent observations in man. In: *Tachycardias: Mechanisms, Diagnosis, Treatment*, p. 113. Ed. by ME Josephson, HJJ Wellens. Lea & Febiger: Philadelphia, Pa

Waldo AL, Plumb VJ, Henthorn RW. (1984) Observations on the mechanism of atrial flutter. In: *Tachycardias*, p. 213. Ed. by B Surawicz, CP Reddy, EN Prystowsky, Martinus Nijhoff: Boston, Mass

Watson RM, Josephson ME. (1980) Atrial flutter. I. Electrophysiologic substrates and modes of initiation and termination. *American Journal of Cardiology* **45**, 732

Weisfogel GM, Batsford WP, Paulay KL, Josephson ME, Ogunkelu JB, Akhtar M, Seides SF, Damato AN. (1975) Sinus node reentrant tachycardia in man. *American Heart Journal* **90**, 295

Wellens HJJ, Janse MJ, van Dam RT, Durrer D. (1971) Epicardial excitation of the atria in a patient with atrial flutter. *British Heart Journal* **33**, 233

Wells HL, MacLean WAH, Hames TN, Waldo AL. (1979) Characteristics of atrial flutter; studies in patients after open heart surgery using fixed electrodes. *Circulation* **60**, 665

Wu D, Amat-y-Leon F, Denes P, Dhingra R, Pietras RJ, Rosen KM. (1975) Demonstration of sustained sinus and atrial re-entry as a mechanism of paroxysmal supraventricular tachycardia. *Circulation* **51**, 234

Wyndham CRC, Amat-y-Leon F, Wu D, Denes P, Dhingra R, Simpson P, Rosen KM. (1977) Effects of cycle length on atrial vulnerability. *Circulation* **55**, 260

Wyndham CR. (1982) What's wrong with the atrium in patients with atrial fibrillation? *International Journal of Cardiology* **2**, 199

Zipes DP, DeJoseph RL. (1973) Dissimilar atrial rhythms in man and dog. *American Journal of Cardiology* **32**, 618

9

Junctional Tachycardias

There is no standard definition of the term 'junctional' tachycardia. For the purpose of this chapter we have adopted the following definition:

> A junctional tachycardia is any tachycardia which arises in the atrioventricular junctional tissue or is in any way dependent on such tissue for its continuation. The term 'atrioventricular junctional conduction tissue' includes the normal AV node and the upper part of the penetrating His bundle, direct atrioventricular and ventriculoatrial anomalous pathways and accessory pathways with AV nodal-like decremental properties.

This definition, therefore, incorporates the following types of tachycardia:

1. Intra-AV nodal re-entrant tachycardias.
2. AV re-entrant tachycardias involving direct AV anomalous pathways of the typical variety.
3. AV re-entrant tachycardias involving an accessory structure with AV nodal-like properties in the retrograde limb.
4. Tachycardias associated with nodoventricular pathways.
5. Focal His bundle tachycardias.

Junctional tachycardias are especially amenable to study by intracardiac recording and stimulation methods because the AV junction is readily identifiable, both anatomically and physiologically. The His potential signifies activation of the immediately adjacent AV node and acts as an important marker.

Clinical observations in patients with junctional tachycardias

Whereas arrhythmias such as atrial fibrillation, flutter and tachycardia are generally associated with heart disease and are therefore prevalent in the elderly, tachycardias associated with functional or anatomical anomalies of the atrioventricular junction are usually seen in otherwise healthy people without organic heart disease and may occur at all ages. Once the junctional tachycardia has 'declared' itself, episodes tend to recurr throughout life even following treatment. Most patients are not severely disabled by the attacks and find them a nuisance rather than a catastrophic incursion. A cumulative nuisance can, however, amount to a serious interference with daily life.

Table 9.1 ELECTROPHYSIOLOGICAL CHARACTERISTICS OF INTRA-AV NODAL RE-ENTRANT TACHYCARDIA

Normal retrograde atrial activation *

Normal His–ventricular conduction †

Prolonged A'H interval ●

Atrial or ventricular dissociation may occur

Possibly provoked by atrial premature beats which induce critical AH delay §

Possibly provoked by ventricular premature beats

Possibly terminated by atrial or ventricular premature beats

---

* Usually the atrial activation sequence during tachycardia is identical to that in response to ventricular pacing, but there may be slight differences due to selective exit from the AV node.

† His–Purkinje blocks or delays may occur – they do not affect the tachycardia cycle length; associated bystander anomalous pathways may produce pre-excited ventricular complexes.

● In the usual form of AV node re-entrant tachycardia the A'H interval is longer than that seen in response to atrial pacing, but in the unusual (long RP') variety the AH'interval is shorter than that produced by atrial pacing at the tachycardia rate (note atrial pacing at the tachycardia rate may initiate tachycardia).

§ Functional longitudinal AH dissociation may be demonstrated in about 50 per cent.

Electrophysiological observations in patients with junctional tachycardias

Atrioventricular nodal re-entrant tachycardias (Table 9.1)

The functional basis for atrioventricular nodal re-entrant tachycardias (AVNRT) is re-entrant excitation of dual AV nodal pathways (see Chapter 3). The anatomical basis for these pathways is not known. It has long been debated whether atrial myocardium is a necessary part of the re-entrant circuit or whether this circuit is entirely confined to the AV node itself. In the only reported case in which autopsy studies were undertaken (Scheinman et al., 1982) there appeared to be no connections between the atrial myocardium and the AV node itself, supporting the notion of 'intranodal' rather than 'atrionodal' re-entry.

The precise nature of the dual AV nodal pathways is unknown. The weight of evidence from experimental and clinical electrophysiological studies has suggested that the circuit is located entirely within the AV node and that access to, or egress from, the circuit takes place over 'initial' and 'final' common pathways (Mignone and Wallace, 1966). For example, it is possible to dissociate the atria from the tachycardia cycle by pacing at a rate slightly faster than tachycardia (Josephson and Kastor, 1976). Studies of entrainment of AV nodal tachycardia (see Chapter 7) show a similar phenomenon (Portillo et al., 1984).

These findings appear to indicate that the atria are not involved in the tachycardia circuit. However, it is also possible to dissociate the low right atrium during atrioventricular tachycardia (see below), which undoubtedly has an atrial link in the circuit. Some reports do suggest that only part of the AV node is involved in the re-entry process (Hariman et al., 1983, DiMarco et al., 1984). It may well be that existing techniques are not sufficiently refined to detect atrial involvement close the AV node during AV nodal re-entrant tachycardia. The debate regarding atrial involvement (Scheinman, 1985) has been reopened with the findings of Ross et al. (1985), who distinguished two types of AV 'junctional' re-entry at surgery (see Chapter 14) in patients with apparent AV nodal re-entrant tachycardia associated with dual pathways. In one form, type A, the earliest atrial activation during tachycardia was anterior and medial to the AV node with a short retrograde 'conduction' time (HA interval <40 msec). In type B tachycardias, the earliest atrial activation was posterior to the node and the HA intervals exceeded 40 msec. These findings are consistent with those of Sung et al. (1981) in a series of patients with dual anterograde and retrograde AV nodal pathways. Using intracardiac methods, these authors noted a change in the retrograde activation sequence consequent upon the transition from retrograde fast to slow pathway conduction. During retrograde fast pathway conduction, earliest atrial activation was observed in the low right atrium, whereas it occurred in the proximal coronary sinus region when the slow pathway was used. It does seem, therefore, that retrograde slow pathway conduction may have several anatomical substrates. Ross et al. (1985) have reported that surgical dissection of the posterior perinodal area in type B patients abolished or impaired retrograde conduction without damaging anterograde fast pathway conduction but slow pathway conduction was abolished. In type A patients the dissection was directed to the central fibrous body, anteromedially to the node. Similarly, in these patients anterograde slow pathway conduction was abolished but retrograde conduction remained intact, albeit with a longer HA interval. The authors concluded that these observations implied the involvement of the perinodal atrium in the tachycardia circuit. However, the exact mechanism of the effect of the surgical procedure is not clear.

The tachycardias are initiated by atrial premature stimulation (or rapid atrial pacing to the point of second degree block) often (but not always) in association with a sudden increase in the AH interval (Fig. 9.1). The increase in the AH interval is a result of block in the faster pathway and slowed conduction in another pathway with a shorter ERP. Thus, two conditions for re-entry have been met. If re-entry is sustained by retrograde excitation of the faster pathway, tachycardia results. The tachycardia circuit therefore comprises an anterograde slow pathway and a retrograde faster pathway. In about one-third of these patients, the tachycardia may also be initiated by ventricular extrastimulation (Wu et al., 1984). Retrograde refractoriness of the His–Purkinje system appears to be an important limiting factor with respect to initiation by ventricular pacing.

During tachycardia the AH interval measured on the His bundle recording tends to be long and the HA interval is short (Fig.9.1). However, these intervals do not represent linear 'conduction' times but rather relative activation times, because the tachycardia impulse conducts towards the His bundle at the same time as the retrograde fast pathway is being activated. Thus, neither the AH

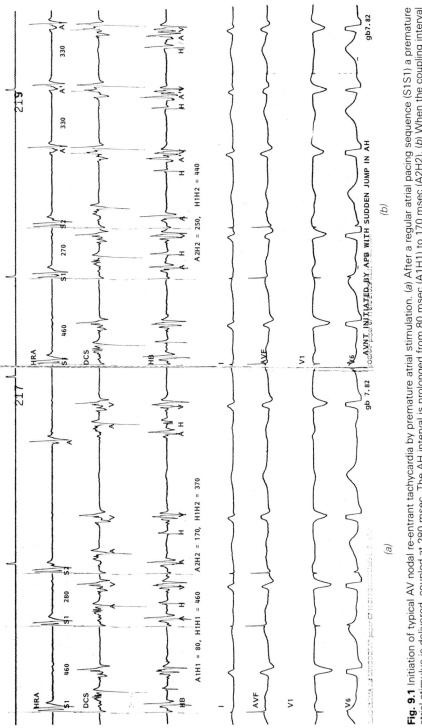

Fig. 9.1 Initiation of typical AV nodal re-entrant tachycardia by premature atrial stimulation. (*a*) After a regular atrial pacing sequence (S1S1) a premature atrial stimulus is delivered, coupled at 280 msec. The AH interval is prolonged from 80 msec (A1H1) to 170 msec (A2H2). (*b*) When the coupling interval S1S2 is reduced by 20 msec the premature beat conducts with a sudden increase in the A2H2 interval (250 msec) and an atrial echo beat is followed by sustained tachycardia. Paper speed 100 mm/sec. DCS = distal coronary sinus; HB = His bundle region; HRA = high right atrium.

interval nor the HA interval during the typical form of AV nodal re-entrant tachycardia truly reflects anterograde slow pathway or, respectively, retrograde fast pathway conduction times. Nevertheless, in patients with AV nodal re-entrant tachycardia there appears to be a direct relationship between the minimum anterograde slow pathway conduction time (defined during atrial extrastimulus testing) and tachycardia cycle length (Bauernfiend et al., 1980b).

The cardiac activation sequence of AV nodal re-entrant tachycardia is shown in Fig. 9.1. The origin of the tachycardia is essentially from a 'point' source, and, because the anterograde conduction time is relatively slow (slow pathway) and the retrograde conduction time is relatively fast (fast pathway), the atria are depolarized at the same time as the ventricles. Thus the interval between the His potential and the atrial electrogram on the His recording (HA) is short. Occasionally, the atrial electrogram is inscribed before the ventricular electrogram (Fig. 9.1) or the QRS complex (thus excluding atrioventricular re-entry). On the surface ECG the P wave is partially or completely hidden by the QRS complex, a reliable sign of the 'usual' form of AV nodal re-entrant tachycardia. The relationship of the P wave to the QRS complex does not convey any information about the exact anatomical location of the tachycardia circuit (i.e. low, mid or upper node) because conduction times from the site of origin to the atria and ventricles are unknown.

Atrioventricular nodal re-entrant tachycardia may also occur in patients with the short PR interval, normal QRS complex syndrome (Lown–Ganong–Levine (LGL) syndrome; see Chapter 6). An example is shown in Fig. 9.2. The 'AV nodal' re-entrant tachycardias which occur in this condition tend to be faster than those associated with dual AV nodal pathways in the absence of a short PR interval (Benditt et al., 1978; Ward and Camm, 1983). At first it would appear that this finding is paradoxical, because the anterograde fast pathway (i.e. the substrate for the short PR interval during sinus rhythm) becomes the retrograde limb during tachycardia and the slow pathway becomes the anterograde limb. Retrograde conduction characteristics in the LGL syndrome do not appear significantly different from normal. There is evidence, however, that slow pathway (as well as fast pathway) conduction is enhanced in the LGL syndrome (Ward et al., 1983). These factors might account for faster tachycardias in the LGL syndrome. (It should be emphasized, however, that the AH interval and the HA interval during tachycardia cannot be taken as precise indications of the anterograde and retrograde conduction times, respectively, in AV nodal or AV re-entrant tachycardias for the reasons described above).

The main electrophysiological features of the typical form of AV nodal re-entry can be summarized as follows:

1. Demonstration of dual AH pathways in approximately two-thirds of patients.
2. Initiation of tachycardia by premature atrial stimuli after a sudden increase in the AH interval in the majority.
3. A normal retrograde atrial activation pattern during tachycardia.
4. Activation of the atria simultaneous with the QRS, with a short HA interval.
5. Activation of the atria before the His bundle (an AHV sequence on the His recording) in a proportion of patients.
6. Continuation of tachycardia during second degree AV or VA block, a rare phenomenon (this is impossible with atrioventricular re-entry, see over).

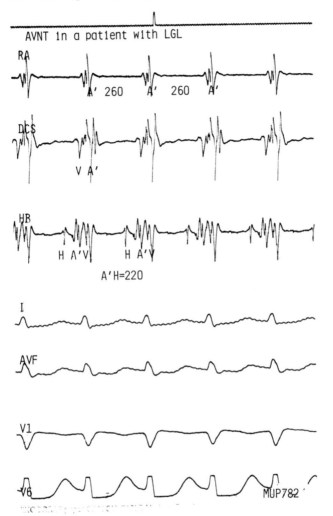

Fig. 9.2 AV nodal re-entrant tachycardia in a patient with the so-called Lown–Ganong–Levine syndrome. The patient had enhanced AV nodal conduction and dual AH pathways. The atrial activation sequence (A′) begins in the low right atrium on the His (HB) recording. The tachycardia is rapid, and intravenous verapamil failed to terminate the arrhythmia. Paper speed 100 mm/sec. DCS = distal coronary sinus; RA = right atrium.

In another form of AV nodal re-entry the P wave is clearly visible before the QRS complex, as shown in Fig. 9.3. In these patients it is supposed that the usual functional circuit is reversed, with anterograde conduction over the faster pathways and retrograde conduction over the slower pathway, resulting in delayed atrial activation relative to the QRS complex. This type of tachycardia may be initiated by premature atrial stimuli which block in the slow pathway, but conduct to the His bundle via the fast pathway (whose ERP is shorter than

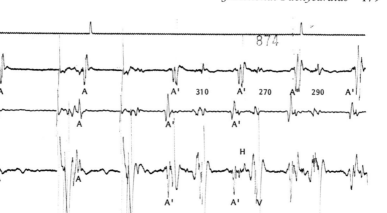

INITIATION OF AVNT (FAST-SLOW) BY RETROGRADE SLOW PATHWAY CONDUCTION

KB1.82

Fig. 9.3 Recordings showing initiation of the atypical form of AV nodal re-entry in a 6-year-old girl. A ventricular premature stimulus (V2) is introduced 300 msec after a regular paced sequence (S1S1) at a cycle length of 400 msec. This resulted in a sudden increase in the VA interval with no change in the atrial activation pattern. This was followed by sustained tachycardia. The RP interval is 200 msec. (RP/RR 0.68) and the P wave clearly precedes the QRS. There was no evidence of an atypical (slowly conducting) anomalous pathway in this patient. Paper speed 100 mm/sec. HB = His bundle region; HRA = high right atrium; PA = pulmonary artery; RVA = right ventricular apex.

the slow pathway) and return via the slow pathway. They may also be initiated by ventricular extrastimulation, with block in the retrograde fast pathway but with conduction to the atria over the slow pathway, thus initiating the sequence of fast anterograde conduction followed by slow retrograde conduction (Fig. 9.3). For this reason they are sometimes referred to as 'fast–slow' AV nodal re-entrant tachycardias. They are also known as the 'unusual' or 'atypical' form. The clinical presentation, surface ECG appearances and electrophysiological findings of this mechanism may closely resemble those of tachycardias caused by anomalous pathways with long conduction times (see later in this chapter).

Retrograde conduction times have revealed dual retrograde pathways in some patients. It has been thought that this represents dual intranodal pathways analogous to those demonstrated by atrial extrastimulus testing. That this is probably true in some instances is suggested by the observation that anterograde dual AV nodal pathways and retrograde dual pathways can be shown in the same patient. However, it is now clear that an almost identical pattern can be revealed in those patients with tachycardias associated with the presence of a paraseptal anomalous direct ventriculoatrial connection with AV nodal-like properties and slow retrograde conduction. This is discussed below.

Tachycardias caused by these mechanisms tend to be frequently repetitive or incessant and were originally described by Coumel et al. (1967) as 'permanent'. Although they may be initiated by premature stimulation, onset of tachycardia is often the result of slight increases in heart rate, presumably sufficient to cause block in the slow pathway. Sometimes no antecedent events are discernible, especially in those patients with the accessory AV nodal-like pathway. Interestingly, these pathways are not known to conduct anterogradely. The combination of permanent anterograde block and slow retrograde conduction in the abnormal pathway may be sufficient to generate incessant or repetitive tachycardias.

The main electrophysiological features of the unusual type of AV nodal tachycardia are:

1. Dual retrograde pathways.
2. Initiation by minor increases in atrial pacing rate without marked anterograde AH delay (cf. the usual type).
3. Initiation by a sudden increase in the retrograde conduction time (dual VA pathways).
4. A normal retrograde atrial activation sequence.
5. Atrial activation well after the QRS complex with a long HA interval (corresponding to a long RP' interval on the ECG).

It should be appreciated that these features are also observed in the long RP' tachycardias associated with an anomalous pathway with AV nodal properties (see below). In this setting, however, features of paraseptal anomalous retrograde conduction may also be demonstrated (see later in this chapter).

Both varieties of AV nodal re-entrant tachycardia can be terminated by atrial or ventricular premature stimulation. The latter is more likely to be successful. Termination by a ventricular premature stimulus that fails to reach the atrium excludes an atrial origin of the tachycardia (Fig. 9.4). Termination of the unusual type is often followed by immediate spontaneous reinitiation.

Atrioventricular re-entrant tachycardias (Table 9.2)

These tachycardias are the most common type in patients with the Wolff–Parkinson–White (WPW) syndrome (see Chapter 6). The anatomical basis for the syndrome is an anomalous pathway directly connecting atrial to ventricular myocardium (see Chapter 6). These pathways may be capable of conducting in

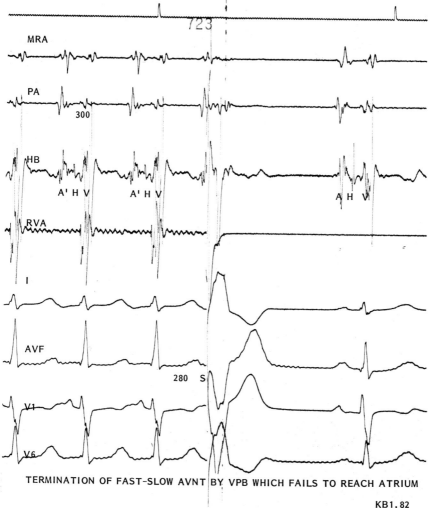

TERMINATION OF FAST–SLOW AVNT BY VPB WHICH FAILS TO REACH ATRIUM

KB1.82

Fig. 9.4 Termination of AV nodal tachycardia (unusual type) by ventricular stimulation in a 6-year-old child with paroxysmal palpitations. The ventricular extrastimulus (S) coupled at 280 msec (20 msec before the next expected His potential) to the preceding QRS terminates the tachycardia without conducting to the atria, thereby excluding an atrial tachycardia. There was no evidence of a retrogradely operating slowly conducting anomalous pathway (another possible substrate for this type of long RP' tachycardia) in this patient. Paper speed 100 mm/sec. HB = His bundle region; MRA = mid-right atrium; PA = pulmonary artery; RV = right ventricle.

anterograde, retrograde or both directions. The directional conduction properties of these pathways to some extent determine the types of tachycardias they can support. There are several different mechanisms of atrioventricular re-entrant tachycardia (AVRT), of which orthodromic tachycardia is by far the most common. In this form, anterograde AV conduction is over the normal pathway and the retrograde limb is the anomalous pathway. The QRS complexes are therefore normal or may show bundle branch aberration (see below). It is evident that for these tachycardias to occur there must be intact anomalous conduction from the ventricles to the atria. Thus, if during ventricular pacing there is retrograde block atrioventricular re-entry can virtually be excluded (beware of accidental trauma to the pathway by catheter manipulation; see Chapter 2). If tachycardia is inducible despite retrograde VA block, it is either atrial or AV nodal in origin.

Table 9.2 ELECTROPHYSIOLOGICAL CHARACTERISTICS OF ORTHODROMIC RE-ENTRANT ATRIOVENTRICULAR TACHYCARDIA

Atrial activation abnormal *

Normal atrioventricular conduction †

Neither total atrial nor ventricular dissociation possible ●

Atrial reset follows ventricular reset §

Possibly provoked by atrial premature beats:

1. critical AV delay
2. specific range of coupling intervals

Possibly provoked by ventricular premature beats which conduct to the atria over the accessory pathway

Possibly terminated by atrial or ventricular premature beats

HV prolongation or ipsilateral bundle branch block prolongs HA′ time

---

* Atrial activation may be similar to normal retrograde activation if anomalous pathway is close to the AV node.

† His–Purkinje blocks or delays may occur; the A′H time is similar to that seen in response to atrial pacing at a similar rate.

● Both atria and ventricles are essential components of the re-entrant circuit; intra-atrial block may produce apparent atrial dissociation.

§ 'Exact atrial capture' is a variety of this phenomenon.

Fig. 9.5 Initiation of AVRT by atrial extrastimulation. (*a*) Recordings from a patient with a left free wall anomalous pathway. During regular right atrial pacing (S1S1) at a cycle length of 600 msec there is ventricular pre-excitation. An atrial premature stimulus coupled at 290 msec blocks in the anomalous pathway and conducts via the AV node with a normal QRS complex and HV interval. This normally conducted beat returns to the atria over the anomalous pathway as evidenced by the early atrial activation in the distal coronary sinus (DCS) recording. Stable tachycardia ensues at a cycle length of 310 msec. (*b*) Recordings from a middle-aged patient with chronic coronary artery disease and a posteroseptal anomalous pathway. During atrial pacing at a cycle length of 460 msec, the QRS complexes are widened to 170 msec. Tachycardia is initiated by an extrastimulus which blocks in the anomalous pathway, revealing underlying left bundle branch block and a markedly prolonged HV interval of 100 msec. These abnormalities persisted during tachycardia and reflected intraventricular conduction system disease. Earliest atrial activation during tachycardia is in the region of the ostium of the coronary sinus. Ablation of the right bundle branch using 100 joules (see Chapter 15) abolished re-entrant tachycardia. Paper speed 100 mm/sec. DCS and PCS = distal and proximal coronary sinus; HB = His bundle region; RA = right atrium.

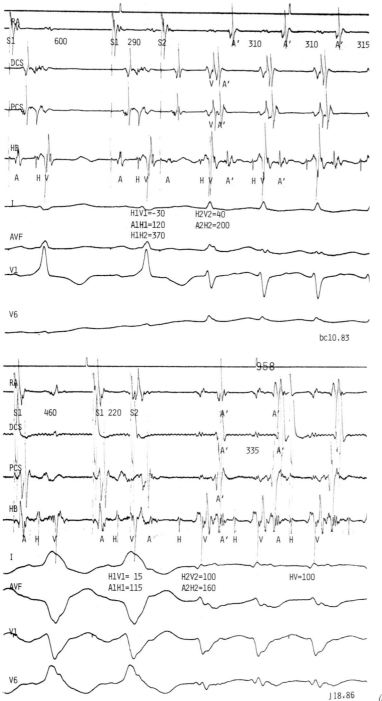

The mode of initiation of these tachycardias is analogous to that of AV nodal tachycardias. An atrial premature stimulus (or spontaneous beat) blocks in the anomalous pathway but conducts slowly through the AV node to the His bundle and ventricles. Slowed anterograde conduction allows retrograde re-entry over the anomalous pathway, causing an atrial echo beat (Fig. 9.5). Sustained tachycardia occurs if the AV node has recovered to allow anterograde conduction and re-entry into the anomalous pathway. The site of atrial stimulation may be critical in the initiation of tachycardia. The echo zone (see Chapter 6) is 'smaller' with a remote stimulation site but wider with a site close to the anomalous pathway.

Ventricular extrastimulation can initiate tachycardia by retrograde block in the normal pathway with VA conduction over the anomalous pathway and anterograde re-entry (Fig. 9.6). Induction of tachycardia by the extrastimulus

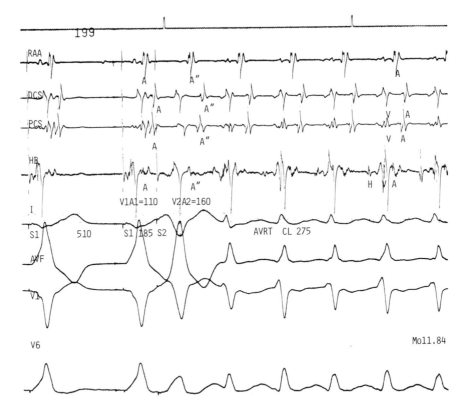

Fig. 9.6 Initiation of AVRT in a patient with a right free wall anomalous pathway. During regular ventricular pacing (S1S1) at a cycle length of 510 msec there is retrograde conduction to the atria over the AV node (in the low right atrium V1V1 = 110 msec). A ventricular premature stimulus S2 conducts to the atria over the right free wall anomalous pathway with a longer VA interval of 160 msec, early low right atrial activation and a change in the atrial activation sequence (A'') with the distal coronary sinus (DCS) atrial electrogram now much later than the right atrial appendage (RAA) electrogram. Thereafter, tachycardia ensues with an unchanged atrial pattern. The retrograde limb of tachycardia is the right-sided anomalous pathway. Paper speed 100 mm/sec. AA = atrial cycle length; CS = coronary sinus.

method is determined by several factors, including the basic drive rate, the site of stimulation, and the relative conduction times and refractory periods of the normal and anomalous pathways. Many different mechanisms of initiation have been observed.

Intracardiac recordings during orthodromic tachycardia may provide useful information about the site of the anomalous connection. Electrodes disposed at various sites around the AV annulus (low right atrium, His bundle region, coronary sinus) allow identification of the earliest site of atrial activation during

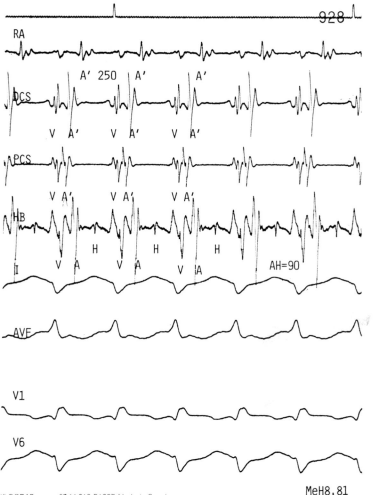

Fig. 9.7 Atrioventricular re-entrant tachycardia in a patient with Lown–Ganong–Levine syndrome. The tachycardia is rapid (cycle length = 250 msec) due to anterograde conduction via the atrio–His pathway (AH = 90 msec) and retrograde conduction over a direct VA posteroseptal anomalous connection. Paper speed 100 mm/sec. DCS and PCS = distal and proximal coronary sinus; HB = His bundle region; RA = right atrium.

tachycardia, thereby localizing the abnormal tract. Wherever the site of the anomalous pathway, the circuit is a relatively large one compared to that of AV nodal re-entry. Thus the ventricles and atria are activated in a sequential manner. The P wave is, therefore, almost always visible after the QRS complex. This fact offers a useful method of distinguishing AV nodal from atrioventricular re-entry on the surface ECG. Atrioventricular re-entrant tachycardia is a common mechanism in patients with the short PR interval/normal QRS syndrome, because a high proportion of these patients have a concealed anomalous pathway. The short AH conduction time persists during tachycardia and the tachycardia rate is correspondingly faster than that seen in patients without enhanced AH conduction (Fig. 9.7). They are also rarely repsonsive to verapamil, a drug which readily terminates AV tachycardia in the absence of enhanced AH conduction.

The mere confirmation of anomalous conduction by extrastimulus methods does not necessarily mean that it supports re-entrant tachycardias – proof of this requires meticulous demonstration. The participation of an anomalous pathway in the retrograde limb of tachycardia is suggested by several observations.

1. *Eccentric atrial activation* – that is, an activation sequence which begins at a site remote from the low right atrium or coronary sinus ostium (see Fig. 9.5) – indicates an atrial insertion of the anomalous pathway remote from the atrionodal junction (the normal exit point during ventriculoatrial conduction). However, anomalous septal pathways may show a normal retrograde sequence. Detailed mapping of the AV ring is essential to demonstrate eccentric atrial activation. The posterior mitral ring can be mapped using the coronary sinus electrode catheter. The tricuspid ring is more difficult to map because there are no easily accessible markers of the location of the annulus. Purpose-designed steerable catheters are available for mapping the tricuspid annulus but they are difficult to use. The right coronary artery offers a channel for mapping. Using small flexible pacing wires or angioplasty guide wires it is possible to record from the right coronary artery to locate anomalous pathways more accurately (Figs. 9.8 and 9.9). This approach may be particularly useful in patients considered

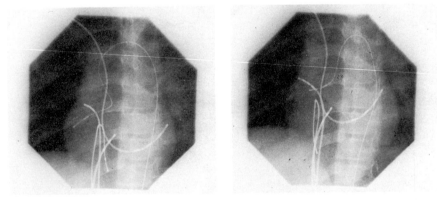

Fig. 9.8 Intracardiac electrodes and a right intracoronary electrode in a patient with right ventricular pre-excitation. The fine pacing wire was introduced into the right coronary artery, and atrial bipolar signals were mapped during atrioventricular re-entrant tachycardia and ventricular pacing. In this way the atrial insertion of the pathway could be accurately localized (see Fig. 9.9).

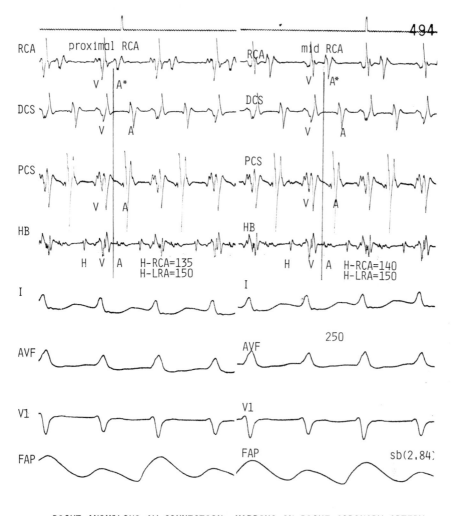

RIGHT ANOMALOUS AV CONNECTION. MAPPING IN RIGHT CORONARY ARTERY

Fig. 9.9 Recordings from the right coronary artery (RCA) during AVRT involving a right free wall anomalous pathway. The coronary artery electrode was used to map atrial activity (A*) via the right coronary artery. Earliest right atrial activation was recorded in the proximal RCA. Paper speed 100 mm/sec.

suitable for transvenous electrical ablation of right AV anomalous pathways (Chapter 15). It has been suggested that recordings during mapping the AV rings should be taken from multiple sites approximately 1 cm apart. This may be very difficult to achieve.

2. *Functional bundle branch block* is common during supraventricular tachycardias, especially those involving an anomalous pathway (see also Chapter 3). The occurrence of bundle branch block during AVRT can provide important diagnostic information. The effect of bundle branch block on the His–atrial (HA)

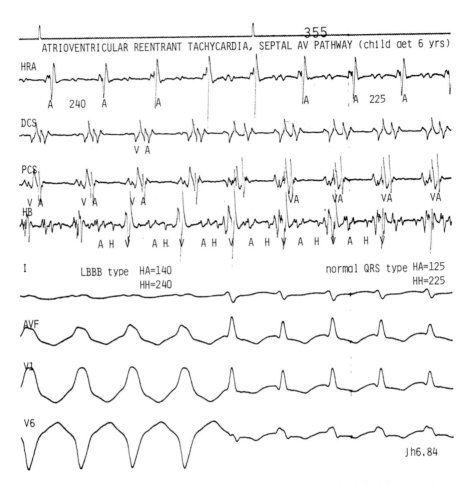

Fig. 9.10 The effect of bundle branch block on AVRT cycle length. The left of the recording shows orthodromic AVRT with functional left bundle branch block. Retrograde atrial activation begins in the proximal coronary sinus (PCS). When bundle branch block disappears the VA interval shortens by 15 msec and there is corresponding shortening of the cycle length (see also Fig. 9.11). Paper speed 100 mm/sec.

Table 9.3 INFLUENCE OF BUNDLE BRANCH BLOCK ON HA' INTERVAL DURING ATRIOVENTRICULAR RE-ENTRANT TACHYCARDIA

Location of AP	RBBB	LBBB
Right free wall	+ ≥ 30 msec	0
Anteroseptal	+ ≤ 30 msec	0
Posteroseptal	0	+ ≤ 30 msec
Left free wall	0	+ ≥ 30 msec

AP = anomalous pathway.

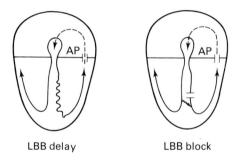

LBB delay LBB block

Fig. 9.11 The effect of bundle branch block on AVRT cycle length. During left bundle branch block, the anterograde tachycardia wavefront activates the left ventricle after traversing the septum from the right bundle branch territory. This adds time to the retrograde limb of the tachycardia cycle. Similarly, right bundle branch block would add time to the cycle of an AV re-entrant tachycardia utilizing a right-sided pathway.

component of the tachycardia cycle depends on the location of the anomalous pathway and the side of the bundle branch block (Figs. 9.10 and 9.11). If these are in the same ventricle the HA interval increases with the development of bundle branch block because the anomalous pathway is activated slightly later. Usually, the increase in HA interval is reflected by a corresponding increase in the tachycardia cycle length (Table 9.3). Contralateral bundle branch block (e.g. RBBB in the presence of orthodromic tachycardia involving a left anomalous pathway) has no effect on tachycardia cycle length. Branch block or delay caused by class 1 antiarrhythmic drugs used during the study may help to provide this information if bundle branch block cannot be induced during conventional attempts at tachycardia initiation. If bundle branch block cannot be induced, and in the absence of other evidence for an anomalous pathway, it may be useful to 'mimic' right and left bundle branch block by pacing the left and right ventricles and examining changes in the VA conduction pattern.

3. *Atrial capture*. The proof that an anomalous pathway is used in the VA limb of tachycardia is provided by the effect of ventricular extrastimulation at the time of His bundle depolarization. If no other retrograde VA pathway is available, conduction to the atria cannot occur because the His bundle is refractory. If an anomalous pathway is present, the atria can be pre-excited by VA conduction over this pathway. The atrial activation pattern will be unchanged but earlier than expected. This is referred to as 'exact atrial capture' (Figs. 9.12 and 9.13). If the site of ventricular extrastimulation is remote from the anomalous pathway, this effect may not be observed. For example, right ventricular stimulation may have no effect on atrial activation during AVRT involving a left free wall pathway. In such cases, stimulation in the left ventricle will usually reveal exact atrial capture. Table 9.4 summarizes the indications for left ventricular pacing during electrophysiological study of patients with the WPW syndrome. As with intranodal re-entrant tachycardia, termination of the tachycardia with a ventricular extrastimulus which fails to conduct to the atria excludes an atrial origin of re-entry.

Using ventricular extrastimulation during tachycardia, Miles et al. (1986) have derived a method which aids in distinguishing between AV nodal and AV re-

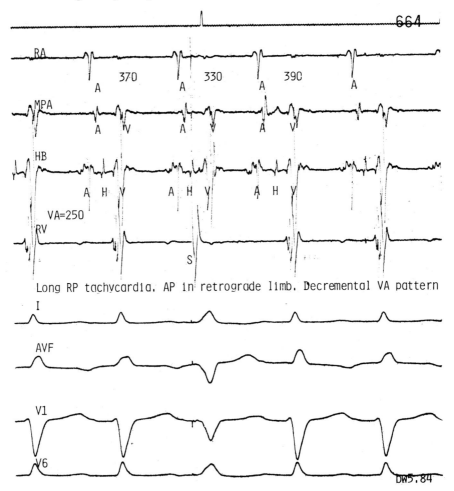

Long RP tachycardia. AP in retrograde limb. Decremental VA pattern

Fig. 9.12 Exact atrial capture by a ventricular extrastimulus (S). These recordings show AVRT due to a slowly conducting anomalous pathway with AV nodal properties. The tachycardia has a long RP' interval (VA = 250 msec). A ventricular premature stimulus delivered synchronously with the His potential (H) advances the atrial electrogram (A) by 40 msec without a change in the atrial activation sequence. This sequence is normal because the anomalous pathway is located in the septum in close proximity to the normal atrionodal junction. This phenomenon proves that the AV node is not part of the retrograde limb of tachycardia. Paper speed 100 mm/sec. MPA = main pulmonary artery; RA = right atrium.

Table 9.4 INDICATIONS FOR LEFT VENTRICULAR PACING IN THE STUDY OF WPW SYNDROME

Revelation of left lateral direct VA pathway conduction

Pre-excitation of the left atrium during AVRT

Location of left-sided direct VA pathway conduction

VA = ventriculoatrial; AVRT = atrioventricular re-entrant tachycardia

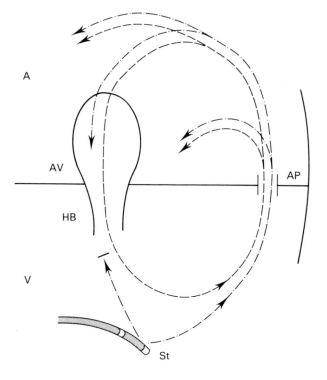

A

AV

HB

V

AP

St

Fig. 9.13 The exact atrial capture phenomenon. Ventricular (V) stimulation (St) coincident with His bundle (HB) depolarization during AVRT may result in retrograde anomalous pathway (AP) conduction to the atria (A) (with an identical activation sequence), which advances the tachycardia cycle. AV = AV node.

entrant tachycardia. A ventricular premature stimulus (V2) introduced late in the tachycardia cycle (V1V1) does not affect the atrial cycle in either form of tachycardia. When the coupling interval of the extrastimulus (V1V2) is reduced, atrial depolarization may be advanced or, in the authors' terminology, the atria are 'pre-excited'. The longest coupling interval (V1V2) which has this effect is used to derive two 'pre-excitation indices' (PI), defined as PI1 = V1V1 − V1V2, and PI2 = V1V2/V1V1. Only a very small proportion (14 per cent) of AV nodal tachycardias demonstrated atrial pre-excitation whereas 90 per cent of AV re-entrant tachycardias showed the phenomenon. The PI was longest in AVNT (PI1 = 108 msec, PI2 = 0.75) and in AVRT utilizing a left free wall pathway (PI1 = 88 msec, PI2 = 0.75). Shorter values were noted for tachycardias involving septal anomalous pathways (PI1 = 17–38 msec, PI2 = 0.88–0.95). Thus, these indices may also be useful in localizing the site of the retrograde limb of orthodromic AVRT.

The main electrophysiological features of orthodromic re-entry (see Table 9.2) are:

1. Initiation by an atrial premature stimulus which blocks in the anomalous pathway.

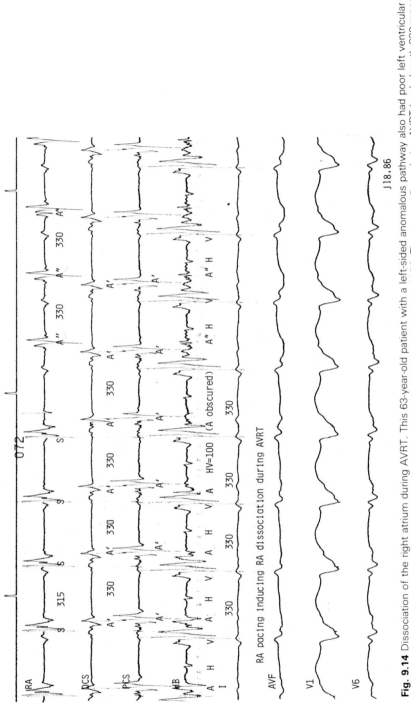

Fig. 9.14 Dissociation of the right atrium during AVRT. This 63-year-old patient with a left-sided anomalous pathway also had poor left ventricular function and intraventricular conduction defects (left bundle branch block and prolonged HV). These recordings during AVRT (cycle length 330 msec) show the effect of right atrial pacing (S) at a cycle length of 315 msec. The high right atrium and the low right atrium, in the region of the AV node–His bundle (A), are dissociated from the coronary sinus atrial electrograms (A′), which remain at the cycle length of tachycardia during pacing. The low right atrial electrogram gradually advances relative to the QRS and is eventually obscured by the ventricular electrogram. When pacing is switched off, the high and low right atrial electrograms (A″) return to a fixed position in the cycle. This phenomenon indicates that the right atrium in the region of the AV node is not an essential part of the tachycardia circuit, possibly because the input to the AV node during a rhythm emanating from the left atrium is different from that during a right atrial rhythm. Paper speed 100 mm/sec. DCS and PCS = distal and proximal coronary sinus; HB = His bundle region; RA = right atrium.

2. Initiation by a ventricular premature stimulus which blocks in the normal retrograde pathway (His–Purkinje system or AV node).
3. Eccentric atrial activation during tachycardia (may not be eccentric with septal pathways).
4. Atrial activation after the QRS in the first half of the RR cycle (VA interval longer than in AV nodal tachycardia).
5. Atrial capture during tachycardia by a ventricular stimulus delivered synchronously with the His spike.
6. Increase in tachycardia cycle length (or HA interval) with the development of functional bundle branch block on the same side as the anomalous pathway and, conversely, a decrease with disappearance of bundle branch block (septal pathways may not exhibit these phenomena).

Recently, it has become apparent that only part of the atrial mass is required to support AVRT (Morady et al., 1983). For example, it is possible, using right atrial pacing, to demonstrate dissociation of the high and the low right atrium (adjacent to the AV node) from the coronary sinus recording of left atrial activation during tachycardia utilizing a left-sided pathway (Fig. 9.14). This finding further suggests that the site of input to the AV node during the tachycardia may not be the same as that during sinus rhythm (see Chapter 2).

In a small proportion (about 10 per cent) of patients with the WPW syndrome the tachycardia circuit is reversed, with anterograde conduction over the anomalous pathway and retrograde conduction over the normal VA pathway (Table 9.5). This type is referred to as 'antidromic' atrioventricular re-entrant tachycardia (Fig. 9.15). The QRS complexes show full pre-excitation because there is no fusion with anterograde conduction over the normal pathway. The retrograde atrial activation sequence is normal unless there is another anomalous pathway participating in the retrograde limb (Fig. 9.16). There are several different mechanisms for these tachycardias. The simplest is anterograde anomalous conduction with retrograde AV nodal conduction. In patients with

Table 9.5 ELECTROPHYSIOLOGICAL CHARACTERISTICS OF ANTIDROMIC ATRIOVENTRICULAR RE-ENTRANT TACHYCARDIA

Normal retrograde atrial activation

Fully pre-excited QRS complex *

Ventricular reset follows atrial reset †

Neither atrial nor ventricular dissociation is possible

Possibly provoked by ventricular premature beats which encounter anomalous pathway VA block

Possibly provoked by atrial premature beats, within critical range of coupling intervals, which conduct with full pre-excitation

Possibly terminated by atrial or ventricular premature beats

* The form of the QRS complex may be affected by the presence of more than one anomalous pathway

† AV conduction during tachycardia is 'non-decremental'

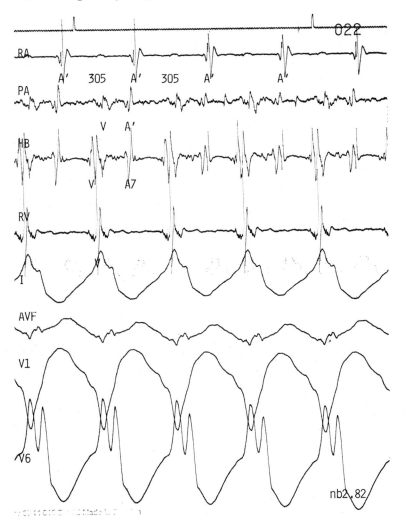

Fig. 9.15 Antidromic tachycardia in a 6-year-old boy with WPW syndrome type B. During tachycardia (cycle length = 305 msec) the QRS complexes are fully pre-excited and there is a normal retrograde atrial activation sequence. Paper speed 100 mm/sec. RA = right atrium; PA = pulmonary artery; HB = His bundle region; RV = right ventricle.

multiple anomalous pathways, several possible circuits can generate these tachycardias. (In the presence of multiple junctional substrates for tachycardias it is often possible, at electrophysiological study, to observe one form of tachycardia converting to another.) Anterograde conduction in an isolated posteroseptal pathway is unusual, perhaps because the potential circuit is too small to sustain tachycardia. Sometimes the AV node–His bundle is completely excluded from the circuit (Fig. 9.16). This finding is of great importance with regard to treatment because drugs acting on the AV node (effective in the usual type of AVRT) will have no benefit.

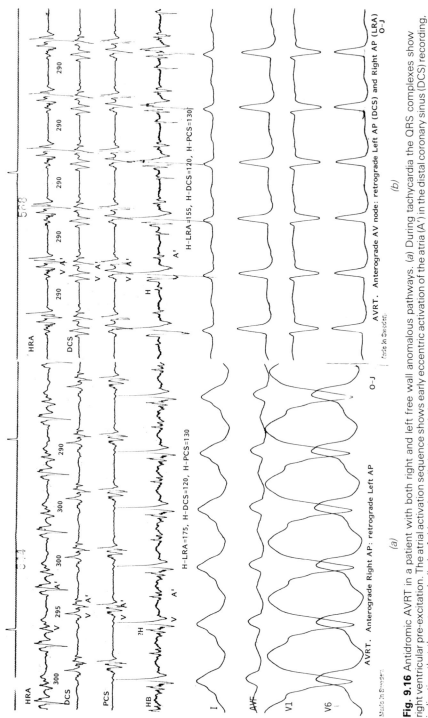
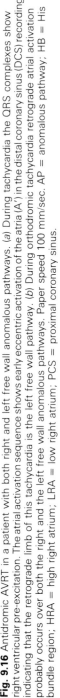

Fig. 9.16 Antidromic AVRT in a patient with both right and left free wall anomalous pathways. (*a*) During tachycardia the QRS complexes show right ventricular pre-excitation. The atrial activation sequence shows early eccentric activation of the atria (A') in the distal coronary sinus (DCS) recording, indicating that the retrograde limb of this tachycardia is the left free wall pathway. (*b*) During orthodromic tachycardia retrograde atrial activation probably occurs over both the right and the left free wall anomalous pathways. Paper speed 100 mm/sec. AP = anomalous pathway; HB = His bundle region; HRA = high right atrium; LRA = low right atrium; PCS = proximal coronary sinus.

Table 9.6 TYPES OF WIDE QRS COMPLEX TACHYCARDIA

Supraventricular

Aberration:
1. Bundle branch block or delay
2. Myocardial delay

Pre-excitation:
1. Direct atrioventricular pathway:
   a. bystander (atrial or AV nodal tachycardia)
   b. antidromic atrioventricular re-entry
2. Nodoventricular pathway:
   a. bystander (atrial or AV nodal tachycardia)
   b. nodoventricular macrore-entry

Ventricular

This tachycardia must be distinguished from other types with wide, 'pre-excited' QRS complexes (Table 9.6). Use of antiarrhythmic drugs with known effects may be of value in this respect (see Chapter 12). For example, termination of pre-excited tachycardia by verapamil-induced retrograde block is highly suggestive of AV re-entry. Continuation of tachycardia after drug- or pacing-induced block in the anomalous pathway excludes AV re-entry and suggests an atrial or intranodal origin. The precise diagnosis of the re-entrant mechanism can be made only by detailed electrophysiological investigations.

Atrioventricular nodal re-entrant tachycardias may also be found in patients with the WPW syndrome. In the presence of anterogradely conducting anomalous AV connection intranodal tachycardias may result in ventricular pre-excitation (Fig. 9.17). In this setting the anomalous pathway does not participate in the tachycardia circuit but is a 'bystander', and pre-excitation is due to 'incidental' anomalous conduction. The features which suggest bystander status are summarized in Table 9.7. Occasionally, AV nodal re-entry and AVRT may coexist and interact with each other. Other settings in which bystander anomalous conduction can result in wide QRS complex junctional tachycardias include AV nodal re-entry with incidental nodoventricular conduction and

Fig. 9.17 Recordings during tachycardia in a patient with a left free wall anomalous pathway showing 'bystander' pre-excitation during AVNT. The recordings to the left of the figure show tachycardia with right bundle branch block. The retrograde atrial activation sequence is normal, beginning in the low right atrium (A') which is inscribed before the QRS. This tachycardia was initiated with a sudden AH jump and reflects intranodal re-entry. Four paced ventricular beats (S1234) have no effect on the atrial cycle or activation sequence but result in the emergence of pre-excitation with a change in the QRS shape. The relationship between the His potential (H) and A' is unchanged, as is the atrial activation sequence, but the ventricular electrogram is advanced by pre-excitation. Presumably, anterograde expression of anomalous pathway conduction prior to ventricular stimulation was prevented by retrograde concealed conduction into the anomalous pathways during tachycardia. Ventricular pacing resulted in abolition of concealed conduction by rephasing the refractory period of the anomalous pathway, thus allowing anterograde expression to become manifest. Paper speed 100 mm/sec. DCS and PCS = distal and proximal coronary sinus; HB = His bundle; HRA = high right atrium.

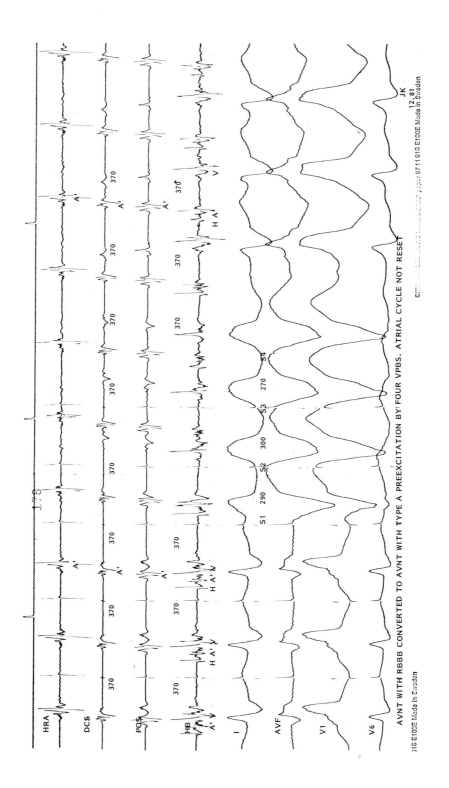

AVNT WITH RBBB CONVERTED TO AVNT WITH TYPE A PREEXCITATION BY FOUR VPBS. ATRIAL CYCLE NOT RESET

orthodromic AV re-entry with anomalous nodoventricular conduction (see below).

Termination of tachycardia may be achieved by atrial or ventricular pacing. The factors which determine the ease of termination are proximity of the pacing site to the circuit, the number of stimuli used and the rate of pacing with several stimuli (see Chapter 13).

Atrioventricular re-entrant tachycardia with a long RP′ interval

This type of anomalous pathway was first reported by Gallagher and Sealy in 1978. They found evidence for such a pathway in a patient with an incessant or 'permanent' tachycardia. The features of this form of tachycardia were described by Coumel et al. in 1967, and it was thought that the underlying mechanism was AV nodal re-entry of the 'fast–slow' type. So convincing is the evidence for the presence of these atypical anomalous pathways that some have claimed that the intranodal mechanism does not exist. It is now clear, however, that either mechanism may be responsible for the permanent form of junctional tachycardia.

The prevalence of slowly conducting anomalous pathways is not known. Anterograde anomalous conduction does not occur, so the anomalous pathways are not manifest during sinus rhythm or atrial pacing (but may be after attempted electrical ablation; see below). Extrastimulus testing by ventricular pacing reveals that these pathways possess decremental conduction properties and are always located in the posteroseptal region. During the retrograde conduction study, the atrial activation pattern may be persistently eccentric until block occurs in the anomalous pathway. These phenomena have led to the suggestion that these anomalous pathways may be accessory AV nodal structures close to the normal conduction axis (Ward and Camm, 1982). In one study, however, left free wall pathways with decremental properties were the substrate for 'long RP′ atrioventricular re-entrant tachycardia'. Interestingly, these pathways were also sensitive to verapamil (Okumura et al., 1986). Dual retrograde pathways may be demonstrated during ventricular extrastimulation when slow pathway conduction is exposed by retrograde fast pathway block. Tachycardia is often initiated with this change in conduction pathway.

Table 9.7 DIAGNOSIS OF BYSTANDER * ANOMALOUS PATHWAY

No proof of participation in re-entrant circuit †
plus
Incomplete pre-excitation (in direction of conduction) during tachycardia
or
Continuation of tachycardia despite abolition of pre-excitation §

* Bystander = presence but not participation in re-entrant circuit

† For example, prolongation of HA′ time in consequence of ipsilateral bundle branch block in atrioventricular re-entrant tachycardia.

§ Pre-excitation may be abolished by: (1) catheter trauma; (2) cardioactive drugs; (3) spontaneously.

During tachycardia the retrograde conduction time is long, with the P wave occurring late in the cycle (see Fig. 9.12). The RP′ interval is longer than the PR interval and these tachycardias are often referred to as 'long RP′ tachycardias'. The atrial activation sequence during tachycardia begins in the low right atrium on the His bundle catheter recording or near the coronary sinus ostium, indicating a septal location of the anomalous pathway. This correlates with an inverted P wave in the inferior frontal leads.

The participation of the anomalous pathway in the retrograde limb of tachycardia is confirmed using the criteria applied to typical retrogradely conducting anomalous pathways (see above). Dual retrograde pathways may be demonstrated during ventricular extrastimulation when slow pathway conduction is exposed by retrograde fast pathway block. Tachycardia is often initiated with this change in conduction pathway. An interesting variation of the 'exact' atrial capture phenomenon may be seen. In patients with a typical VA anomalous pathway the atrial capture is accompanied by advancement of the atrial electrogram whereas delay may be observed if VA conduction during tachycardia involves an atypical pathway (Bardy et al., 1985). It should be added that failure to demonstrate the typical features of anomalous retrograde conduction during tachycardia does not exclude its presence.

Unexplained emergence of ventricular pre-excitation has been noted in several patients who have undergone attempted ablation (see Chapter 14) of the anomalous pathway, in most instances with first degree AV block. The mechanism of this effect is unknown. Histological confirmation of a paraseptal pathway has been found in a patient with permanent junctional tachycardia.

Junctional tachycardias associated with anomalous nodoventricular pathways

These pathways insert the right ventricular septum and produce ventricular pre-excitation with QRS complexes of 'LBBB' type (see Chapter 6). Some patients with these pathways are prone to develop tachycardias. The central question is whether or not the anomalous pathway supports a re-entrant mechanism in any way. The tachycardias typically show QRS complexes of LBBB morphology. This has been interpreted as indicating anterograde participation of the nodoventricular pathway in the tachycardia circuit or incidental bystander nodoventricular conduction during some other mechanism of tachycardia. Many of these patients have demonstrable AV nodal pathways, and it may be shown that intranodal re-entry is a mechanism of tachycardia in some of these patients (Figs. 9.18 and 9.19). Gallagher and associates have presented strong arguments for the 'macrore-entry' mechanism (Table 9.8). The strongest evidence is the observation of atrioventricular dissociation during tachycardia in several patients. This phenomenon is also known to occur, albeit rarely, in AV nodal re-entrant tachycardia.

The His potential can often be recorded coincident with the onset of the broad QRS complex (HV interval = zero) (Fig. 9.19). To explain this finding by macrore-entry the anomalous pathway would have to be inserted directly into the right bundle branch with simultaneous anterograde conduction to the myocardium and retrograde conduction to the His bundle (Fig. 9.20). With an HV interval of zero during sinus rhythm, it is unnecessary to postulate this

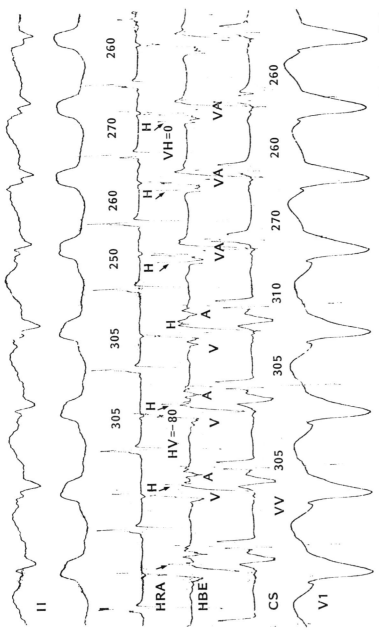

Fig. 9.19 Recordings during tachycardia in a patient with an anomalous nodoventricular pathway and dual AV nodal pathways. During atrial pacing at 100 b.p.m. the HV interval was −20 msec. The recordings to the left show stable tachycardia with a cycle length of 305 msec. The QRS complexes are broad and show a 'left bundle branch block' morphology. The His spike (arrowed) is seen well after the QRS (HV = −80 msec, or VH = 80 msec). In the middle of the recording, the His spike suddenly changes its position relative to the QRS (HV = zero). This event is followed by a shortening of the VA interval and atrial cycle length (to 250 msec) and subsequently the ventricular cycle length and tachycardia are again stable. The H to HRA interval increases transiently immediately after the change of the HV interval to zero, but returns to its prior state in the faster tachycardia. The AV interval increases from 115 to 145 msec. On other occasions a transient lesser change in the HV interval and cycle length was observed. Paper speed 100 mm/sec. CS = coronary sinus; HBE = His bundle region; HRA = high right atrium.

Table 9.8 ELECTROPHYSIOLOGICAL CHARACTERISTICS OF NODOVENTRICULAR OR FASCICULOVENTRICULAR MACRORE-ENTRANT TACHYCARDIA

1. Normal retrograde atrial activation *

2. (a) Fully pre-excited QRS complexes (antidromic tachycardia), with negative H'V interval †

   or

   (b) Normal ventricular activation (orthodromic tachycardia), with normal or prolonged HV interval

3. Possibly provoked and terminated by ventricular premature beats

4. Possibly initiated by atrial premature beats which conduct to the ventricles with full pre-excitation (2a) or normal conduction (2b)

5. Possibly terminated by atrial premature beats which conduct to the ventricles

6. Atrial dissociation possible

---

* Simultaneous atrial arrhythmia or sinus rhythm may be present.

† In antidromic tachycardia the His bundle is depolarized retrogradely; the His depolarization may be masked by the ventricular electrogram.

Fig. 9.18 Initiation of tachycardia by premature atrial extrastimulation in a patient with nodoventricular pre-excitation. (*a*) After regular atrial pacing (S1S1) at a cycle length of 520 msec, an atrial premature stimulus (S2) is introduced at a coupling interval of 360 msec. During the regular paced rhythm the AH interval is 115 msec and the HV interval is 55 msec. In response to S2, the AV interval increases but not as much as the AH interval. Thus the HV interval is shortened by 70 msec to −15 msec. This disparate lengthening in the AV and AH intervals is caused by the emergence of ventricular pre-excitation as a result of nodoventricular conduction. The QRS complex in response to S2 shows the typical 'left bundle branch block' pattern of right ventricular septal pre-excitation. (*b*) When the coupling interval of A2 is reduced by 20 msec, there is a sudden increase in the AH and AV intervals, with the HV interval remaining unchanged at −15 msec. An atrial echo beat (A') is followed by sustained tachycardia with QRS complexes identical to that seen in response to A2. The retrograde atrial sequence (A') is normal. The mechanism of initiation of this tachycardia implies the presence of dual AV nodal pathways and intranodal re-entrant tachycardia. That the HV interval and QRS complex during anterograde conduction in response to S2 are identical to those seen during tachycardia suggests that the His bundle is depolarized anterogradely, not retrogradely, during the tachycardia (i.e. excluding macrore-entry involving anterograde anomalous conduction and retrograde His–Purkinje conduction). This conclusion is supported by the observation that, on some occasions, the atrial echo in response to S2 occurred after a partially pre-excited QRS, reflecting fusion between anterograde conduction in the anomalous and normal pathways. The latter pathway could not therefore be used for retrograde conduction. Paper speed 100 mm/sec. CS = coronary sinus; HB = His bundle region; RA = right atrium; RV = right ventricle.

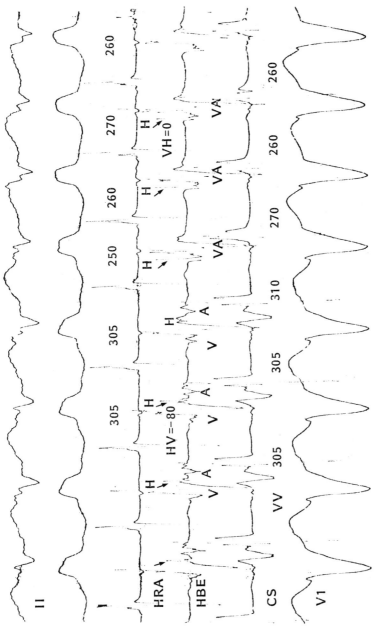

Fig. 9.19 Recordings during tachycardia in a patient with an anomalous nodoventricular pathway and dual AV nodal pathways. During atrial pacing at 100 b.p.m. the HV interval was −20 msec. The recordings to the left show stable tachycardia with a cycle length of 305 msec. The QRS complexes are broad and show a 'left bundle branch block' morphology. The His spike (arrowed) is seen well after the QRS (HV = −80 msec, or VH = 80 msec). In the middle of the recording, the His spike suddenly changes its position relative to the QRS (HV = zero). This event is followed by a shortening of the VA interval and atrial cycle length (to 250 msec) and subsequently the ventricular cycle length and tachycardia are again stable. The H to HRA interval increases transiently immediately after the change of the HV interval to zero, but returns to its prior state in the faster tachycardia. The AV interval increases from 115 to 145 msec. On other occasions a transient lesser change in the HV interval and cycle length was observed. Paper speed 100 mm/sec. CS = coronary sinus; HB = His bundle region; HRA = high right atrium.

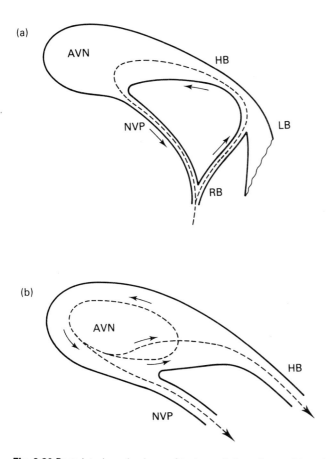

Fig. 9.20 Postulated mechanisms of tachycardia in patients with nodoventricular pre-excitation. (a) The 'subjunctional' macrore-entrant circuit in which the anomalous nodoventricular pathway (NVP) forms the anterograde limb of the re-entrant tachycardia circuit. If the pathway inserts directly into the right bundle branch (RB) it is possible for the HV interval to be slightly positive, zero or slightly negative during tachycardia, depending on the relative anterograde (to myocardium) and retrograde (to His bundle, HB) conduction times in the right bundle from the point of insertion of the anomalous pathway. AVN = atrioventricular node; LB = left bundle branch. (b) Possible circuits of the tachycardia shown in Fig 9.18 during the changing HV interval. The initial event is advancement of the His potential independent of a change in the ventricular cycle. The sudden advancement of the His potential must therefore have occurred after engagement of the nodoventricular pathway (NVP). A possible explanation is that a faster intra-AV nodal (AVN) pathway distal to the origin of the anomalous pathway accounts for the shorter HV interval followed by the earlier timing of the next atrial and ventricular events. As the His bundle is not on circuit in this mechanism the changes in the HV interval need not be reflected exactly by changes in the cycle length (as would be the case in the subjunctional mechanism).

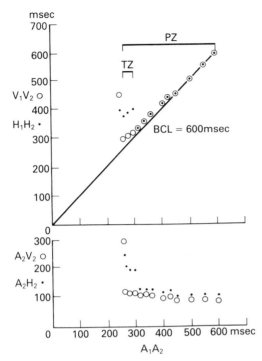

Fig. 9.21 Anterograde conduction curves from the patient shown in Fig. 9.19. The H1H2 and V1V2 intervals are plotted against the coupling interval of the test beat (A1A2). During atrial pacing there is ventricular pre-excitation with HV = −20. As the test stimulus is advanced the AV interval and the AH interval are prolonged slightly. A sudden jump in the AH interval is seen when A1A2 is 300 msec. The A2V2 increases to a much smaller degree. Thus the His potential is delayed sufficiently to appear after the QRS. Tachycardia is initiated coincident with this sudden AH jump. At very short test beat intervals the anomalous pathway blocked, revealing normal conduction. These findings are best explained by intranodal re-entrant tachycardia on the basis of dual AV nodal pathways and incidental or 'bystander' anomalous ventricular pre-excitation. PZ = pre-excitation zone; TZ = tachycardia zone; BCL = basic cycle length.

mechanism. The patient shown in Fig. 9.19 also has evidence of dual AV nodal pathways (Fig. 9.21). Although macrore-entry using the nodoventricular pathway in the anterograde limb of the circuit probably accounts for some of the tachycardias in this setting, proof of this mechanism by electrophysiological techniques is difficult to obtain. This type of tachycardia is best referred to as 'subjunctional' or as a form of ventricular tachycardia during which the QRS complexes show a left bundle branch block pattern. Anomalous nodoventricular conduction may also be observed during atrioventricular tachycardias involving a typical direct anomalous VA pathway.

Focal His bundle tachycardia

This rare form of tachycardia, thought to be due to an abnormal automatic focus, was first described by Coumel et al. (1975) and is found almost exclusively in

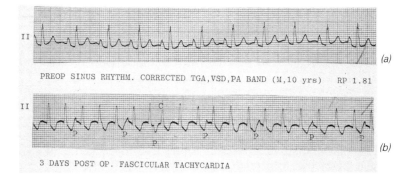

PREOP SINUS RHYTHM. CORRECTED TGA,VSD,PA BAND (M,10 yrs)   RP 1.81

(a)

3 DAYS POST OP. FASCICULAR TACHYCARDIA

(b)

Fig. 9.22 Focal His bundle tachycardia in a 10-year-old boy 3 days after complex surgery to repair multiple intracardiac defects. (*a*) Preoperative sinus rhythm. (*b*) Three days after operation, there is a tachycardia with QRS complexes identical to those recorded before surgery (this was shown in all 12 leads). There is AV dissociation with clearly inscribed P waves and occasional capture beats (C). The arrhythmia caused severe haemodynamic disturbances. It was controlled with intravenous flecainide. Paper speed 25 mm/sec.

children. It is also known as junctional ectopic tachycardia (JET). It may be congenital or may emerge after cardiac surgery. The ectopic focus arises in the lower AV node or the His bundle with normal ventricular activation (narrow QRS complex). Atrioventricular dissociation is often present (Fig. 9.22). The rapid tachycardias can precipitate pulmonary oedema and are notoriously resistant to drug therapy. Electrical ablation of the His bundle has been effective in some cases.

Clinical electrophysiological studies in patients with junctional tachycardias

The main indications for study of patients with junctional tachycardias are:

1. Confirmation of the diagnosis and mechanism of tachycardia where this is relevant to management of the patient.
2. Investigation of serious symptoms (e.g. syncope) possibly caused by junctional tachycardia in a patient known to suffer from the arrhythmia.
3. Formal assessment of drug treatment in patients who have failed to respond to empirical therapy with conventional agents.
4. Formal assessment of alternative therapies such as ablation (surgical or percutaneous catheter methods) and pacemakers in patients unresponsive to drugs.
5. Assessment of risk, especially in patients with the WPW syndrome.

The strategy of study (see Chapter 11) in these patients depends to some extent on the reasons for study and the type of tachycardia. In essence, formal anterograde and retrograde conduction studies are performed at the beginning of the study. During the course of these studies tachycardias are often induced and should be studied rather than terminated in favour of the conduction studies. For obvious reasons, drug studies are performed last of all.

The aims of study in patients with junctional tachycardias are:

1. Definition of the mechanism of re-entrant junctional tachycardia.
2. Localization of the re-entrant pathways (this is especially important in patients with the WPW syndrome who may be suitable for surgical or electrical ablation of the anomalous pathway; see Chapters 14 and 15).
3. Evaluation of the functional properties of the re-entrant pathways. In patients with anomalous AV conduction and ventricular pre-excitation this includes initiation of atrial fibrillation (see Chapter 6).
4. Investigation of the efficacy of pacemaker termination, especially in patients who may be candidates for this option (see Chapter 13).
5. Establishment of effective drug treatment (see Chapter 12).

References and further reading

Akhtar M, Damato AN, Batsford WP, Ruskin JN, Caracta AR, Weisfogel GM, Lau SH. (1975) Induction of atrioventricular nodal reentrant tachycardia after atropine. *American Journal of Cardiology* **36**, 288

Akhtar M, Damato AN, Ruskin JN, Batsford WP, Reddy CP, Ticzon AR, Dhatt MS, Gomes JAC, Calon AH. (1978) Antegrade and retrograde conduction characteristics in three patterns of paroxysmal junctional reentrant tachycardia. *American Heart Journal* **95**, 22

Akhtar M. (1983) Electrophysiologic bases for wide QRS tachycardias. *Pacing and Clinical Electrophysiology* **6**, 81

Bar FW, Brugada P, Dassen WRM, Wellens HJJ. (1984) Differential diagnosis of tachycardia with narrow QRS complex (shorter than 0.12 second). *American Journal of Cardiology* **54**, 555

Bardy GH, Packer DL, German LD, Gallagher JJ. (1984a) Preexcited reciprocating tachycardia in patients with the Wolff–Parkinson–White syndrome: incidence and mechanisms. *Circulation* **70**, 377

Bardy GH, German LD, Packer DL, Coltorti F, Gallagher JJ. (1984b) Mechanism of tachycardia using a nodofascicular Mahaim fiber. *American Journal of Cardiology* **54**, 110

Bardy GH, Fedor JM, German LD, Packer DL, Gallagher JJ. (1984c) Surface electrocardiographic clues suggesting the presence of a nodoventricular Mahaim fiber. *Journal of the American College of Cardiology* **3**, 1161

Bardy GH, Packer DL, German LD, Coltorti F, Gallagher JJ. (1985) Paradoxical delay in accessory pathway conduction during long R'P tachycardia after interpolated ventricular premature complexes. *American Journal of Cardiology* **55**, 1223

Barold SS, Coumel P. (1977) Mechanisms of atrioventricular junctional tachycardia. Role of reentry and concealed accessory pathways. *American Journal of Cardiology* **39**, 97

Bauernfeind RA, Wyndham CR, Dhingra R, Swiryn SP, Palileo E, Strasberg B, Rosen KM. (1980a) Serial electrophysiologic testing of multiple drugs in patients with atrioventricular nodal tachycardia. *Circulation* **62**, 1341

Bauernfeind RA, Ayres BF, Wyndham CR, Dhingra R, Swiryn S, Strasberg B, Rosen KM. (1980b) Cycle length in atrioventricular nodal reentrant paroxysmal tachycardia with observations on the Lown–Ganong–Levine syndrome. *American Journal of Cardiology* **45**, 1148

Benditt DG, Pritchett ELC, Smith WM, Wallace AG, Gallagher JJ. (1978) Characteristics of atrioventricular conduction and the spectrum of arrhythmias in Lown–Ganong–Levine syndrome. *Circulation* **57**, 454

Benditt DG, Epstein ML, Benson DW. (1982) Dual accessory nodoventricular pathways:

role in paroxysmal wide QRS reciprocating tachycardia. *Pacing and Clinical Electrophysiology* **6**, 577

Brugada P, Vanagt EJ, Dassen WR, Gorgels AP, Bar FWHM, Wellens HJJ. (1980) Atrioventricular nodal tachycardia with and without discontinuous anterograde and retrograde atrioventricular conduction nodal curves: a reappraisal of the dual pathway concept. *European Heart Journal* **1**, 399

Brugada P, Farre J, Green M, Heddle B, Roy D, Wellens HJJ. (1983) Observations in patients with supraventricular tachycardia having a PR interval shorter than the RP interval: differentiation between atrial tachycardia and reciprocating atrioventricular tachycardia using an accessory pathway with long conduction times. *American Heart Journal* **107**, 556

Brugada P, Wellens HJJ. (1984) Electrophysiology, mechanisms, diagnosis and treatment of paroxysmal recurrent atrioventricular nodal reentrant tachycardia. In: *Tachycardias*, p. 131. Ed. by B Surawicz, CP Reddy. Martinus Nijhoff: Boston, Mass

Cinca J, Valle V, Figueras J, Gutierrez L, Montoyo J, Ruis J. (1984) Shortening of ventriculoatrial conduction in patients with left-sided Kent bundles. *American Heart Journal* **107**, 912

Coumel P, Cabrol C, Fabiato A, Gourgon R, Slama R. (1967) Tachycardie permanente par rhythme reciproque. I. Preuves du diagnostic par stimulation auriculaire at ventriculaire. *Archives des Maladies du Coeur* **60**, 1830

Coumel P, Attuel P. (1974) Reciprocating tachycardia in overt and latent preexcitation. Influence of functional bundle branch block on the rate of the tachycardia. *European Journal of Cardiology* **1**, 423

Coumel P. (1975) Junctional reciprocating tachycardias. The permanent and paroxysmal forms of AV nodal reciprocating tachycardias. *Journal of Electrocardiology* **8**, 79

Coumel P, Fidelle JE, Attuel P, Brechenmacher C, Batisse A, Bretagne J, Clementy J, Gerard R, Grolleau R, Hualt G, Mouy J, Kachaner J, Ribiere M, Toumieux MC. (1975) Tachycardies focales hissienes congenitales. *Archives des Maladies du Coeur* **69**, 899

Coumel P, Attuel P, Slama R, Curry P, Krikler D. (1976) 'Incessant' tachycardias in Wolff–Parkinson–White syndrome. II. Role of atypical cycle length dependency and nodal–His escape beats in initiating reciprocating tachycardias. *British Heart Journal* **38**, 897

Denes P, Wu D, Amat-y-Leon F, Dhingra R, Wyndham CR, Rosen KM. (1977) The determinants of atrioventricular nodal reentrance with premature atrial stimulation in patients with dual AV nodal pathways. *Circulation* **56**, 253

Denes P, Wu D, Amat-y-Leon F, Dhingra R, Wyndham CR, Kehoe R, Ayres BF, Rosen KM. (1979) Paroxysmal supraventricular tachycardia induction in patients with Wolff–Parkinson–White syndrome. *Annals of Internal Medicine* **90**, 153

DiMarco JP, Sellers TD, Belardinelli L. (1984) Paroxysmal supraventricular tachycardia with Wenckebach block: evidence for reentry within the upper portion of the atrioventricular node. *Journal of the American College of Cardiology* **3**, 1551

Durrer D, Schoo L, Schuilenberg RM, Wellens HJJ. (1967) The role of premature beats in the initiation and the termination of supraventricular tachycardia in the Wolff–Parkinson–White sydrome. *Circulation* **36**, 644

Durrer D, Schuilenberg RM, Wellens HJJ. (1970) Preexcitation revisited. *American Journal of Cardiology* **25**, 690

Farshidi A, Josephson ME, Horowitz LN. (1978) Electrophysiologic characteristics of concealed bypass tracts: clinical and electrocardiographic correlates. *American Journal of Cardiology* **41**, 1052

Gallagher JJ, Sealy WC, Kasell J, Wallace AG. (1976) Multiple accessory pathways in patients with the preexcitation syndrome. *Circulation* **54**, 571

Gallagher JJ, Pritchett ELC, Benditt DG, Tonkin AM, Campbell RWF, Dugan FA,

Bashore TM, Tower A, Wallace AG. (1977) New catheter techniques for analysis of the sequence of retrograde atrial activation in man. *European Journal of Cardiology* **6**, 1

Gallagher JJ, Sealy WC. (1978) The permanent form of junctional reciprocating tachycardia: further elucidation of the underlying mechanism. *European Journal of Cardiology* **8**, 413

Gallagher JJ, Smith WM, Kasell J, Benson DW, Sterba R, Grant AO. (1981) The role of Mahaim fibers in cardiac arrhythmias in man. *Circulation* **64**, 176

Gallagher JJ, German LD, Broughton A, Guarnieri T, Trantham JL. (1983) Variants of the prexcitation syndromes. In: *Frontiers of Cardiac Electrophysiology*, p. 724 Ed. by MB Rosenbaum, MV Elizari. Martinus Nijhoff: The Hague

Gallagher JJ. (1985) Variants of preexcitation. Update 1984. In: *Cardiac Electrophysiology and Arrhythmias*, p. 419. Ed. by D Zipes, J Jalife. Grune & Stratton: Orlando, Fla

Geddes JS. (1976) Wolff–Parkinson–White syndrome. Circus movement tachycardia dependent on procainamide. *British Heart Journal* **38**, 330

Gmeiner R, Ng CK, Hammer I, Becker AE. (1984) Tachycardia caused by an accessory nodoventricular tract: a clinico-pathologic correlation. *European Heart Journal* **5**, 233

Goldreyer BN, Bigger JT. (1971) The site of reentry in paroxysmal supraventricular tachycardia in man. *Circulation* **43**, 15

Goldreyer BN, Damato AN. (1971) The essential role of atrioventricular conduction delay in the initiation of paroxysmal supraventricular tachycardia. *Circulation* **43**, 679

Gomes JA, Dhatt MS, Rubenson DS, Damato AN. (1979) Electrophysiologic evidence for selective retrograde utilization of a specialized conducting system in atrioventricular nodal reentrant tachycardia. *American Journal of Cardiology* **43**, 687

Green M, Heddle B, Dassen W, Wehr M, Abdollah H, Brugada P, Wellens HJJ. (1983) Value of QRS alternation in determining site of origin of narrow QRS supraventricular tachycardia. *Circulation* **68**, 368

Hammill SC, Pritchett ELC, Klein GJ, Smith WM, Gallagher JJ. (1980) Accessory atrioventricular pathways that conduct only in the anterograde direction. *Circulation* **62**, 1335

Hariman RJ, Chen C-M, Caracta AR, Damato AN. (1983) Evidence that AV nodal reentry does not require the participation of the entire AV node. *Pacing and Clinical Electrophysiology* **6**, 1252

Heddle WF, Tonkin AM. (1980) Atrial and His bundle stimulation with an accessory nodoventricular connection. *Pacing and Clinical Electrophysiology* **3**, 286

Jackman WM, Friday KJ, Naccarelli GV. (1983) VT or not VT? An approach to the diagnosis and management of wide QRS complex tachycardia. *Clinical Progress in Pacing and Electrophysiology* **1**, 225

Josephson ME, Kastor J. (1976) Paroxysmal supraventricular tachycardia. Is the atrium a necessary link? *Circulation* **54**, 430

Josephson ME, Kastor JA. (1977) Supraventricular tachycardia in Lown–Ganong–Levine syndrome: atrionodal versus intranodal reentry. *American Journal of Cardiology* **40**, 521

Josephson ME. (1978) Paroxysmal supraventricular tachycardia: an electrophysiologic approach. *American Journal of Cardiology* **41**, 1123

Kerr CR, Gallagher JJ, German LD. (1982) Changes in ventriculoatrial intervals with bundle branch block aberration during reciprocating tachycardia in patients with accessory atrioventricular pathways. *Circulation* **66**, 196

Klein GJ, Prystowsky EN, Pritchett ELC, Davis D, Gallagher JJ. (1979) Atypical patterns of retrograde conduction over acessory atrioventricular pathways in the Wolff–Parkinson–White syndrome. *Circulation* **60**, 1447

Klein GJ, Yee R, Sharma AD. (1984) Concealed conduction in accessory atrioventricular pathways: an important determinant of the expression of arrhythmias in patients with

Wolff–Parkinson–White syndrome. *Circulation* **70**, 402

Krikler D, Curry P, Attuel P, Coumel P. (1976) 'Incessant' tachycardias in Wolff–Parkinson–White syndrome. I. Initiation without antecedent extrasystoles or PR lengthening, with reference to reciprocation after shortening of cycle length. *British Heart Journal* **38**, 885

Lerman BB, Waxman HL, Proclemer A, Josephson ME (1982) Supraventricular tachycardia associated with nodoventricular and concealed atrioventricular bypass tracts. *American Heart Journal* **104**, 1097

Levy S, Clementy J, Lacaze JC, Bemurat M, Choussat A, Bricaud H. (1979) Tachycardias supraventriculaires paroxystiques avec block auriculoventriculaire complet ou dissociation auriculoventriculaire complet. *Archives des Maladies du Coeur* **72**, 615

Mandel WJ, Laks MM, Obayashi K. (1975) Atrioventricular nodal reentry in the Wolff–Parkinson–White syndrome. *Chest* **68**, 321

Mendez C, Moe GK. (1966) Demonstration of a dual AV nodal conduction system in the isolated rabbit heart. *Circulation Research* **19**, 378

Mignone RJ, Wallace AG. (1966) Ventricular echoes: evidence for dissociation of conduction and reentry within the AV node. *Circulation Research* **19**, 638

Miles WM, Yee R, Klein GJ, Zipes DP, Prystowsky EN. (1986) The preexcitation index: an aid in determining the mechanism of supraventricular tachycardia and localizing accessory pathways. *Circulation* **74**, 493

Morady F, Scheinman MM, Gonzalez R, Hess D. (1981) His–ventricular dissociation in a patient with reciprocating tachycardia and a nodoventricular bypass tract. *Circulation* **64**, 839

Morady F, Wang YS, Scheinman MM, Sung RJ, Shen E, Shapiro WA. (1983) Extent of atrial participation in atrioventricular reciprocating tachycardia. *Circulation* **67**, 646

Morady F, Scheinman MM, Winston SA, DiCarlo LA, Davis JC. (1984) Dissociation of atrial electrograms by right and left atrial pacing in patients with atrioventricular reciprocating tachycardia. *Journal of the American College of Cardiology* **4**, 1283

Motte D, Brechenmacher C, Davy JM, Belhassen B. (1980) Association de fibres nodo-ventriculaires et atrio-ventriculaires a l'origine de tachycardias reciproques. *Archives des Maladies du Coeur* **73**, 737

Neuss H, Schlepper M, Thormann J. (1975) Analysis of re-entry mechanisms in three patients with concealed Wolff–Parkinson–White syndrome. *Circulation* **51**, 75

Novick TL, Pritchett ELC, Campbell RWF, Rogers GC, Wallace AG, Gallagher JJ. (1978) Temporary, catheter-induced block in accessory pathways. *Circulation* **58**, 932

Okumura K, Henthorn RW, Epstein AE, Plumb VJ, Waldo AL. (1986) 'Incessant' atrioventricular tachycardia utilizing left lateral bypass pathway with a long retrograde conduction time. *Pacing and Clinical Electrophysiology* **9**, 332

Portillo B, Leon-Portillo N, Zaman L, Myerburg RJ, Castellanos A. (1984) Entrainment of atrioventricular nodal reentrant tachycardias during overdrive pacing from the high right atrium and coronary sinus. *American Journal of Cardiology* **53**, 1570

Pritchett ELC, Gallagher JJ, Wallace AG. (1978) Reentry within the atrioventricular node in man: a reassessment. *European Heart Journal* **6**, 437

Pritchett ELC, Prystowsky EN, Benditt DG, Gallagher JJ. (1980) 'Dual atrioventricular nodal pathways' in patients with Wolff–Parkinson–White syndrome. *British Heart Journal* **43**, 7

Przybylski J, Chaile PA, Halpern S, Lazzari JO, Elizari M, Rosenbaum MB. (1978) Existence of automaticity in anomalous bundle of Wolff–Parkinson–White syndrome. *British Heart Journal* **40**, 672

Reddy CP, McAllister RG. (1984) Effect of verapamil on retrograde conduction in atrioventricular nodal reentrant tachycardia. *American Journal of Cardiology* **54**, 535

Rosen KM, Bauernfeind RA, Wyndham CR, Dhingra R. (1979) Retrograde properties of the fast pathway in patients with proxysmal atrioventricular nodal reentrant tachycardia. *American Journal of Cardiology* **43**, 863

Ross DL, Johnson DC, Denniss AR, Cooper MJ, Richards DA, Uther JB. (1985) Curative surgery for atrioventricular junctional ("AV nodal") reentrant tachycardia. *Journal of the American College of Cardiology* **6**, 1383

Scheinman MM, Gonzalez R, Thomas A, Ullyot D, Bharati S, Lev M. (1982) Reentry confined to the atrioventricular node: electrophysiologic and anatomic findings. *American Journal of Cardiology* **49**, 1814

Scheinman MM. (1985) Atrioventricular nodal or atriojunctional reentrant tachycardia? *Journal of the American College of Cardiology* **6**, 1393

Sellers TD, Gallagher JJ, Cope GD, Tonkin AM, Wallace AG. (1976) Retrograde atrial preexcitation following premature ventricular beats during reciprocating tachycardia in the Wolff–Parkinson–White syndrome. *European Journal of Cardiology* **4**, 283

Smith WM, Broughton A, Reiter MH, Benson DW, Grand AO, Gallagher JJ. (1983) Bystander accessory pathway during AV node reentrant tachycardia. *Pacing and Clinical Electrophysiology* **6**, 537

Spurrell RAJ, Krikler D, Sowton E. (1973) Two or more intra AV nodal pathways in association with either a James or Kent extranodal bypass in 3 patients with paroxysmal supraventricular tachycardia. *British Heart Journal* **35**, 113

Spurrell RAJ, Krikler DM, Sowton E. (1974a) Concealed bypass of the atrioventricular node in patients with paroxysmal supraventricular tachycardia revealed by intracardiac electrical stimulation and verapamil. *American Journal of Cardiology* **33**, 590

Spurrell RAJ, Krikler DM, Sowton E. (1974b) Retrograde invasion of the bundle branches producing aberration of the QRS complex during supraventricular tachycardia studied by programmed electrical stimulation. *Circulation* **50**, 487

Spurrell RAJ. (1976) Reciprocation: a mechanism for tachycardias. *American Heart Journal* **91**, 409

Strasberg B, Swiryn S, Bauernfeind R, Palileo E, Scagliotti D, Duffy CE, Rosen KM. (1981) Retrograde dual atrioventricular nodal pathways. *American Journal of Cardiology* **48**, 639

Sung RJ, Gelband H, Castellanos A, Aranda JM, Myerburg RJ. (1977) Clinical and electrophysiologic observations in patients with concealed accessory bypass tracts. *American Journal of Cardiology* **40**, 839

Sung RJ, Styperek JL, Myerburg RJ, Castellanos A. (1978) Initiation of two distinct forms of atrioventricular nodal reentrant tachycardia during programmed ventricular stimulation in man. *American Journal of Cardiology* **42**, 404

Sung RJ, Styperek JL. (1979) Electrophysiologic identification of dual atrioventricular nodal pathway conduction in patients with reciprocating tachycardia using anomalous bypass tracts. *Circulation* **60**, 1464

Sung RJ, Waxman HL, Saksena S, Juma Z. (1981) Sequence of retrograde atrial activation in patients with dual atrioventricular nodal pathways. *Circulation* **64**, 1059

Sung RJ. (1983) Incessant supraventricular tachycardia. *Pacing and Clinical Electrophysiology* **6**, 1306

Touboul P, Huerta F, Arnaud P, Porte J, Delahaye JP (1975) Etude electrophysiologique de deux cas de preexcitation ventriculaire compatibles avec la presence de fibres de Mahaim. *Archives des Maladies du Coeur* **68**, 841

Touboul P, Vexler RM, Chatelain MT. (1978) Re-entry via Mahaim fibres as a possible basis for tachycardia. *British Heart Journal* **40**, 806

Ward DE, Camm AJ, Spurrell RAJ. (1978) Reentrant tachycardia using two bypass tracts and excluding AV node in short PR interval, normal QRS syndrome. *British Heart Journal* **40**, 1127

Ward DE, Camm AJ, Spurrell RAJ. (1979a) Ectopic ventricular tachycardia in association with a concealed accessory pathway. *European Journal of Cardiology* 9, 473

Ward DE, Camm AJ, Spurrell RAJ. (1979b) Ventricular preexcitation due to anomalous nodoventricular pathways: report of 3 cases. *European Journal of Cardiology* 9, 111

Ward DE, Camm AJ, Spurrell RAJ. (1979c) Patterns of atrial activation during right ventricular pacing in patients with concealed left-sided Kent pathways. *British Heart Journal* 42, 192

Ward DE, Camm AJ, Cory-Pearce R, Fuenmayor I, Rees GM, Spurrell RAJ. (1979d) Ebstein's anomaly in association with anomalous nodoventricular conduction. Preoperative and intraoperative electrophysiological studies. *Journal of Electrocardiology* 12, 227

Ward DE, Camm AJ. (1982) Ventriculo-atrial conduction over accessory pathways exhibiting decremental properties. *European Heart Journal* 3, 267

Ward DE, Camm AJ. (1983) Mechanisms of junctional tachycardia in the Lown–Ganong–Levine syndrome. *American Heart Journal* 105, 169

Ward DE, Bexton RS, Camm AJ. (1983) Characteristics of atrio–His conduction in the short PR interval, normal QRS complex syndrome. Evidence for enhanced slow pathway conduction. *European Heart Journal* 4, 882

Ward DE, Bennett DH, Camm AJ. (1984) Mechanisms of junctional tachycardia showing ventricular preexcitation. *British Heart Journal* 52, 369

Waxman MB, Bonet JF, Finley JP, Wald RW. (1980a) Effects of respiration and posture on paroxysmal supraventricular tachycardia. *Circulation* 62, 1011

Waxman MB, Wald RW, Sharma AD, Huerta F, Cameron DA. (1980b) Vagal techniques for termination of paroxysmal supraventricular tachycardia. *American Journal of Cardiology* 46, 655

Weiss J, Cabeen WR, Roberts NK. (1981) Nodoventricular accessory atrioventricular connection with dual atrioventricular pathways: a case report and review of the literature. *Journal of Electrocardiology* 14, 185

Wellens HJJ, Durrer D. (1968) Supraventricular tachycardia with left aberrant conduction due to retrograde invasion into the left bundle branch. *Circulation* 36, 673

Wellens HJJ, Schuilenberg RM, Durrer D. (1971) Electrical stimulation of the heart in patients with Wolff–Parkinson–White syndrome, type A. *Circulation* 43, 99

Wellens HJJ, Durrer D. (1973) Combined conduction disturbances in two AV pathways in patients with Wolff–Parkinson–White syndrome. *European Journal of Cardiology* 1, 23

Wellens HJJ, Durrer D. (1974a) Patterns of ventriculoatrial conduction in the Wolff–Parkinson–White syndrome. *Circulation* 49, 22

Wellens HJJ, Durrer D. (1974b) Wolff–Parkinson–White syndrome and atrial fibrillation: relation between refractory period of accessory pathway and ventricular rate during atrial fibrillation. *American Journal of Cardiology* 34, 777

Wellens HJJ, Durrer D. (1975) The role of an accessory atrioventricular pathway in reciprocal tachycardia. Observations in patients with and without the Wolff–Parkinson–White syndrome. *Circulation* 52, 58

Wellens HJJ, Wesdorp JC, Duren DR, Lie LK. (1976) Second degree block during reciprocal atrioventricular nodal tachycardia. *Circulation* 53, 595

Wellens HJJ. (1979) The electrophysiological properties of the accessory pathway in the Wolff–Parkinson–White syndrome. In: *Conduction System of the Heart*, p. 567. Ed. by HJJ Wellens, KI Lie, MJ Janse. Lea & Febiger, Philadelphia, Pa

Wellens HJJ, Farre J, Bar FW. (1979) Wolff–Parkinson–White syndrome: value and limitations of programmed electrical stimulation. In: *Cardiac Arrhythmias: Electrophysiology, Diagnosis and Management*, p. 589. Ed. by O Narula. Williams & Wilkins, Baltimore, Md

Wellens HJJ, Ross DL, Farre J, Brugada P. (1985) Functional bundle branch block during supraventricular tachycardia in man: observations on mechanisms and their incidence. In: *Cardiac Electrophysiology and Arrhythmias*, p. 435. Ed. by D Zipes, J Jalife. Grune & Stratton: Orlando, Fla

Wu D, Denes P, Amat-y-Leon F, Wyndham CR, Dhingra R, Rosen KM. (1977) An unusual variety of atrioventricular nodal reentry due to retrograde dual atrioventricular nodal pathways. *Circulation* **56**, 50

Wu D, Denes P, Amaty-y-Leon F, Dhingra R, Wyndham CRC, Bauernfeind R, Latif P, Rosen KM. (1978) Clinical, electrocardiographic and electrophysiologic observations in patients with paroxysmal supraventricular tachycardia. *American Journal of Cardiology* **41**, 1045

Wu D. (1983) A-V nodal reentry. *Pacing and Clinical Electrophysiology* **6**, 1190

Wu D, Hwai-Cheng K, San-Jou Y, Fun-Chung L, Jui-Sung H. (1984) Determinants of tachycardia induction using ventricular stimulation in dual pathway atrioventricular nodal reentrant tachycardia. *American Heart Journal* **108**, 44

Zaman L, Garcia N, Luceri RM, Castellanos A, Myerburg RJ. (1983) Ectopic left atrial rhythm that produces QRS changes in absence of Wolff–Parkinson–White syndrome. *Circulation* **68**, 701

Zipes DP, DeJoseph RL, Rothbaum DA. (1974) Unusual properties of accessory pathways. *Circulation* **49**, 1200

10

Ventricular Tachycardias

Ventricular tachycardias are a complex group of arrhythmias of diverse mechanisms, multifarious aetiologies and protean clinical manifestations, ranging from palpitations to sudden death. In Europe and North America the commonest cause of this arrhythmia is chronic ischaemic myocardial disease. The mechanisms, investigation and prognostic implications of ventricular tachycardia in association with acute myocardial ischaemia and reperfusion of ischaemic muscle are distinctly different from recurrent ventricular tachycardias associated with myocardial scarring, and electrophysiological investigations are generally not indicated in these groups of patients. These aspects of ventricular tachycardias will not be discussed.

In most cases of chronic recurrent ventricular tachycardia, organic heart disease of some form or another is present. Thus, in addition to ventricular disease related to coronary artery disease, other causes include the 'dilated' cardiomyopathies, hypertrophic cardiomyopathy, right ventricular dysplasia and ventricular surgery for congenital heart disease.

Ventricular tachycardias also occur in the absence of cardiac disease and there are several distinct types described by the QRS morphology. Two forms have been well studied.

1. Tachycardia with right bundle branch block and left axis deviation which presents as recurrent paroxysmal tachycardia.
2. Tachycardia with left bundle branch block pattern and inferior or right axis deviation often paroxysmal and precipitated by exertion.

Ventricular tachycardia may be sustained or non-sustained. This distinction is relevant in that the value of electrophysiological studies is more clearly defined for the sustained variety, and the outlook for non-sustained tachycardia may be better than for sustained ventricular tachycardia.

Diagnosis of ventricular tachycardia

No other arrhythmia has given rise to so much electrocardiographic confusion. The currently accepted diagnostic criteria for ventricular tachycardias comprise four basic groups of ECG features which provide important information:

1. Atrioventricular dissociation.
2. QRS duration >140 msec.
3. QRS axis more negative than −30 degrees.
4. Specific QRS morphologies.

These phenomena are best appreciated on a 12-lead ECG of tachycardia and it is essential that this is recorded if the patient is not haemodynamically unstable.

Atrioventricular dissociation is a strong indicator of ventricular tachycardia. There are several electrocardiographic clues of its being present:

1. The presence of an atrial rhythm which has no causal relationship with the tachycardia complexes; this is described as AV dissociation (the atrial rhythm may be sinus rhythm or any atrial tachycardia).
2. As a result of AV dissociation, capture beats and fusion beats may occur but they are not an inevitable consequence of AV dissociation because other factors (tachycardia rate, ventricular refractoriness) may prevent their expression.
3. Ventriculoatrial conduction during tachycardia is not uncommon and may cause confusion if there is a 1:1 correspondence. On occasions, variable or blocked VA conduction is observed when the retrograde P waves have a clear relationship with the tachycardia complexes, confirming a ventricular origin. The cycle length of ventricular tachycardia is often variable (by ±40 msec). When changes in atrial cycle length follow changes in QRS cycle length, a ventricular origin is most likely. An exception is atrioventricular re-entrant tachycardia (see Chapter 8).

If the QRS duration is greater than 140 msec this indicates markedly slowed intramyocardial conduction, and ventricular tachycardia is much more likely than supraventricular tachycardia with bundle branch block – a notorious source of confusion. The wider the QRS, the more likely the tachycardia is to be of ventricular origin.

A change of axis from the normal range to markedly leftward or rightward at the onset of tachycardia is also strongly suggestive of ventricular tachycardia. This is very uncommon with supraventricular tachycardias unless they show ventricular pre-excitation (Chapter 9). In patients with pre-existing bundle branch block a different QRS morphology during tachycardia suggests a ventricular origin.

Certain types of QRS morphology are characteristic of ventricular tachycardia. Uniformly positive or negative complexes in the chest leads (concordant patterns) strongly indicate a ventricular tachycardia. Particular types of QRS are also more commonly found in ventricular tachycardia than in supraventricular tachycardia with bundle branch aberration. An Rsr' in lead V1 or a deep S wave (rS) in V6 are especially useful and easily remembered. The presence of separate episodes with multiple QRS types or a changing QRS morphology during tachycardia is strongly indicative of ventricular tachycardia. The QRS morphology cannot be used to ascribe the source of tachycardia to right or left ventricles, a commonly held but incorrect assumption. A 'right bundle branch block' pattern is usually of left ventricular origin but a 'left bundle branch block' pattern may arise from either the right ventricle or the interventricular septum.

Mechanisms of ventricular tachycardia

Several investigators in the late nineteenth and early twentieth centuries had suspected that ventricular tachycardia (and fibrillation) was probably caused by circus movement. Experimental and clinical evidence for this as the most important mechanism for clinical ventricular tachycardia was not forthcoming until quite recently. Whereas Garrey (1914) and Mines (1913, 1914) had thought a 'circulating rhythm' responsible, Lewis (1925) initially favoured the concept of 'ectopic impulses'. In 1972 Wellens and associates demonstrated repeated initiation of ventricular tachycardia in 5 patients with organic heart disease (old infarction in 4 patients). They also noted that termination of the arrhythmias by either one or two timed stimuli was possible in all patients. They interpreted these findings as strongly suggestive of re-entrant excitation. In a later communication Wellens and colleagues (1976) demonstrated the role of slowed conduction in the initiation of the tachycardia, further supporting the re-entry theory. These observations have now been confirmed by many investigators, and other evidence for clinical re-entrant ventricular excitation has been adduced – in particular,

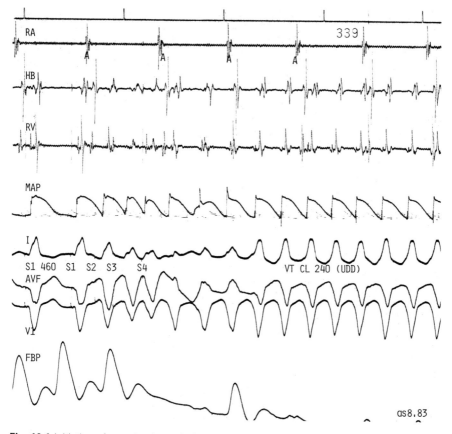

Fig. 10.1 Initiation of sustained ventricular tachycardia by ventricular pacing (S1S1) at a cycle length of 460 msec and triple ventricular extrastimulation (S2S3S4). The systemic arterial pressure in the femoral artery (FBP) falls dramatically but recovers within several seconds (not shown). Paper speed 50 mm/sec. A = atrial electrogram; MAP = monophasic action potential; UDD = 'up, down, down' indicating the direction of the QRS in leads I, AVF and V1 (see also Fig. 12.5).

localized delayed activitation (late potentials) during sinus rhythm and continuous electrical activity during ventricular tachycardia demonstrated by endocardial mapping (see below). The concept of 'entrainment' (see Chapter 7) has also been used to prove the re-entrant basis of many ventricular tachycardias (MacLean et al., 1981; Waldo et al., 1984).

Although the subject of great speculation, the importance of triggered automaticity in the generation of clinical ventricular tachycardias is unknown (see Chapter 8). Abnormal automaticity may account for some ventricular arrhythmias in the acute phase of myocardial ischaemia. It is not sufficient to conclude that automatic mechanisms of tachycardia are more likely and re-entrant excitation less likely, merely because the accepted classic features of re-entry cannot be demonstrated, for reasons determined by other factors (e.g. site and intensity of stimulation, rate or coupling interval of stimulation, etc.).

Electrophysiological observations in patients with recurrent ventricular tachycardias

Ventricular tachycardia associated with chronic coronary artery disease

The initiation and termination of ventricular tachycardia by extrastimulation has been referred to above and is taken as strong evidence for a re-entrant mechanism (Fig. 10.1). This observation has laid the foundation for electrophysiologically based drug, pacemaker and ablation therapies for ventricular tachycardia. Ventricular tachycardia can be induced in the laboratory in over 90 per cent of

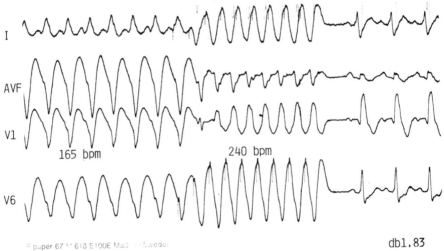

Fig. 10.2 Termination of ventricular tachycardia by rapid left ventricular pacing. In this patient, right ventricular pacing at a similar rate was not effective in terminating the tachycardia. Pacing the left ventricle close to the endocardially mapped origin of the arrhythmia resulted in prompt and safe termination. Paper speed 25 mm/sec.

patients with spontaneous ventricular tachycardia associated with previous myocardial infarction or chronic coronary disease. Termination by premature stimulation is likely to succeed in only two-thirds of instances. Two or more premature stimuli are usually needed, and often (in more than 85 per cent) only a rapid burst of pacing is effective. This is, unfortunately, associated with a high risk of tachycardia acceleration or degeneration to ventricular fibrillation (Fig. 10.2). The electrophysiological characteristics of re-entrant ventricular tachycardia are listed in Table 10.1.

Endocardial mapping studies

Using a multipolar electrode catheter it is possible to explore the endocardial surface and to determine the activation sequence by timing electrograms. The origin of tachycardia is closest to the earliest site of endocardial activation during tachycardia. The earliest detectable electrogram often precedes the onset of the surface QRS complex by 20–40 msec (Fig. 10.3). In many instances localized, prolonged and 'fractionated electrograms' can be recorded during sinus rhythm (Fig. 10.4). These abnormal electrograms probably represent areas of slow conduction in abnormal myocardium. Delayed potentials can also be detected using signal-averaged surface electrocardiography. Using the ventricular extrastimulus method, these fractionated electrograms may become increasingly fragmented as the coupling interval of the extrastimulus is decreased or the pacing rate increased (Fig. 10.4). This phenomenon may reflect the development of slowed conduction necessary to initiate re-entrant excitation. It has been suggested that it is artefactual (Waxman and Sung, 1980), generated as a result of a catheter movement and technical aspects of the recording system. With the weight of evidence from transvenous and operative endocardial studies now available (Josephson and Wit, 1984), this seems improbable.

Table 10.1 ELECTROPHYSIOLOGICAL CHARACTERISTICS OF RE-ENTRANT VENTRICULAR TACHYCARDIA

Provoked and terminated by ventricular, but not atrial, premature beats *

Atrial dissociation may be present, or may be induced

Abnormal ventricular activation †

His dissociation or negative HV time ●

Normal atrial activation patterns §

---

* Atrial premature beats which provoke ventricular tachycardia must conduct to the ventricles.

† Ventricular activation may resemble an aberrant beat if tachycardia arises from, or close to, the His–Purkinje fascicles.

● The His depolarization may be enveloped within the ventricular electrogram.

§ Atrial activation may be retrograde (VA conduction) or abnormal (concomitant atrial arrhythmia, retrograde conduction via a bystander anomalous pathway).

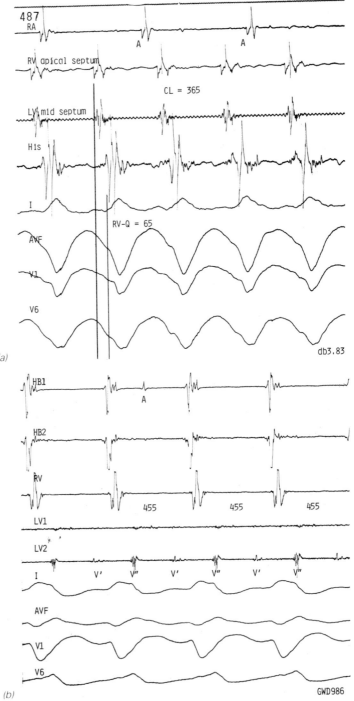

(a)

487
RA
          A   A

RV apical septum

CL = 365

LV mid septum

H1s

I

RV-Q = 65

AVF

V1

V6

db3.83

(b)

HB1
        A

HB2

RV
        455   455   455

LV1

LV2

I
V' V'' V' V'' V' V''

AVF

V1

V6

GWD986

During sustained tachycardia, in localized areas close to its origin, the duration of the fragmented signals may be markedly prolonged (Fig. 10.4), occasionally extending throughout the tachycardia cycle. This 'continuous electrical activity' (Josephson et al., 1978c) was thought to reflect activation of the entire microre-entrant loop. The meaning of continuous activity during tachycardia is debated. Recently, Brugada and colleagues (1985) have shown that similar activity may appear or disappear spontaneously or can be disturbed by stimulation without affecting continued tachycardia, implying that it can be recorded from areas of electrically abnormal myocardium not needed to sustain tachycardia (e.g. from loops not on the circuit). Another phenomenon seen occasionally during endocardial mapping is localized double potential electrograms (see Fig. 10.3). This is thought to represent activation of adjacent parts of myocardium which are electrically separated. For example, activation of 'blind loops' of tissue in the centre of a wavefront circulating around an area of functional block may result in double potentials in a recording close to such loops. An alternative explanation advanced by Olshansky (1986, personal communication) is that these double potentials may reflect conduction across an area of slowed conduction. Thus, the closely coupled components (say, A and B) of the double potential do not reflect the same impulse, but successive impulses. That is, B is the deflection recorded prior to slowed conduction and A after propagation through the area of slowed conduction. Thus, B is linked with A (rather than A with B) but separated from it by a long isoelectric segment. It is likely that double potentials may be produced by several different unrelated mechanisms.

Recent evidence has demonstrated that re-entry over large areas of myocardium (re-entry over a 'continuous loop') is a mechanism of sustained ventricular tachycardia in some patients (Miller et al., 1985b). In this setting, endocardial mapping from the entire area of the loop shows electrograms throughout the cycle and the concept of 'earliest site of activation' becomes less meaningful. It may be arbitrarily defined as activity occurring within 20–40 msec of the onset of the QRS. Gessman et al. (1983) defined earliest activation of a

---

Fig. 10.3 Endocardial mapping of ventricular tachycardia. (*a*) Right and left ventricular electrode catheters were used to map this tachycardia in a patient with a left ventricular aneurysm after myocardial infarction. Earliest endocardial activation was located in the region of the apical part of the septum on the right ventricular aspect 65 msec before the onset of the QRS complex (not easy to determine). The left ventricular mid-septal electrodes recorded activity 10 msec later. The local electrograms at both sites are abnormal, that at the right ventricular apical septum being distinctly split into two components. (*b*) Right and left endocardial mapping in this tachycardia (also associated with a left ventricular aneurysm) revealed earliest activation in the septum near the left ventricular apex (LV2). The recordings from this site showed two distinct electrograms in each cycle. One (V') precedes the onset of the QRS by 70 msec and the second (V'') occurs late in the QRS. The origin of these double potentials is not clear. Possible explanations include (1) recordings from different parts of the re-entrant loop, (2) recordings from vortices or blind loops within a re-entrant circuit, or (3) a combination of these (i.e. one reflecting the re-entrant impulse and another being an 'epiphenomenon'). In this particular example the earliest deflection (V') could be entrained but not the later electrogram (V''), which was activated orthodromically from the pacing site. Termination of tachycardia during entrainment was associated with block towards V'. Thus, V' probably reflects early activity on or near to the circuit and V'' is incidental depolarization of tissue not on circuit but close to the electrodes. Paper speed 100 mm/sec. HB = His bundle region; LV = left ventricle; RV = right ventricle. (*Kindly supplied by Dr D. W. Davies*)

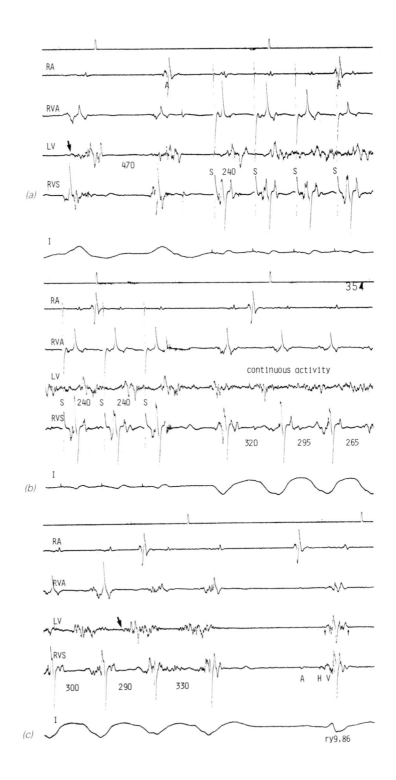

macrore-entrant loop tachycardia in dogs as the earliest electrogram recorded within 10 msec of the start of the QRS. This was found at the zone of transition from the slow conducting, late diastolic part of the circuit to the fast, early systolic part of the circuit. These authors successfully terminated canine macrore-entrant tachycardias using cryosurgery at a point remote from the 'site of origin'. Mason et al. (1985) have emphasized that mapping techniques may not provide enough information to distinguish between focal re-entry with centrifugal spread and macrore-entry over a large loop. However, in their study, only 24 sites were mapped, whereas Miller et al. (1985b) sampled up to 120 sites.

The presence of endocardial fractionated electrograms during sinus rhythm was proposed as a marker of the tachycardia substrate, especially as such signals could be recorded in areas generating continuous activity during tachycardia. Further studies of this phenomenon (Kienzle et al. 1984) have shown, however, that fractionation is recorded from the site of earliest endocardial activation (the supposed origin of tachycardia) in only a small proportion of patients. It is a specific but insensitive indicator of the tachycardia origin.

The electrophysiological responses to stimulation and the detailed data from endocardial mapping studies have shown that most ventricular tachycardias associated with coronary artery disease arise from small areas of damaged endocardium on the borders of a myocardial scar (localized re-entry). If this is so, it should be possible to mimic the QRS morphology of the tachycardia by pacing at the supposed site of origin (described as 'pacemapping') of tachycardia determined by the methods discussed above (Fig. 10.5). To some extent the method achieves this, presumably because the tachycardia origin is localized to a small area (effectively a point source).

Intramyocardial or epicardial origin of tachycardia cannot be accurately localized by this technique. Also, pacing at several different sites within a small area can produce similar morphologies, which is unhelpful. Pacing at higher

---

Fig. 10.4 Fractionated and continuous electrical activity. (*a*) Initiation of right ventricular (RV) pacing (S1S1 = 240 msec) during ventricular tachycardia of cycle length 470 msec. The left ventricular (LV) recording site shows fractionated and prolonged electrograms during tachycardia (arrowed). At the start of pacing the fractionation becomes more marked and extends throughout the cycle. (*b*) Pacing is turned off and a different, faster, tachycardia emerges (cycle length 320 msec). The LV recording site now reveals continuous electrical activity. When this tachycardia terminates spontaneously, there is abrupt disappearance of continuous electrical activity (*c*). Immediately prior to termination, the continuous electrical activity seems to become more organized but still extends through most of the cycle (large arrow). The electrogram recorded from this site during sinus rhythm is also fractionated and prolonged, with onset to termination (small arrows) separated by 140 msec. For convenience, only one surface lead is shown.

The interpretation of these findings is not straightforward. The observation that pacing results in a change from non-continuous to continuous electrical activity with emergence of a new, faster tachycardia might suggest that a different substrate is activated. Whether or not the continuous activity directly reflects re-entrant excitation is not known. The transition from continuous to non-continuous activity (bottom) without any change in the tachycardia rate or morphology is consistent with the idea that this type of electrical activity is incidentical to the tachycardia (an 'epiphenomenon'). On the other hand, the transition preceded (by two cycles) termination of the tachycardia. Although rapid pacing during the slower tachycardia did result in continuous activity (top), it was only when this activity was sustained after termination of pacing that the faster tachycardia emerged. Paper speed 100 mm/sec. A = atrial electrogram; RVA = right ventricular apex; RA = right atrium; RVS = right ventricular septum.

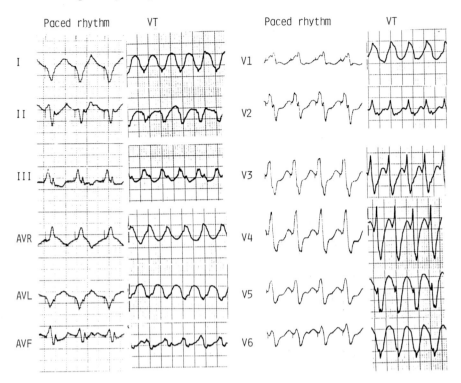

Fig. 10.5 Recordings illustrating the principle of 'pacemapping' in a 55-year-old male patient with refractory ventricular tachycardia (VT). The spontaneous tachycardia is shown to the right of each panel. Pacing the left ventricle at several sites on the septum and free wall resulted in different QRS morphologies. The paced QRS (shown to the left of each panel) which most closely matched the spontaneous tachycardia QRS was obtained by stimulation of the left free wall mid-way between the aortic valve and the apex. An identical match in all 12 leads could not be achieved despite detailed mapping in a small area. Nevertheless, transarterial catheter ablation in this region was successful in the long term.

energies may recruit more myocardium, with consequent changes of QRS shape without a change of pacing site. Simultaneous multiple lead recordings of some ventricular tachycardias may show marked phase shifts between one lead and another (QRS onset in one lead is markedly delayed compared to another). Presumably this is a reflection, in part, of concealed depolarization vectors, and also of phasic activation. In such a setting pacemapping cannot be expected to imitate tachycardia.

Because rate may also have an effect on intramyocardial conduction velocity and hence the QRS shape, pacemapping should be performed at the rate of tachycardia. There is no doubt, however, that it is an important corroborative method of localizing the tachycardia origin and is likely to be of considerable importance in the application of transvascular ablation to ventricular tachycardias (Chapter 15).

With larger circuits of the type mentioned above, this type of pacemapping would not be expected to reproduce the QRS morphology of tachycardia because it is not possible to mimic activation emanating from a large re-entrant circuit by pacing at a point unless there is sustained unidirectional block during pacing such that the circuit is activated in the same manner as in tachycardia. This latter phenomenon is known as entrainment.

The phenomenon of entrainment was first described in relation to atrial flutter (see Chapter 7) but it is becoming increasingly important in the study of ventricular tachycardia. Using this method, it may be possible to demonstrate re-entry as the mechanism of a ventricular tachycardia and to define the area of slow conduction necessary for re-entry to continue (Josephson et al., 1985).

Ventricular tachycardias associated with other forms of heart disease

Arrhythmogenic right ventricular dysplasia

This condition is a form of cardiomyopathy affecting localized areas of the right ventricle or, in severe forms, the entire heart. The characteristic pathological feature is fatty infilatrion and fibrosis of the myocardium in the outflow tract and at the base and the apex of the right ventricle (and occasionally affecting the left ventricle). This provides a substrate for re-entry, a mechanism which is strongly suggested by the electrophysiological features of this condition. During sinus rhythm delayed excitation is sometimes obvious even on the conventional surface ECG ('epsilon' waves). Endocardial mapping may show pronounced late potentials. Wide potentials are also seen.

The tachycardias arise from the right ventricle. During tachycardia the QRS complexes show left bundle branch block pattern with variable abnormal axes (i.e. rightward or leftward axis deviation). Different episodes of tachycardia may show multiple QRS morphologies. Tachycardias are commonly inducible by extrastimulus techniques but the induced tachycardias may be of different QRS morphology from spontaneous tachycardias.

Ventricular surgery for congenital heart disease

Ventricular tachycardias after correction of congenital heart disease are a recognized complication of surgery. The condition in which these tachycardias have been studied most is tetralogy of Fallot. In these cases it has been observed that tachycardias may be induced and terminated by stimulation. During tachycardia, which in most instances is localized to the region of a ventricular incision scar, continuous electrical activity has been recorded. Re-entry around the scar tissue has been postulated.

Dilated cardiomyopathies

There is a high incidence of sustained and non-sustained ventricular tachycardias in these conditions. Late potentials may sometimes be recorded and tachycardias are often inducible during electrophysiological study. Tachycardias may have multiple morphologies or may be monomorphic. The value of serial drug testing with conventional antiarrhythmic drugs in this clinical context is not known (see below).

Other diseases

In hypertrophic cardiomyopathy ventricular tachycardia is ominous. Such tachycardias may sometimes be provoked but there is little electrophysiological information about this condition. Some have said that electrophysiological investigation of hypertrophic cardiomyopathy patients is dangerous. In any case, the value of the findings is open to question (see below).

Mitral valve prolapse is associated with non-sustained ventricular arrhythmias. Only in patients with documented ventricular tachycardia can a ventricular arrhythmia be provoked at study. These are often polymorphic and non-sustained, and their electrophysiologic basis is not known.

Ventricular tachycardia not associated with heart disease

Fascicular tachycardia

This form of tachycardia, which may be provoked by exertion, tends to occur in otherwise healthy, young people with no evidence of structural heart disease. During sinus rhythm the QRS complex is usually normal, but minor repolarization changes are seen in most patients. During tachycardia the QRS complexes are relatively narrow (<140 msec) and resemble right bundle branch block (Fig. 10.6) At the onset of tachycardia there is almost always a significant leftward axis shift.

The electrophysiological features of this tachycardia include:

1. Initiation by ventricular extrastimulation and often characteristically by rapid atrial pacing.
2. Termination by premature stimulation and rapid pacing in either the atrium or the ventricle.
3. AV dissociation is usual but a His (or fascicular) potential is associated with each QRS complex. This potential may be inscribed shortly before, simultaneous with or shortly after the onset of the QRS but the 'HV' interval is always less than during sinus rhythm (Fig. 10.7).
4. Atrial stimulation during tachycardia may result in capture of the His bundle alone or both the His bundle and the ventricles with a normal HV interval (i.e. longer than that during tachycardia). The QRS complex which results is usually identical to that during sinus rhythm (Fig. 10.8).

These characteristics suggest a re-entrant basis of fascicular tachycardia. In most cases it would appear that the re-entry does not involve the proximal His–Purkinje system but is localized (microre-entry) to the territory of the left posterior fascicle.

Sustained fascicular tachycardia due to macrore-entry around the major bundle branches is extremely rare. It differs in that capture of the ventricles by a supraventricular beat resulting in a complex identical to that seen during sinus rhythm is impossible unless tachycardias associated with nodoventricular pathways may involve retrograde re-entrant excitation of the His–Purkinje system following anterograde activation of the nodoventricular pathway. This

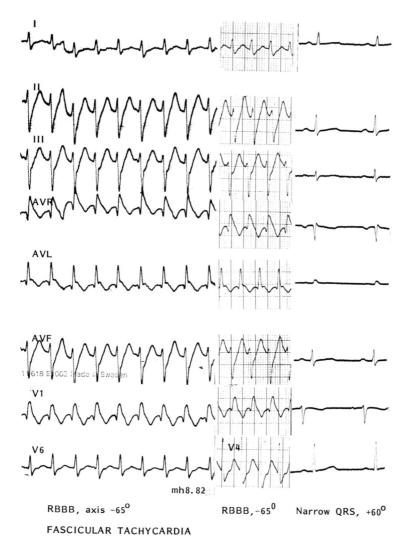

RBBB, axis -65°   RBBB, -65°   Narrow QRS, +60°

FASCICULAR TACHYCARDIA

Fig. 10.6 Surface ECG recordings of fascicular tachycardia. This patient had recurrent episodes of tachycardia which could be repeatedly terminated be verapamil and were regarded as 'SVT'. These recordings show the typical features of fascicular tachycardia. The axis during tachycardia is shifted to the left compared with sinus rhythm. The QRS complexes show right bundle branch block morphology. Left panel: tachycardia induced at electrophysiological study. Centre panel: spontaneous tachycardia. Right panel: sinus rhythm. Paper speed 25 mm/sec.

would therefore be a form of fascicular tachycardia. Because these anomalous pathways insert into the right ventricular septum, this type of anomalous conduction shows a 'left bundle branch block' pattern which is present during tachycardia. Other mechanisms for these tachycardias are also possible (see Chapter 8).

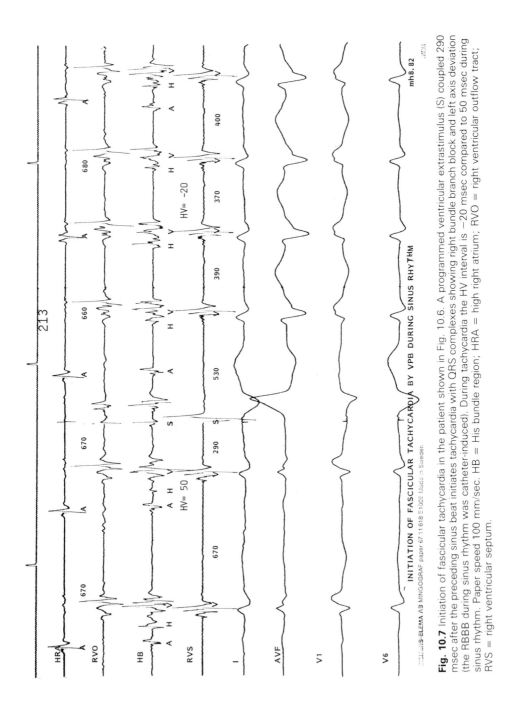

Fig. 10.7 Initiation of fascicular tachycardia in the patient shown in Fig. 10.6. A programmed ventricular extrastimulus (S) coupled 290 msec after the preceding sinus beat initiates tachycardia with QRS complexes showing right bundle branch block and left axis deviation (the RBBB during sinus rhythm was catheter-induced). During tachycardia the HV interval is –20 msec compared to 50 msec during sinus rhythm. Paper speed 100 mm/sec. HB = His bundle region; HRA = high right atrium; RVO = right ventricular outflow tract; RVS = right ventricular septum.

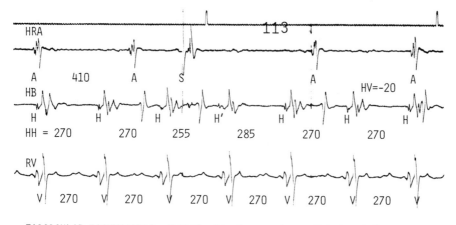

FASCICULAR TACHYCARDIA. Atrial stimulus captures H but not V.

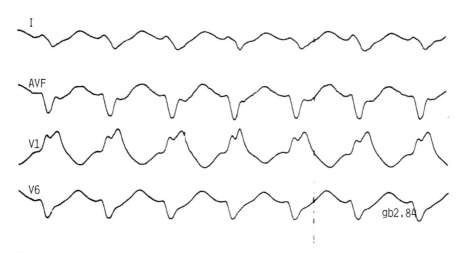

Fig. 10.8 The effect of an atrial premature stimulus during fascicular tachycardia in 30-year-old man. The recordings show the typical features of the tachycardia. An atrial premature stimulus (S) conducts to the His bundle, advancing the His bundle electrogram by 15 msec without altering the timing of the QRS. This phenomenon excludes participation of the His bundle in the re-entry circuit, which is most probably located in the left posterior fascicle. Paper speed 100 mm/sec. HRA = high right atrium; HB = His bundle region; RV = right ventricle.

Exercise-induced right ventricular tachycardia

Approximately 50 per cent of patients with ventricular tachycardias which may be induced by exercise have ischaemic heart disease. Of the remainder, most have cardiomyopathy, particularly minor forms of right ventricular dysplasia (see above), or fascicular tachycardia.

A small proportion, some of whom are trained athletes, have tachycardia which can be localized to the right ventricular outflow tract. The ECG during

Induced VT   Spontaneous VT

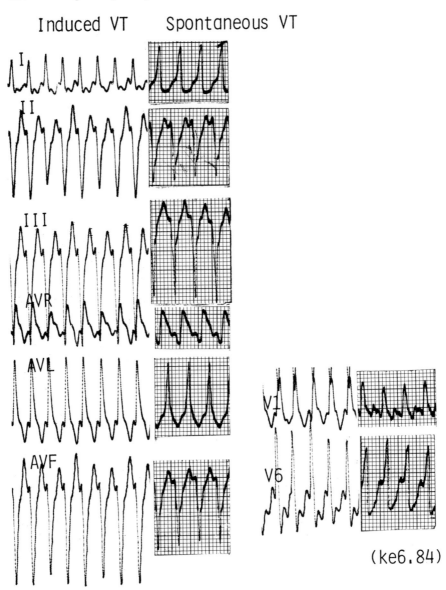

(ke6.84)

Fig. 10.9 Comparison of induced (left) and spontaneous (right) ventricular tachycardia (VT) in each of eight leads. The QRS morphology and rate of the induced tachycardia are virtually identical to that of the spontaneous clinically occurring episodes. This indicates a single mechanism and location of both tachycardias. Paper speed 25 mm/sec.

tachycardia shows left bundle branch block and rightward axis. Sometimes these tachycardias can be induced by electrical stimulation techniques, but about one-third to one-half are provoked by isoprenaline infusion, supporting the notion that they are catetholamine-dependent. Their mechanism is obscure.

Table 10.2 BASIC STUDY PLAN FOR VENTRICULAR TACHYCARDIA

Record conduction intervals during sinus rhythm (search for late potentials, etc.)

Determine anterograde and retrograde conduction characteristics

Provoke tachycardia (Table 10.4)

Prove ventricular origin of tachycardia (Table 10.1)

Map earliest activation and explore ventricles for fractionated activity

Terminate tachycardia with:
    Pacing techniques
    Internal cardioversion
    Drugs *or*
    external cardioversion

Administer intravenous antiarrrhythmic drugs

Reassess inducibility of tachycardia, etc.

Clinical electrophysiological studies of patients with ventricular tachycardia

The use of intracardiac studies for the assessment of ventricular tachycardia is based on several principles derived from the study of sustained ventricular tachycardias in patients with coronary artery disease:

1. Inducible monomorphic tachycardia is rare in patients without spontaneous ventricular tachycardia.
2. Tachycardia can be induced in over 90 per cent of patients with spontaneous recurrent sustained monomorphic ventricular tachycardia.
3. Usually the arrhythmia provoked in the laboratory is morphologically (similar QRS complexes in three or more leads, and at a similar rate) identical to the spontaneous episodes (Fig. 10.9).
4. A favourable long-term prognosis is associated with suppression (non-inducibility) of tachycardia with an antiarrhythmic drug (see Chapter 12).
5. When tachycardia remains inducible, the risk of spontaneous recurrence is high.

A possible plan for the clinical electrophysiological study of a patient with ventricular tachycardia is summarized in Table 10.2.

Limitations of the principles of study

There is considerable debate about the principles enumerated above. Although it has been shown that inducible stable monomorphic tachycardia is rare in patients without spontaneous episodes, it is now emerging that this finding may be largely a function of the protocol used to stimulate the ventricular myocardium. For example, 'aggressive' burst pacing or large numbers (three or more) of extrastimuli can induce ventricular fibrillation or polymorphic

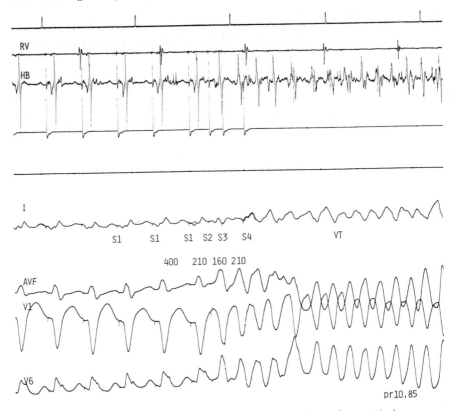

Fig. 10.10 A non-specific response to ventricular stimulation. Aggressive ventricular extrastimulation (three closely coupled beats following rapid (cycle length = 400 msec)), regular right ventricular drive (S1S2) results in sustained polymorphic ventricular tachycardia (VT). Even if this response is produced by one or two ventricular extrastimuli, it is likely to be non-specific (Mahmud et al., 1986). Paper speed 50 mm/sec. HB = His bundle region; RV = right ventricle.

ventricular tachycardia in normal hearts (Fig. 10.10). Furthermore, these aggressive methods are more likely to induce such arrythmias in patients with ventricular disease but without spontaneous tachycardias. It has been pointed out by Brugada and Wellens (1985b) that the sensitivity and specificity of the stimulation method should relate to the presence or absence of spontaneous tachycardia in patients with a comparable extent of disease ('substrate' for tachycardia). Thus, many of the studies claiming high sensitivity and specificity have failed to distinguish between presence or absence of inducible arrhythmia and the presence or absence of a substrate for the arrhythmia (e.g. a myocardial scar). These studies are diminished in value by the fact that they compared patients with myocardial disease and tachycardia with disease-free patients without tachycardia (Vandepol et al., 1980).

Another problem relates to the significance of an induced response. In this context, derivation of sensitivity and specificity, etc., requires comparison of the test result with spontaneously occurring phenomena. In many settings, however, such a comparison is difficult or not possible. Most investigators agree that induction of sustained monomorphic ventricular tachycardia is an important and meaningful endpoint of the study. This is especially so when it can be shown by electrocardiographic comparison that the induced tachycardia closely resembles a previously documented spontaneous tachycardia. Such tachycardias are usually long-lived and stable, allowing documentation. In settings such as spontaneous symptomatic transient (non-sustained) ventricular tachycardia, sudden out-of-hospital cardiac arrest (failed sudden death) and syncope, definitions demanding such comparisons are not possible. Thus the induction of ventricular arrhythmias of any type in these settings has not (directly) been shown to be clinically important. Furthermore, Wellens et al. (1985) have emphasized that reponses such as polymorphic ventricular tachycardia or ventricular fibrillation are not uncommonly induced in patients without spontaneous episodes, especially if aggressive protocols are employed. It has also been shown that the characteristics (rate, mode of initiation, etc.) of polymorphic tachycardia induced in patients with prior mycocardial infarction are not substantially different from those of tachycardias induced in patients with normal hearts (Stevenson et al. 1986b). Monomorphic non-sustained tachycardia can also be induced in a large proportion of patients with ventricular disease but free from the arrhythmia, and as an endpoint of study is subject to similar limitations.

The constraints outlined above limit the value of provocation studies to assess risk (potential substrate for arrhythmia). They are also relevant to the use and interpretation of such studies to establish effective antiarrhythmic therapy (see Chapter 12). If the induced arrhythmias cannot be shown to be clinically relevant, it follows that therapy which suppresses these induced arrhythmias may not suppress spontaneous ones, and the long-term clinical effect is not easily predictable. In patients with recurrent sustained monomorphic tachycardia secondary to coronary artery and left ventricular disease, drug suppression of inducible arrhythmias has been shown to be associated with improved survival when compared to patients in whom no effective suppressive agent was identified (Swerdlow et al., 1983a) (see Chapter 12). Nevertheless, it is still not known whether treatment with an 'ineffective' drug (tachycardia still inducible) other than amiodarone will provide as reliable long-term suppression as an 'effective' drug (tachycardia not inducible). Wellens et al. (1985) have correctly stated that ineffective drugs as well as effective drugs must be used in the long term (a protocol referred to as 'parallel testing') if the true predictive accuracy and clinical value of electrophysiological drug testing is to be established (Brugada and Wellens, 1986) (Fig. 10.11). Such a scheme, however, potentially deprives some patients of 'effective' treatment and subjects them to invasive testing from which no benefit is gained. Unfortunately, there is, as yet, no method of selecting a drug *a priori*. Which patients are likely to benefit from treatment or be harmed by it cannot be predicted without testing. The criteria for defining effective drug treatment using electrophysiological testing are also the subject of controversy (see Chapter 12).

A further concern which has been voiced by several investigators relates to the reproducibility of an induced ventricular tachycardia. This issue is of central importance to the use of provocation testing to assess drug efficacy. Bigger et al. (1986) noted that 87 per cent of patients with inducible tachycardia at a baseline

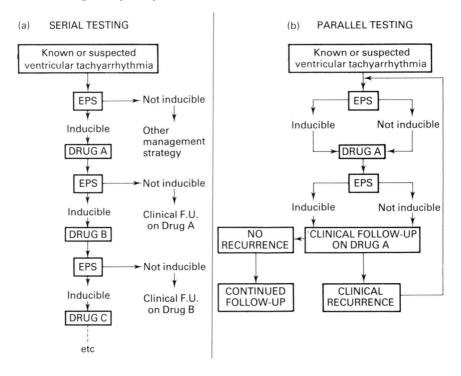

Fig. 10.11 Schematic representation of two methods of formally assessing drug efficacy for long-term treatment of ventricular tachycardia. (*a*) The serial methods which has been widely adopted for clinical purposes. (*b*) An alternative scheme proposed by Wellens et al. (1985). This protocol generates information from which it is possible to derive formally the true sensitivity, specificity and predictive accuracy of electrophysiological testing of a particular drug with respect to long-term clinical outcome (Friedman and Yusuf, 1986).

study could be induced at a subsequent study within 4 days, with a similar QRS type in all but 2 per cent of these patients. In most of these (78 per cent) the same stimulation protocol was effective. Kudenchuk et al. (1986) found the arrhythmias induced by three or more stimuli at initial study were less likely to be reproduced (in terms of rate and mode of initiation) at a subsequent study. Thus, in 27 per cent of 114 patients who had tachycardias induced by quadruple stimuli, the same tachycardia was not induced at a subsequent study. Similar conclusions were reached by Lombardi et al. (1986).

These limitations make interpretation of induced polymorphic tachycardias even more difficult, especially during the course of serial drug testing. The study of Kudenchuk et al. (1986) did not, however, take into account the QRS morphology. In patients with sustained monomorphic ventricular tachycardia (those most likely to benefit from drug testing), reproducibility is less likely to prevent interpretative and clinical difficulties. Buitleir et al. (1986) investigated the immediate (at the time of study) reproducibility of tachycardia induction. They found that 9 per cent of clinical and 23 per cent of non-clinical tachycardias could not be reinduced a few minutes after the initial induction. These findings also have a bearing on the interpretation of apparent drug effects. Furthermore, it would seem that reproducibility *per se* is not an indicator of clinical rather than non-clinical arrhythmias.

The principles enumerated above must therefore be interpreted in the light of the stimulation protocol (see below) and the clinical setting. Since most studies have been based largely on patients with coronary disease, it is important to appreciate that the principles may not apply to the study of ventricular tachycardia associated with other forms of ventricular disease.

Indications for electrophysiological study

The major indication for clinical electrophysiological study of ventricular tachycardia is for the prescription of optimum therapy rather than solely for diagnosis. The indications for study include:

1. Recurrent paroxysmal sustained ventricular tachycardia.
2. Inadequate response to thearpy.
3. Consideration of alternative treatments (including alternative drug treatment, pacemaker, ablation and implantable defibrillator).
4. Electrocardiographic diagnostic difficulties when the surface ECG is confusing, missing or unhelpful.
5. Clinical presentations very suggestive of a ventricular tachycardia, such as syncope of unknown cause, sudden out-of-hospital cardiac arrest and palpitations in a patient with bifascicular block (see Chapter 5).

Several investigators have searched for features which may be used to predict the outcome of electrophysiological drug testing in patients with sustained ventricular arrhythmias (Table 10.3). An easily measurable or derivable indicator which could be used to select patients likely to benefit from the electrophysiological approach and identify those unlikely to gain would be of considerable value. Using discriminant analysis methods, Spielman et al. (1983) were not able to identify a single factor which consistently predicted outcome.

Table 10.3 PREDICTION OF SUCCESSFUL ELECTROPHYSIOLOGICALLY GUIDED DRUG TREATMENT FOR VENTRICULAR TACHYCARDIA

Demographic	*Functional status*
Female Young (<45 years)	Low New York Heart Association grade

Arrhythmia	*Anatomy*
Short history Few unsuccessful drug trials Few spontaneous episodes Inducible only with more than one extrastimulus	Ejection fraction >50% Few coronary stenoses No aneurysms

Modified from Spielman et al. (1983), Swerdlow et al. (1983b) and Anderson and Mason (1986).

Poor left ventricular systolic function (ejection fraction <50 per cent) was the best single variable for prediction of failure. Patients of advanced age with extensive coronary artery disease and poor left ventricular function who have had numerous empirical drug trials seem least likely to benefit from electrophysiological investigation. Unfortunately, these include the patients at highest risk from sudden death after myocardial infarction.

Electrophysiological studies in patients with spontaneous, non-sustained tachycardias

Non-sustained ventricular tachycardia (the definition varies from paper to paper) is often found during ambulatory monitoring, especially in patients with underlying organic heart disease. The prognostic significance of this arrhythmia is probably determined by the presence or absence of important organic heart disease (especially that which causes impairment of left ventricular function). Thus, in patients with non-sustained ventricular tachycardia following myocardial infarction, mortality at one year may be as high as 40 per cent (Bigger et al., 1983). Data from patients with other forms of heart disease are limited. In patients with idiopathic dilated cardiomyopathy, non-sustained ventricular tachycardia appears to have a similar poor prognosis in some studies (Meinertz et al., 1984) although others do not support this conclusion (Huang et al., 1983).

Electrophysiological testing may demonstrate sustained tachycardia in up to one-third of patients with spontaneous non-sustained tachycardia (Breithardt et al., 1986) and may be a risk factor for sudden death (Buxton et al., 1984b). Gomes et al. (1984) performed electrophysiological studies in patients with high grade ventricular ectopic activity but without sustained tachycardia. Survival in patients with inducible sustained tachycardias was significantly less than in those with no sustained tachycardia. In contrast, Veltri et al. (1985) found that inducibility of tachycardia did not predict late morbidity. Thus, there is conflicting evidence for use of invasive electrophysiological provocation studies in this setting. Although some studies have addressed the effect of suppressve therapy, none has been adequately designed. It must be concluded, therefore, that the place of electrophysiological drug testing in patients with non-sustained tachycardia is far from clear and further, larger studies, using control groups and randomization of treatment, are needed.

Non-sustained monomorphic tachycardia in a repetitive pattern usually occurs in patients without organic heart disease. There is limited information about the use of electrophysiological testing in this setting. Rahilly et al. (1982) induced tachycardia in only 2 of 9 patients, none of whom had evidence of coronary artery disease. Buxton et al. (1984a) were able to induce tachycardia in a much higher proportion of patients. Interestingly, they suggested that the outlook for this pattern of ventricular arrhythmia is benign, even in patients with previous remote myocardial infarction, contrasting with their conclusions from another study (Buxton et al., 1984b) mentioned above.

Definitions of inducible ventricular arrhythmias

The terminology of clinical electrophysiology is nowhere more confused than in respect of ventricular tachycardias. A policy meeting (Waldo et al., 1985) of the North American Society of Pacing and Electrophysiology (NASPE) established several important definitions, quoted here.

1. Sustained ventricular tachycardia: a sustained ventricular tachycardia lasting 30 seconds or more, or requiring intervention (on clinical grounds) to terminate the tachycardia.
2. Non-sustained ventricular tachycardia: a ventricular tachycardia lasting at least six beats up to a maximum of 30 seconds, terminating spontaneously and not requiring intervention on a clinical basis.
3. Monomorphic ventricular tachycardia: ventricular tachycardia with stable morphology of the QRS complexes in at least three simultaneously recorded ECG leads, with a constant relationship of inscription of the QRS complexes in the three recorded leads.
4. Multiple monomorphic ventricular tachycardias: two or more monomorphic ventricular tachycardias in the same patient. The use of the term 'pleomorphic' ventricular tachycardia is discouraged.
5. Polymorphic ventricular tachycardia: ventricular tachycardia with an unstable (continuously varying) QRS complex morphology in any recorded ECG lead.
6. Ventricular fibrillation: a ventricular tachyarrhythmia with absence of clearly defined QRS complexes in the surface ECG. It may be indistinguishable from sustained polymorphic ventricular tachycardia in some cases.
7. Single ventricular response: one non-stimulated ventricular beat in response to a paced premature beat or beats.
8. Repetitive ventricular responses: two to five ventricular beats in response to a paced premature beat or beats.
9. Bundle branch re-entrant beat: this is difficult to distinguish from a single ventricular response. An attempt to differentiate between them can be made using the definition and techniques described by Akhtar et al. (1974).

Stimulation protocols for the induction of ventricular tachycardia

The response to ventricular stimulation is dependent upon the stimulation protocol (Table 10.4). The simplest protocol consists of a single premature ventricular stimulus, introduced during sinus rhythm, with a gradual reduction in the coupling interval in order to scan diastole (in 10–20 msec steps) until the ventricular refractory period is reached. Stimulation may be more 'aggressive' by introducing additional extrastimuli, pacing the ventricles (basic drive of at least 8 beats) prior to extrastimulation, increasing the rate of basic drive and changing the site of stimulation (using additional right and left ventricular sites).

As more aggressive stimulation protocols are applied, the likelihood of finding clinical tachycardias (spontaneously occurring) is increased but there is also an increasing tendency to induce non-clinical responses (not occurring spontaneously) and other responses of indeterminate significance. Thus, sensitivity (for induction of clinical tachycardia) increases and specificity decreases. The maximum predictive accuracy is achieved with protocols most

Table 10.4 STIMULATION PROTOCOLS FOR INDUCTION OF VENTRICULAR TACHYCARDIA

Extrastimulus technique during sinus rhythm (S2), (S2S3), (S2S3S4)

Extrastimulus technique during V pacing:
    Slow drive, (S1S2), (S1S2S3), (S1S2S3S4)
    Fast drive, (S1S2S3), (S1S2S3S4)

Incremental ventricular pacing to exit block
Right ventricular outflow tract pacing
Left ventricular pacing
2 × diastolic threshold and higher energy pacing Isoprenaline infusion (and at surgery hyperthermia) AC current stimulation

likely to induce clinical tachycardias and least likely to induce other responses. Current information suggests that the use of four or more stimuli, or rapid ventricular pacing, yields a high incidence of non-clinical responses and these methods of induction are now discouraged. In a large proportion of patients with documented tachycardias, two stimuli suffice but a third is necessary in a small proportion.

Thus, protocols acceptable to the NASPE committee can be derived from the following recommendations:

1. Single, double and triple ventricular extrastimuli following at least two basic drive cycle lengths at two ventricular sites (e.g. right ventricular apex and outflow tract).
2. Single, double and triple ventricular extrastimuli following at least three basic drive cycle lengths at one ventricular site (e.g. the right ventricular apex).

In patients without documented clinical ventricular tachycardias the provocation of a polymorphic ventricular tachycardia in response to the introduction of a third extrastimulus is of dubious significance but a monomorphic tachycardia must be considered as clinically relevant.

Wellens et al. (1985) have suggested the following 12-stage structured protocol for the investigation of patients with documented sustained ventricular tachycardia (Fig. 10.12):

1. Single and double ventricular premature stimuli during sinus rhythm.
2. Single and double ventricular premature stimuli during right ventricular apical pacing at 100, 120 and then 140 b.p.m.
3. Triple ventricular premature stimuli during sinus rhythm and right ventricular apical pacing at 100, 120 and then 140 b.p.m.

The above protocol is currently undergoing detailed prospective evaluation. In preliminary reports, it has a sensitivity of 95 per cent in patients with sustained tachycardia and 40 per cent in those with non-sustained tachycardia (Wellens et al., 1985). The specificity falls with stages 9–12 and there is a very small improvement of sensitivity (Fig. 10.12). When more than one extrastimulus is

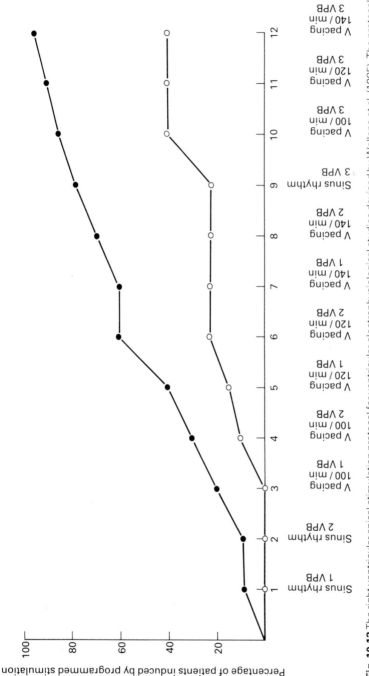

Fig. 10.12 The right ventricular apical stimulation protocol for ventricular electrophysiological studies devised by Wellens et al. (1985). The protocol comprises 12 steps, indicated on the horizontal axis in the sequence they are used. The vertical axis indicates the cumulative number of patients in whom tachycardia was induced. The graph shows that in 95 per cent of patients with sustained VT the tachycardia could be induced at study. The addition of a second stimulus at a rate of 140 b.p.m. did not increase the yield whereas a second stimulus at 120 b.p.m. resulted in marked increase in yield. VPB = ventricular premature beat. Closed circles = sustained VT; open circles = nonsustained VT. (Based on Wellens et al., 1985).

used, it is conventional to insert the first stimulus close to the refractory period (within 50 msec). This may be inappropriate in some settings because of concealed penetration of the circuit by the first extrastimulus which occurs too early to complete its re-entrant circulation. On the whole, it would seem that this theoretical consideration does not jeopardize the sensitivity of the method.

Other protocols include the routine use of isoprenaline, right ventricular outflow tract stimulation, left ventricular stimulation, accelerating (ramp) pacing and high energy stimulation (greater than twice diastolic threshold). Their relative merits and demerits are not known. It is believed that pacing at other sites and stimulation during isoprenaline infusion may increase the sensitivity of the technique without diminishing its specificity.

The value of higher energy stimulation (to achieve shorter coupling intervals of the extrastimulus) is not known. Herre et al. (1986) observed that a protocol using this modification was more likely to induce non-clinical tachycardias. This idea is supported by the observation by Morady et al. (1986a) that the coupling intervals of extrastimuli initiating non-clinical arrhythmias is significantly shorter than those required to initiate clinical forms of tachycardia. They suggest that the specificity of provocation studies can be improved without compromising sensitivity (see above) by avoiding very short coupling intervals. In an earlier study, the same group (Morady et al., 1986b) observed that high current stimulation may fail to initiate ventricular tachycardia which had been induced with extrastimuli at twice diastolic threshold. The mechanism of this apparent 'suppressive' effect is not clear.

The basic drive cycle length of ventricular stimulation has also been the subject of formal investigation by Estes et al. (1986). They found that right ventricular extrastimulation using a range of basic drive cycle lengths (covering a range of 200 msec) increased the sensitivity of the procedure and suggested that this method should be used before resorting to procedures whose sensitivity and specificity (e.g. left ventricular stimulation and use of isoprenaline) are not known.

Electrophysiological testing in specific high risk conditions

Provocation studies have been applied in several settings where ventricular tachycardias are suspected as a cause of symptoms or to expose a potential substrate for tachycardia. These uses of clinical electrophysiology include:

1. Investigation of patients who have suffered sudden cardiac arrest outside hospital.
2. Investigation of patients with unexplained syncope.
3. Assessment of the risk of sudden death after myocardial infarction.
4. Assessment of risk after correction of Fallot's tetralogy.
5. Investigation of prolonged QT interval syndromes.
6. Hypertrophic cardiomyopathy.
7. Mitral value prolapse.
8. Dilated cardiomyopathy.

Investigation of out-of-hospital cardiac arrest

The exact incidence of this important problem is difficult to ascertain because of confused definitions. It has been estimated, however, to be about 450 000 cases per annum in the USA and 50 000 per annum in the UK. Almost all have coronary artery disease but only a minority of those rescued from sudden death have sustained an acute myocardial infarction. It is therefore supposed that the cause of the arrest in the majority of this particular group of patients is a primary electrical event. Electrophysiological studies have shown that ventricular tachycardias (ventricular fibrillation is not often induced as a primary event and when it does occur at study it is usually the result of degeneration of ventricular tachycardia) can be provoked in about two-thirds of cases. It is likely that many of these responses to stimulation are non-specific (see above) and non-clinical. Drug suppression of inducible tachycardia is possible in about 50 per cent of patients with a survival rate of about 80 per cent, compared to 60 per cent in patients in whom arrhythmias were still inducible. It is noteworthy, however, that the survival rate in patients given no treatment (no tachycardia induced) is about 80 per cent. Thus, although the collective information from several studies suggests that there is impressive evidence for the electrophysiological approach to treatment of survivors of out-of-hospital arrest, it should be noted that the studies are uncontrolled and the predictive accuracy of electrophysiological testing in this setting is not known.

Investigation of unexplained syncope

Unexplained syncope may be defined as syncope without any apparent cause after physical examination, neurological investigation and 24-hour tape ECG monitoring. In up to 50 per cent of patients investigated for syncope no cause can be found. In about half of the remainder a cardiovascular abnormality is found. It is likely that cardiovascular disease is directly or indirectly responsible for unexplained syncope in a significant proportion of these patients. Ambulatory monitoring is not of value in the vast majority of patients because it is improbable that syncope will occur at the time of recording, and the more common, related symptoms such as dizziness have many possible causes and are difficult to interpret.

Electrophysiological provocation testing has recently been used to improve

Table 10.5 ELECTROPHYSIOLOGY STUDY OF SYNCOPE IN 490 PATIENTS *

	Pacemaker	Drug treatment	Total	Blind treatment
Treatment	26	102	182 †	58
Recurrence of symptoms	8(31%)	18(18%)	49(27%)	19(33%)

* Abnormal EPS result, $N=269$; Normal EPS result, $N=221$.

† Includes 54 unspecified treatments.

Compiled from Brandenburg et al, (1981), DiMarco et al. (1981), Gulamhusein et al. (1982), Hess et al. (1982), Akhtar et al. (1983), Morady et al. (1983a), Doherty et al. (1985) and Olshansky et al. (1985).

diagnostic accuracy in these patients. The collated results of several studies are shown in Table 10.5. Abnormal electrophysiological findings were observed in about 55 per cent. The most common abnormality was ventricular tachycardia. The recurrence rate in patients who undergo electrophysiologically guided therapy is about 13 per cent compared to 37 per cent of those with normal electrophysiological findings. These data suggest that invasive electrophysiological study is valuable in the management of this problem but closer inspection exposes limitations. The so-called electrophysiological abnormalities included 'soft' endpoints such as prolonged sinoatrial recovery time or conduction time, prolonged AV nodal refractoriness, abnormal HV interval, etc. The meaning of inducible polymorphic or non-sustained ventricular tachycardias in this setting is not known. It is not possible to derive the sensitivity and specificity of tachycardia induction (with respect to induction of clinical arrhythmia) in this context because, by definition, the spontaneous rhythm disturbance is not observed. Furthermore, there is a high rate of spontaneous remission in untreated patients. The role of electrophysiological testing in these patients has yet to be determined.

Assessment of the risk of sudden death after myocardial infarction

Several years ago, repetitive ventricular responses to single ventricular extrastimuli (during atrial pacing) after myocardial infarction were thought to indicate a higher risk of sudden death. It soon became clear, however, that this finding was non-specific. Recently there has been renewed interest in this application of provocation testing using different stimulation protocols and different criteria for a positive test. One study (Richards et al., 1983) using up to two extrastimuli during ventricular pacing with a high current (20 mA) showed that induction of ventricular tachycardia (more than 20 seconds) or fibrillation was 86 per cent sensitive and 83 per cent specific for prediction of sudden death or spontaneous tachycardia in otherwise well patients. Another study (Marchlinski et al., 1983) using a similar protocol failed to show that induction of tachycardia was of predictive value. The specificity of a negative test was similar to the previous study at 75 per cent. Other studies have identified a high false positive rate (high incidence of inducible tachycardia in survivors). It must be concluded, therefore, that the value of provocation testing to identify a risk of sudden death after myocardial infarction is far from clear and cannot be recommended as a standard clinical investigation.

The question of time-related changes of inducibility of ventricular tachycardia after myocardial infarction has been studied by Stevenson et al. (1986a). In patients with spontaneous sustained monomorphic ventricular tachycardia soon (3 days or more) after the acute myocardial infarction, sustained tachycardias (but not necessarily of the same QRS morphology) could be induced at 1–3 weeks and 6–18 months after the acute event. Roy et al. (1986) found similar results using strict criteria for reproducibility. Of 9 patients with inducible monomorphic tachycardia at the initial study soon after infarction, 7 had monomorphic tachycardia at the second, remote study. In 3 of these the QRS configuration was similar. Thus, although a potential substrate for late-onset ventricular tachycardia may be revealed early after myocardial infarction, the clinical significance of these results is unclear.

Assessment of risk after correction of Fallot's tetralogy

It is now recognized that ventricular tachycardias are responsible for a significant proportion of sudden deaths after correction of Fallot's tetralogy. Electrophysiological studies in patients with spontaneous episodes have shown that the tachycardias are inducible and are re-entrant in type (see above). It has also been shown that such tachycardias can be induced in patients who have not suffered from spontaneous tachycardia. Furthermore, in some studies aggressive induction protocols have been applied and non-clinical tachycardias may therefore have been induced (see Chapter 16). Thus the value of provocative testing to expose a substrate for tachycardia is not clear. Symptomatic patients may, however, benefit from such studies. Deanfield et al. (1985), using a different approach, performed endocardial mapping of the right ventricle in 22 patients with corrected tetralogy. They detected fractionation of the electrogram at one or more sites in 12 patients. Ventricular arrhythmias were more common in these patients than in those without fractionation. Fractionation was observed at several right ventricular endocardial sites not associated with the ventriculotomy scar. The left ventricular apical signal was normal in all patients. These findings suggest that diffuse myocardial abnormalities unrelated to surgery may also be important in the formation of a substrate for sustained ventricular tachycardia in these patients.

The argument is that fractionation and delay during sinus rhythm reflect slow conduction and this may predispose to the emergence of re-entrant excitation. The evidence for this argument is based on numerous studies in adults with established ventricular tachycardia (see above). There is hardly any information about the predictive value (with respect to spontaneous tachycardia) of fractionation and delay of endocardial electrograms in patients without spontaneous ventricular tachycardia. Klein et al. (1982), using epicardial operative mapping methods, found fractionation in 20 of 21 patients with documented arrhythmias but in only 2 of 17 without arrhythmias. It remains to be shown whether or not these abnormalities of endocardial activation after correction of Fallot's tetralogy can predict patients at risk.

Investigation of abnormal repolarization syndromes (congenitally prolonged QT interval) and atypical ventricular tachycardia

There are several congenital and acquired syndromes characterized by prolonged (long QT interval) or deranged repolarization and associated atypical ventricular tachycardia, also known as 'torsade de pointes'. These tachycardias are distinctive: their rate and axis vary continuously, they are usually transient and self-terminating but occasionally degenerate to ventricular fibrillation, and they initiate spontaneously after late-coupled ventricular extrasystoles. Conventional electrophysiological studies are of limited value in these syndromes because:

1. Tachycardias can rarely be provoked by ventricular electrical stimulation (Fig. 10.13).
2. There is no consistently demonstrable abnormality of cardiac electrophysiology (occasional late potentials are detected).
3. Tachycardias, which are sometimes provoked by isoprenaline, are unsuitable for detailed study because they are short lived and unstable.

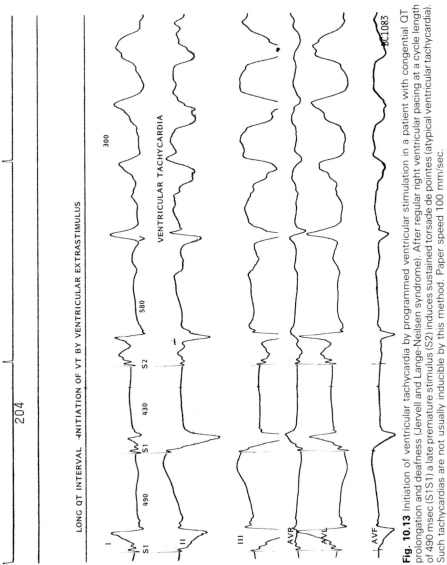

Fig. 10.13 Initiation of ventricular tachycardia by programmed ventricular stimulation in a patient with congenital QT prolongation and deafness (Jervell and Lange-Neilsen syndrome). After regular right ventricular pacing at a cycle length of 490 msec (S1S1) a late premature stimulus (S2) induces sustained torsade de pointes (atypical ventricular tachycardia). Such tachycardias are not usually inducible by this method. Paper speed 100 mm/sec.

Provocation studies in hypertrophic cardiomyopathy

A preliminary report by Geibel et al. (1986) investigated the use of a standardized stimulation protocol in 18 patients with hypertrophic cardiomyopathy, of whom 7 had had documented ventricular arrhythmias or syncope. Sustained monomorphic tachycardia was induced by two ventricular extrastimuli only in the 2 patients with clinical documentation of such episodes. Using a third extrastimulus, a variety of ventricular arrhythmias were induced in the 11 patients without documented ventricular arrhythmias which the investigators regarded as non-specific. Many of these arrhythmias were haemodynamically unstable, requiring cardioversion. Similar results were found by Kunze et al. (1986). In patients presenting with syncope of unknown origin, electrophysiological studies may reveal atrial arrhythmias which may be the cause of spontaneous symptoms (Schiavone et al., 1986). The induction of ventricular fibrillation in these patients (Kowey et al., 1984; Watson et al., 1985) is difficult to interpret because this response may be non-specific, even if only one or two extrastimuli were used during the provocation test (see above). Thus the value of provocative studies in the prediction of risk and assessment of therapy in this setting has yet to be determined.

Mitral value prolapse

There are limited data concerning the value of stimulation studies in this group of patients. A recent report by Rosenthal et al. (1985) describes the results of such studies in 20 patients with the condition. No patient had sustained monomorphic ventricular tachycardia and only 9 had either non-sustained tachycardia (5 patients) or ventricular fibrillation (4 patients). The responses to provocation in these 9 patients (using up to three extrastimuli) were non-sustained polymorphic tachycardia or ventricular fibrillation, which are considered by most investigators to be non-specific responses (at least in the context of myocardial disease due to scarring from infarction). Furthermore, the result of the study did not seem to have any bearing on subsequent outcome. Thus, provocation studies appear to be of limited value in this group of patients.

Dilated cardiomyopathy

Ventricular arrhythmias are frequent in this group of patients and are probably the single most important cause of sudden death. In one study of the value of ventricular provocation testing (Poll et al., 1984b), sustained tachycardia was induced in all patients. After the introduction of antiarrhythmic drug therapy, sustained tachycardia could be induced (albeit slower and better tolerated in some patients) in 81 per cent of patients. Even this effect did not seem to confer a prognostic advantage. Meinertz et al. (1985) studied a group of patients with frequent ventricular arrhythmias on ambulatory monitoring but were unable to induce sustained monomorphic tachycardias in any patient. Late potentials were recordable in only 1 of 42 patients. This suggests that the anatomical substrate for tachycardia in this condition might be different from that found in patients with chronic myocardial scarring due to coronary artery disease. Endocardial

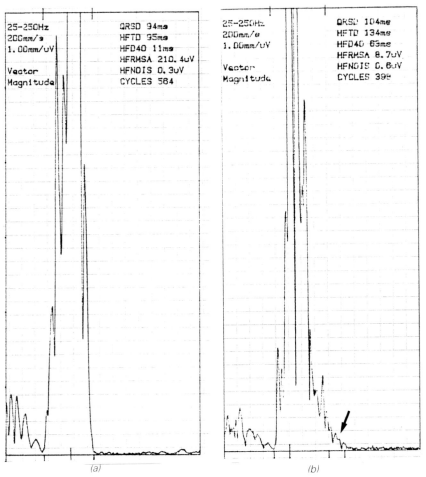

Fig. 10.14 Signal-averaged surface electrocardiograms. (*a*) Recordings from a normal subject. The QRS complex is greatly amplified (1.0 mm/μV). The end of the unfiltered QRs is indicated by the third vertical bar and coincides with the end of the filtered QRS. (*b*) A recording from a patient 3 months after a myocardial infarction. The unfiltered QRS (end marked by third vertical bar) is followed by low-amplitude activity (arrowed) typical of delayed potentials. These last for 63 msec at a root-mean-square amplitude of 8.7 μV.

catheter mapping in this setting (Cassidy et al., 1986) fails to reveal fractionated electrograms and slow conduction, phenomena characteristic of scar-related tachycardias. Operative procedures (see Chapter 14) aimed solely at the endocardium in patients with dilated cardiomyopathy are not likely to be effective.

The role of signal-averaged surface electrocardiography in risk assessment

The presence of low-amplitude, high-frequency electrical activity in the terminal part of the QRS complex was described by Uther et al. and Fontaine et al. in 1978.

These potentials are thought to reflect the same substrate as the delayed and fractionated potentials observed at electrophysiological study and are therefore markers of slowed intramyocardial conduction, a prerequisite for the development of re-entrant tachycardias, as described above. It is not surprising that these potentials have been the subject of study by several groups, especially in relation to their use as an indicator of the risk of developing ventricular tachycardia. These signals are recorded using computer-averaging techniques (Fig. 10.14) to remove noise artefact. Some systems are capable of beat-to-beat analysis. Simson (1981) has defined late potentials as present when the terminal 40 msec of the QRS is less than 25 μV in amplitude (Fig. 10.14). Numerous other definitions have been suggested (Breithardt and Borggrefe, 1986).

There is a significantly higher incidence of late potentials in patients with old myocardial infarction and with spontaneous ventricular tachycardia than in those without the arrhythmia. Several studies, reviewed in detail by Breithardt and Borgreffe (1986), have shown that the presence of late potentials is a strong predictor of the spontaneous occurrence of ventricular tachycardia after myocardial infarction. There are few data from patients in the other high risk groups described above. Poll et al. (1984) studied a group of patients with dilated cardiomyopathy and concluded that late potentials occur more often in those with ventricular tachycardia. Kuchar et al. (1984) applied the technique to patients with recurrent syncope and found late potentials in 70 per cent of patients who had documented ventricular tachycardia compared to none of the patients with syncope due to other causes. These data suggest that late-potential recording may be used as a method of selecting patients with a potentially 'high-risk' substrate for invasive studies. Breithardt and Borggrefe (1986b) have shown the feasibility of this approach in the setting of post-myocardial infarction.

References and further reading

Akhtar M, Damato AN, Batsford WP, Ruskin JN, Ogunkelu BB, Vargas G. (1974) Demonstration of re-entry within the His–Purkinje system in man. *Circulation* **50**, 1150

Akhtar M, Shenasa M, Denker S, Gilbert CJ, Rizwi N. (1983) Role of cardiac electrophysiologic studies in patients with unexplained recurrent syncope. *Pacing and Clinical Electrophysiology* **6**, 192

Akhtar M. (1984) Clinical application of rapid ventricular burst pacing versus extrastimulation for induction of ventricular tachycardia. *Journal of the American College of Cardiology* **4**, 305

Anderson KP, Mason JW. (1986) Criteria for selection of patients for programmed electrical stimulation. *Circulation* **73**, suppl. II, 50

Belhassen B, Caspi A, Miller H, Shapira I, Laniado S. (1984) Extensive endocardial mapping during sinus rhythm and ventricular tachycardia in a patient with arrhythmogenic right ventricular dysplasia. *Journal of the American College of Cardiology* **6**, 1302

Benditt DG, Benson DW, Klein GJ, Pritzker MR, Kriett JM, Anderson RW. (1983) Prevention of recurrent sudden cardiac arrest: role of provocative electropharmacologic testing. *Journal of the American College of Cardiology* **2**, 418

Bhandari AK, Shapiro W, Morady F, Shen EN, Mason J, Sheinman MM. (1985) Electrophysiologic testing in patients with the long QT syndrome. *Circulation* **71**, 63

Bigger JT, Weld FM, Rolnitzky LM, Coromilas J. (1983) Prevalence and significance of nonsustained ventricular tachycardia after myocardial infarction. *Clinical Progress in Pacing and Electrophysiology* **1**, 3

Bigger JT, Reiffel J, Livelli FD, Wang PJ. (1986) Sensitivity, specificity, and reproducibility of programmed ventricular stimulation. *Circulation* **73**, suppl. II, 73

Brandenburg RO, Holmes DR, Hartzler GO. (1981) The electrophysiologic assessment of patients with syncope. *American Journal of Cardiology* **47**, 443

Breithardt G, Seipel L, Abendroth RR, Loogen F. (1980) Serial electrophysiological testing of antiarrhythmic drug efficacy in patients with recurrent ventricular tachycardia. *European Heart Journal* **1**, 11

Breithardt G, Borggrefe M. (1986) Pathophysiological mechanisms and clinical significance of ventricular late potentials. *European Heart Journal* **7**, 364

Breithardt G, Borggrefe M, Podczeck A. (1986) Electrophysiology and pharmacology of asymptomatic nonsustained ventricular tachycardia. *Clinical Progress in Electrophysiology and Pacing* **4**, 81

Brugada P, Green M, Abdollah H, Wellens HJJ. (1984) Significance of ventricular arrhythmias initiated by programmed ventricular stimulation: the importance of the type of response and the number of premature stimuli. *Circulation* **69**, 87

Brugada P, Wellens HJJ. (1985a) Comparison in the same patient of two programmed ventricular stimulation protocols to induce ventricular tachycardia. *American Journal of Cardiology* **55**, 380

Brugada P, Wellens HJJ. (1985b) Programmed electrical stimulation of the heart in ventricular arrhythmias. *American Journal of Cardiology* **56**, 187

Brugada P, Abdollah H, Wellens HJJ. (1985) Continuous electrical activity during sustained monomorphic ventricular tachycardia. Observations on its dynamic behaviour during the arrhythmia. *American Journal of Cardiology* **55**, 402

Brugada P, Wellens HJJ. (1986) Need and design of a prospective study to assess the value of different strategic approaches for management of ventricular tachycardia or fibrillation. *American Journal of Cardiology* **57**, 1180

Buitleir M, Morady F, DiCarlo LA, Baerman JM, Krol R. (1986) Immediate reproducibility of clinical and nonclinical forms of induced ventricular tachycardia. *American Journal of Cardiology* **58**, 279

Buxton AE, Waxman HL, Marchlinski FE, Simson MB, Cassidy D, Josephson ME. (1983a) Right ventricular tachycardia: clinical and electrophysiologic characteristics. *Circulation* **68**, 917

Buxton AE, Waxman HL, Marchlinski FE, Simson MB, Cassidy D, Josephson ME. (1983a) Right ventricular tachycardia: clinical and electrophysiologic characteristics. *Circulation* **68**, 917

Buxton AE, Marchlinski FE, Doherty JU, Cassidy DM, Vassallo JA, Flores BT, Josephson ME. (1984a) Repetitive monomorphic ventricular tachycardia: clinical and electrophysiologic characteristics in patients with and patients without organic heart disease. *Amerian Journal of Cardiology* **54**, 997

Buxton AE, Marchlinski FE, Waxman HL, Flores BT, Cassidy DM, Josephson ME. (1984b) Prognostic factors in nonsustained ventricular tachycardia. *American Journal of Cardiology* **53**, 1275

Buxton AE. (1985) The use of multiple extrastimuli during programmed ventricular stimulation: how many should be used? *International Journal of Cardiology* **7**, 86

Cassidy DM, Vassallo JA, Buxton AE, Doherty JU, Marchlinski FE, Josephson ME. (1984) The value of catheter mapping during sinus rhythm to localize site of origin of ventricular tachycardia. *Circulation* **69**, 1103

Cassidy DM, Vassallo JA, Buxton AE, Doherty JU, Marchlinski FE, Josephson ME. (1985) Catheter mapping during sinus rhythm: relation of local electrogram duration to ventricular tachycardia cycle length. *American Journal of Cardiology* **55**, 713

Cassidy DM, Vassallo JA, Miller JM, Poll DS, Buxton AE, Marchlinski FE, Josephson

ME. (1986) Endocardial catheter mapping in sinus rhythm: relationship to underlying heart disease and ventricular arrhythmias. *Circulation* 73, 645

Curry PVL, O'Keefe B, Pitcher D, Sowton E, Deverall PB, Yates AK. (1979) Localization of ventricular tachycardia by a new technique – pacemapping. *Circulation* 60, suppl. II, II-25

Dancy M, Ward DE. (1985) Diagnosis of ventricular tachycardia: a clinical algorithm. *British Medical Journal* 291, 1036

Dancy M, Camm AJ, Ward DE. (1985) Misdiagnosis of ventricular tachycardia. *Lancet* 2, 320

Deanfield J, McKenna W, Rowland E. (1985) Local abnormalities of right ventricular depolarization after repair of tetralogy of Fallot: a basis for ventricular arrhythmia. *American Journal of Cardiology* 55, 522

Denes P, Wu D, Dhingra R, Amat-y-Leon F, Wyndham CRC, Mautner RK, Rosen KM. (1986) Electrophysiological studies in patients with chronic recurrent ventricular tachycardia. *Circulation* 54, 229

Denniss AR, Baaijens H, Cody DV, Richards DA, Russell PA, Young AA, Ross DL, Uther JB. (1985) Value of programmed stimulation and exercise testing in predicting one-year mortality after acute myocardial infarction. *American Journal of Cardiology* 56, 213

DiMarco J, Garan H, Harthorne JW, Ruskin JN. (1981) Intracardiac electrophysiologic techniques in recurrent syncope of unknown cause. *Annals of Internal Medicine* 95, 542

Doherty JU, Pembrook-Rogers D, Grogan EW, Falcone RA, Buxton AE, Marchlinski FE, Cassidy DM, Kienzle MG, Almendral JM, Josephson ME. (1985) Electrophysiologic evaluation and follow-up characteristics of patients with recurrent unexplained syncope and presyncope. *American Journal of Cardiology* 55, 703

Dungan WT, Garson A, Gillette PC. (1981) Arrhythmogenic right ventricular dysplasia: a cause of ventricular tachycardia in children with apparently normal hearts. *American Heart Journal* 102, 745

Estes NAM, Garan H, McGovern B, Ruskin JN. (1986) Influence of drive cycle length during programmed ventricular stimulation on induction of ventricular arrhythmias: analysis of 403 patients. *American Journal of Cardiology* 57, 108

Fisher JD. (1978) Ventricular tachycardia – practical and provocative electrophysiology. *Circulation* 58, 1000

Fontaine G, Guiraudon G, Frank R. (1978) Intramyocardial conduction defects in patients prone to chronic ventricular tachycardia. I. The post-excitation syndrome in sinus rhythm. In: *Managment of Ventricular Tachycardia: Role of Mexiletine*, p. 39. Ed. by E Sandoe, DG Julian, JW Bell. Excerpta Medica: Amsterdam

Foale R, Nihoyannopoulos P, Ribeiro P, McKenna WJ, Oakley C, Krikler DM, Rowland E. (1986) Right ventricular abnormalities in ventricular tachycardia of right ventricular origin: relation to electrophysiological abnormalities. *British Heart Journal* 56, 45

Friedman J, Yusuf S. (1986) Does therapy directed by programmed electrical stimulation provide a satisfactory clinical response? *Circulation* 73, suppl. II, 59

Garrey WE. (1914) The nature of fibrillary contraction of the heart. Its relation to tissue mass and form. *American Journal of Physiology* 33, 397

Geibel A, Brugada P, Zehender M, Kersshot I, Wellens HJJ. (1986) Results of a standardized ventricular stimulation protocol in patients with hypertrophic cardiomyopathy. *Journal of the American College of Cardiology* 7, 195A (abstract)

Gessman LJ, Endo T, Gallagher JJ, Hastie R, Maroko PR. (1983) Dissociation of the site of origin from the site of cryo-termination of ventricular tachycardia. *Pacing and Clinical Electrophysiology* 6, 1293

Gomes JAC, Hariman RI, Kang PS, El-Sherif N, Chowdhry I, Lyons J. (1984)

Programmed electrical stimulation in patients with high-grade ventricular ectopy: electrophysiologic findings and prognosis for survival. *Circulation* 70, 43

Gulamhusein S, Naccarelli VC, Ko PT, Prystowsky EN, Zipes DP, Barnett HJM, Heger JJ, Klein GJ. (1982) Value and limitations of clinical electrophysiologic study in assessment of patients with unexplained syncope. *American Journal of Medicine* 73, 700

Hamer A, Vohra J, Hunt D, Sloman G. (1982) Prediction of sudden death by electrophysiological studies in high risk patients surviving acute myocardial infarction. *American Journal of Cardiology* 50, 223

Hartzler GO, Maloney JD. (1977) Programmed ventricular stimulation in management of recurrent ventricular tachycardia. *Mayo Clinic Proceedings* 52, 731

Herre JM, Mann DE, Luck JC, Magro SA, Figali S, Breen T, Wyndham CRC. (1986) Effect of increased current, multiple pacing sites and number of ventricular extrastimuli on induction of ventricular tachycardia. *American Journal of Cardiology* 57, 102

Hess DS, Morady F, Scheinman MM. (1982) Electrophysiologic testing in the evaluation of patients with syncope of undetermined origin. *American Journal of Cardiology* 50, 1309

Holt P, Smallpiece C, Deverall PB, Yates AK, Curry PVL. (1985) Ventricular arrhythmias: a guide to their localisation. *British Heart Journal* 53, 417

Horowitz LN, Josephson ME. (1980) Intracardiac electrophysiologic studies as a method for the optimization of drug therapy in chronic ventricular arrhythmia. *Progress in Cardiovascular Diseases* 23, 81

Horowitz LN, Vetter V, Harken A, Josephson ME. (1980) Electrophysiologic characteristics of sustained ventricular tachycardia occurring after repair of tetralogy of Fallot. *American Journal of Cardiology* 46, 446

Huang SK, Messer JV, Denes P. (1983) Significance of ventricular tachycardia in idiopathic dilated cardiomyopathy: observations in 35 patients. *American Journal of Cardiology* 51, 507

Josephson ME, Horowitz LN, Farshidi A, Kastor J. (1978a) Recurrent sustained ventricular tachycardia. 1. Mechanisms. *Circulation* 57, 431

Josephson ME, Horowitz LN, Farshidi A, Spear JF, Kastor JA, Moore EN. (1978b) Recurrent ventricular tachycardia. 2. Endocardial mapping. *Circulation* 57, 440

Josephson ME, Horowitz LN, Farshidi A. (1978c) Continuous local electrical activity: a mechanism for recurrent ventricular tachycardia. *Circulation* 57, 659

Josephson ME, Horowitz LN, Farshidi A, Spielman SR, Michelson EL, Greenspan AM. (1978d) Sustained ventricular tachycardia: evidence for protected localized reentry. *American Journal of Cardiology* 42, 416

Josephson ME, Horowitz LN. (1979) Electrophysiologic approach to therapy of recurrent sustained ventricular tachycardia. *American Journal of Cardiology* 54, 631

Josephson ME, Spielman GR, Greenspan AM, Horowitz LN. (1979) Mechanism of ventricular fibrillation in man. Observations based on electrode catheter recordings. *American Journal of Cardiology* 44, 623

Josephson ME, Horowitz LN, Greenspan AM, Vandepol C, Harken AH. (1980) Comparison of endocardial catheter mapping with intraoperative mapping of ventricular tachycardia. *Circulation* 61, 395

Josephson ME, Horowitz LN, Waxman HL, Cain ME, Spielman SR, Greenspan AM, Marchlinski FE, Ezri MD. (1981) Sustained ventricular tachycardia: role of the 12 lead electrocardiogram in localizing site of origin. *Circulation* 64, 257

Josephson ME. (1982) *Ventricular Tachycardia: mechanisms and management.* Futura: Mount Kisco, NY

Josephson ME, Wit AL. (1984) Fractionated electrical activity and continuous electrical activity: fact or artefact? *Circulation* **70**, 529

Josephson ME, Marchlinski FE, Buxton AE, Waxman HL, Doherty JU, Kienzle MG, Falcone R. (1984) Electrophysiologic basis for sustained ventricular tachycardia – role of reentry. In: *Tachycardias: Mechanisms, Diagnosis and Treatment*, p. 305. Ed. by ME Josephson, HJJ Wellens. Lea & Febiger, Philadelphia, Pa.

Josephson ME, Buxton AE, Marchlinski FE, Doherty JU, Cassidy DM. Kienzle MG, Vassallo JA, Miller JM, Almendral J, Grogan W. (1985) Sustained ventricular tachycardia in coronary artery disease – evidence for reentrant mechanism. In: *Cardiac Electrophysiology and Arrhythmias*, p. 409. Ed. by D Zipes, J Jalife. Grune & Stratton: Orlando, Fla

Kienzle MG, Miller J, Falcone RA, Harken A, Josephson ME. (1984) Intraoperative endocardial mapping during sinus rhythm: relationship to site of origin of ventricular tachycardia. *Circulation* **70**, 957

Kienzle MG, Doherty JU, Cassidy D, Buxton AE, Marchlinski FE, Waxman HL, Josephson ME. (1986) Electrophysiologic sequelae of chronic myocardial infarction: local refractoriness and electrographic characteristics of the left ventricle. *American Journal of Cardiology* **58**, 63

Klein H, Karp RB, Kouchoukos NT, Zorn GL, James TN, Waldo AL. (1982) Intraoperative electrophysiologic mapping of the ventricles during sinus rhythm in patients with a previous myocardial infarction. Identification of the electrophysiologic substrate of ventricular arrhythmias. *Circulation* **66**, 847

Kowey PR, Eisenberg R, Engel TR. (1984) Sustained arrhythmias in hypertrophic obstructive cardiomyopathy. *New England Journal of Medicine* **310**, 1566

Kuchar DL, Thorburn CW, Sammel NL. (1984) Evaluation of recurrent syncope using signal averaged electrocardiography. *Circulation* **70**, suppl. II, 374 (abstract)

Kudenchuk J, Kron J, Walance CG, Murphy ES, Morris CD, Griffith KK, McAnulty JH. (1986) Reproducibility of arrhythmia induction with intracardiac electrophysiologic testing: patients with clinical sustained ventricular tachyarrhythmias. *Journal of the American College of Cardiology* **7**, 819

Kunze KP, Kuck KH, Geiger M, Bleifeld W. (1986) Programmed electrical stimulation in hypertrophic cardiomyopathy – specificity and sensitivity of different stimulation protocols. *Journal of the American College of Cardiology* **7**, 195A (abstract)

Lewis T. (1925) Ventricular fibrillation. In: *The Mechanisms and Graphic Registration of the Heart Beat*, p. 369. Shaw: London

Livelli FD, Bigger JT, Reiffel JA, Gang ES, Patton JN, Noethling PM, Rolnitzky LM, Gliklich JI. (1982) Response to programmed ventricular stimulation: sensitivity, specificity and relation to heart disease. *American Journal of Cardiology* **50**, 452

Lombardi F, Stein J, Podrid PJ, Graboys TB, Lown B. (1986) Daily reproducibility of electrophysiologic test results in malignant ventricular arrhythmia. *American Journal of Cardiology* **57**, 96

McKenna WJ, Krikler DM. (1984) Arrhythmia in cardiomyopathy. In: *Tachycardias*, p. 373. Ed. by B Surawicz, CP Reddy, EN Prystowsky. Martinus Nijhoff: Boston, Mass

MacLean WAH, Plumb VJ, Waldo AL. (1981) Transient entrainment and interruption of ventricular tachycardias. *Pacing and Electrophysiology* **4**, 358

Mahmud R, Denker S, Lehmann MH, Tchou P, Dongas J, Akhtar M. (1986) Incidence and clinical significance of ventricular fibrillation induced with single and double ventricular extrastimuli. *American Journal of Cardiology* **58**, 75

Marchlinski FE, Buxton AE, Waxman HL, Josephson ME. (1983) Identifying patients at risk of sudden death after myocardial infarction: value of the response to programmed stimulation, degree of ventricular ectopic activity and severity of left ventricular dysfunction. *American Journal of Cardiology* **52**, 1190

Marcus FI, Fontaine GH, Guiraudon G, Frank R, Laurenceau JL, Malergue C, Grosgogeat Y. (1982) Right ventricular dysplasia: a report of 24 adult cases. *Circulation* 65, 384

Mason J, Winkle R. (1978) Electrode catheter arrhythmia induction in the selection and assessment of antiarrhythmic drug therapy for recurrent ventricular tachycardia. *Circulation* 58, 971

Mason JW, Stinson EB, Oyer PE, Winkle RA, Hunt S, Anderson KP. Derby GC. (1985) The mechanisms of ventricular tachycardia in humans determined by intraoperative recording of the electrical activation sequence. *International Journal of Cardiology* 8, 163

Meinertz T, Hofmann T, Kasper W, Treese N, Bechtold H, Stienen U, Pop T, Leitner ER, Andresen D, Meyer J. (1984) Significance of ventricular arrhythmias in idiopathic dilated cardiomyopathy. *American Journal of Cardiology* 53, 902

Meinertz T, Treese N, Kasper W, Geibel A, Hofmann T, Zehender M, Bohn D, Pop T, Just H. (1985) Determinants of prognosis in idiopathic dilated cardiomyopathy as determined by programmed electrical stimulation. *American Journal of Cardiology* 56, 337

Miller JM, Vassallo JA, Hargrove WC, Josephson ME. (1985a) Intermittent failure of local conduction during ventricular tachycardia. *Circulation* 72, 1286

Miller JM, Harken AH, Hargrove WC, Josephson ME. (1985b) Pattern of endocardial activation during sustained ventricular tachycardia. *Journal of the American College of Cardiology* 6, 1280

Mines GR. (1913) On the dynamic equilibrium in the heart. *Journal of Physiology* 46, 349

Mines GR. (1914) On the circulating excitations in heart muscles and their possible relation to tachycardia and fibrillation. *Transactions of the Royal Society of Canada*, series 3, section IV, 8, 43

Morady F, Shen E, Schwartz A, Hess D, Bhandari A, Sung RJ, Scheinmann MM. (1983a) Long-term follow-up of patients with recurrent unexplained syncope evaluated by electrophysiologic testing. *Journal of the American College of Cardiology* 2, 1053

Morady F, Scheinman MM, Hess DS, Sung RJ, Shen E, Shapiro W. (1983b) Electrophysiologic testing in the management of survivors of out-of-hospital cardiac arrest. *American Journal of Cardiology* 51, 85

Morady F, Shen E, Bhandari A, Schwartz A, Scheinman MM. (1984a) Programmed ventricular stimulation in mitral valve prolapse: analysis of 36 patients. *American Journal of Cardiology* 53, 135

Morady F, Shapiro W, Shen E, Sung RJ, Scheinman MM. (1984b) Programmed ventricular stimulation in patients without spontaneous ventricular tachycardia. *American Heart Journal* 107, 875

Morady F, DiCarlo LA, Baerman JM, Buitleir M. (1986a) Comparison of coupling intervals that induce clinical and nonclinical forms of ventricular tachycardia during programmed stimulation. *American Journal of Cardiology* 57, 1269

Morady F, DiCarlo LA, Liem KB, Krol RB, Baerman JM. (1986b) Effects of high stimulation current on the induction of ventricular tachycardia. *American Journal of Cardiology* 56, 73

Naccarelli GV, Prystowsky EN, Jackman WM, Heger JJ, Rahilly GT, Zipes DP. (1982) Role of electrophysiologic testing in managing patients who have ventricular tachycardia unrelated to coronary artery disease. *American Journal of Cardiology* 50, 165

Olshansky B, Mazuz M, Martins JB. (1985) Significance of inducible tachycardia in patients with syncope of unknown origin: a long-term follow-up study. *Journal of the American College of Cardiology* 5, 216

Oseran DS, Gang ES, Hamer AW, Zaher CA, Rosenthal ME, Mandel WJ. (1985) Mode of stimulation versus response: validation of a protocol for induction of ventricular tachycardia. *American Heart Journal* 110, 646

Palileo E, Ashley WW, Swiryn S, Bauernfeind RA, Strasberg B, Petropoulos AT, Rosen KM. (1982) Exercise provocable right ventricular outflow tachycardia. *American Heart Journal* 104, 185

Pietras RJ, Lam W, Bauernfeind R, Sheikh A, Palileo E, Strasberg B, Swiryn S, Rosen KM. (1983) Chronic recurrent right ventricular tachycardia in patients without ischemic heart disease: clinical, hemodynamic and angiographic findings. *American Heart Journal* 105, 357

Platia EV, Reid PR. (1985) Nonsustained ventricular tachycardia during programmed ventricular stimulation: criteria for a positive test. *American Journal of Cardiology* 56, 79

Podrid PJ, Schoenberger A, Lown B, Lambert S, Matos J, Porterfield J, Raeder E, Corrigan E. (1983) Use of nonsustained ventricular tachycardia as a guide to antiarrhythmic drug therapy in patients with malignant ventricular arrhythmia. *American Heart Journal* 105, 181

Poll DS, Marchlinski FE, Falcone RA, Simson MB. (1984a) Abnormal signal averaged ECG in nonischemic congestive cardiomyopathy: relationship to sustained ventricular arrhythmias. *Circulation* 70, 253 (abstract)

Poll DS, Marchlinski FE, Buxton AE, Doherty JU, Waxman HL, Josephson ME. (1984b) Sustained ventricular tachycardia in patients with idiopathic dilated cardiomyopathy: electrophysiological testing and lack of response to antiarrhythmic drug therapy. *Circulation* 70, 451

Rahilly GT, Prystowsky EN, Zipes DP, Naccarelli GV, Jackman WM, Heger JJ. (1982) Clinical and electrophysiologic findings in patients with repetitive monomorphic ventricular tachycardia and otherwise normal electrocardiogram. *American Journal of Cardiology* 50, 459

Richards DA, Cody DV, Denniss AR, Russell PA, Young AA, Uther JB. (1983) Ventricular electrical instability: a predictor of death after acute myocardial infarction. *American Journal of Cardiology* 51, 75

Rinkenberger RL, Prystowsky EN, Jackman WM, Naccarelli GV, Heger JJ, Zipes DP. (1982) Drug conversion of nonsustained ventricular tachycardia to sustained ventricular tachycardia during serial electrophysiologic studies: identification of drugs that exacerbate tachycardia and potential mechanisms. *American Heart Journal* 103, 177

Rosenthal ME, Hamer A, Gang ES, Oseran DS, Mandel WJ, Peter T. (1985) The yield of programmed ventricular stimulation in mitral valve prolapse patients with ventricular arrhythmias. *American Heart Journal* 110, 970

Roy D, Waxman HL, Kienzle MG, Buxton AE, Marchlinski FE, Josephson ME. (1983) Clinical characteristics and long-term follow-up in 119 survivors of cardiac arrest: relation to inducibility at electrophysiologic testing. *American Journal of Cardiology* 52, 969

Roy D, Marchand E, Theroux P, Waters DD, Pelletier GB, Cartier R, Bourassa MG. (1986) Long-term reproducibility and signifiance of provocable ventricular arrhythmias after myocardial infarction. *Journal of the American College of Cardiology* 8, 32

Scheinman MM. (1978) Induction of ventricular tachycardia: a promising new technique or clinical electrophysiology gone awry? *Circulation* 58, 998

Schiavone WA, Maloney JD, Lever HM, Castle LW, Sterba R, Morant V. (1986) Electrophysiologic studies of patients with hypertrophic cardiomyopathy presenting with syncope of undetermined origin. *Pacing and Clinical Electrophysiology* 9, 476

Schoenfeld MH, McGovern B, Garan H, Kelly E, Grant G, Ruskin J. (1985) Determinants of outcome of electrophysiologic study in patients with ventricular tachyarrhythmias. *Journal of the American College of Cardiology* 6, 298

Silver M. (1986) Morphologic substrates of ventricular arrhythmias. *Clinical Progress in Electrophysiology and Pacing* **4**, 1

Simson MB. (1981) Use of signals in the terminal QRS complex to identify patients with ventricular tachycardia after myocardial infarction. *Circulation* **64**, 235

Spielman SR, Farshidi A, Horowitz LN, Josephson ME. (1978) Ventricular fibrillation during programmed electrical stimulation: incidence and clinical implications. *American Journal of Cardiology* **42**, 913

Spielman SR, Schwartz JS, McCarthy DM, Horowitz LN, Greenspan AM, Sadowski LM, Josephson ME, Waxman HL. (1983) Predictors of the success or failure of medical therapy in patients with chronic recurrent sustained ventricular tachycardia: a discriminant analysis. *Journal of the American College of Cardiology* **1**, 401

Spielman SR, Greenspan AM, Kay HR, Discigil KF, Webb CR, Sokoloff N, Rae AP, Morganroth J, Horowitz LN. (1985) Electrophysiologic testing in patients at high risk for sudden cardiac death. I. Nonsustained ventricular tachycardia and abnormal ventricular function. *Journal of the American College of Cardiology* **6**, 31

Spurrell RAJ, Sowton E, Deuchar DC. (1973) Ventricular tachycardia in 4 patients evaluated by programmed electrical stimulation of the heart and treated in 2 patients by surgical division of anterior radiation of left bundle branch. *British Heart Journal* **35**, 1014

Stevenson WG, Brugada P, Kersschot I, Waldecker B, Zehender M, Geibel A, Wellens HJJ. (1986a) Electrophysiologic characteristics of ventricular tachycardia or fibrillation in relation to age of myocardial infarction. *American Journal of Cardiology* **57**, 387

Stevenson WG, Brugada P, Waldecker B, Zehender M, Wellens HJJ. (1986b) Can potentially significant polymorphic ventricular arrhythmias initiated by programmed stimulation be distinguished from those that are nonspecific? *American Heart Journal* **111**, 1073

Sung RJ, Shen EN, Morady F, Scheinmann MM, Hess D, Botvinick EH. (1983) Electrophysiologic mechanism of exercise-induced sustained ventricular tachycardia. *American Journal of Cardiology* **53**, 525

Swerdlow CD, Blum J, Winkle RA, Griffin JC, Ross DL, Mason JW. (1982) Decreased incidence of antiarrhythmic drug efficacy at electrophysiologic study associated with the use of a third extrastimulus. *American Heart Journal* **104**, 1004

Swerdlow CD, Winkle RA, Mason JW. (1983a) Determinants of survival in patients with ventricular tachyarrhythmias. *New England Journal of Medicine* **308**, 1436

Swerdlow CD, Gong G, Echt DS, Winkle RA, Griffin JC, Ross DL, Mason JW. (1983b) Clinical factors predicting successful electrophysiologic–pharmacologic study in patients with ventricular tachycardia. *Journal of the American College of Cardiology* **1**, 409

Swerdlow CD, Winkle RA, Mason JW. (1983c) Prognostic significance of the number of induced ventricular complexes during assessment of therapy for ventricular tachyarrhythmias. *Circulation* **68**, 400

Swerdlow CD, Freedman RA, Peterson J, Clay D. (1986) Determinants of prognosis in ventricular tachyarrhythmia patients without induced sustained arrhythmias. *American Heart Journal* **111**, 433

Teichman SL, Felder SD, Matos JA, Kim SG, Waspe LE, Fisher JD. (1985) The value of electrophysiologic studies in syncope of undetermined origin: report of 150 cases. *American Heart Journal* **110**, 469

Touboul P, Kirkorian G, Atallah G, Moleur G. (1983) Bundle branch reentry: a possible mechanism of ventricular tachycardia. *Circulation* **67**, 674

Untereker WJ, Spielman SR, Waxman HL, Horowitz LN, Josephson ME. (1985) Ventricular activation in normal sinus rhythm: abnormalities with recurrent sustained tachycardia and a history of myocardial infarction. *American Journal of Cardiology* **55**, 974

Uther JB, Dennett CJ, Tan A. (1978) The detection of delayed activation potentials of low amplitude in the vector cardiogram of patients with recurrent ventricular tachycardia by signal averaging. In: *Management of Ventricular Tachycardia: Role of Mexiletine*, p. 80. Ed. by E Sandoe, DG Julian, JW Bell, Excerpta Medica: Amsterdam

Vandepol CJ, Farshidi A, Spielman SR, Horowitz LN, Josephson ME. (1980) Incidence and clinical significance of induced ventricular tachycardia. *American Journal of Cardiology* 45, 725

Velebit V, Podrid P, Lown B, Cohen BH, Graboys T. (1982) Aggravation and provocation of ventricular arrhythmias by antiarrhythmic drugs. *Circulation* 65, 886

Veltri EP, Platia EV, Griffith LSC, Reid PR. (1985) Programmed ventricular stimulation and long-term follow-up in asymptomatic, nonsustained ventricular tachycardia. *American Journal of Cardiology* 56, 309

Waldo AL, Kaiser GA. (1973) Study of ventricular arrhythmias associated with acute myocardial infarction in the canine heart. *Circulation* 47, 1222

Waldo AL, MacLean WAH, Karp RB, Kouchoukos NT, James TN. (1977) Entrainment and interruption of atrial flutter with atrial pacing: studies in man following open heart surgery. *Circulation* 56, 737

Waldo AL, Plumb V, Arciniegas JG, MacLean WAH, Cooper TB, Priest MF, James TN. (1983) Transient entrainment and interruption of the atrioventricular bypass type of paroxysmal atrial tachycardia: a model for understanding and identifying reentrant arrhythmias. *Circulation* 67, 73

Waldo AL, Henthorn RW, Plumb VJ, MacLean WAH. (1984) Demonstration of the mechanism of transient entrainment of ventricular tachycardia with rapid atrial pacing. *Journal of the American College of Cardiology* 3, 422

Waldo AL, Akhtar M, Brugada P, Henthorn RW, Scheinman MM, Ward DE, Wellens HJJ. (1985) The minimally appropriate electrophysiologic study for the initial assessment of patients with documented sustained monomorphic ventricular tachycardia. *Journal of the American College of Cardiology* 6, 1174

Ward DE, Nathan AN, Camm AJ. (1984) Fascicular tachycardia sensitive to calcium antagonists. *European Heart Journal* 5, 896

Ward DE, Camm AJ. (1985) Recurrent ventricular tachycardia. *British Medical Journal* 290, 1926

Ward DE. (1986) The management of arrhythmias in children. Are electrophysiological studies of value? *International Journal of Cardiology* 11, 149

Ward DE, Cheesman M, Dancy M. (1986) Effect of intravenous and oral flecainide on ventricular tachycardia. *International Journal of Cardiology* 10, 251

Waspe LE, Seinfeld D, Ferrick E, Kim SG, Matos JA, Fisher JD. (1985) Prediction of sudden death and spontaneous ventricular tachycardia in survivors of complicated myocardial infarction: value of the response to programmed stimulation using a maximum of three ventricular extrastimuli. *Journal of the American College of Cardiology* 5, 1292

Watson RM, Liberati JM, Tucker E, Cannon RO, Rosing DR, Epstein SE, Josephson ME. (1985) Inducible ventricular fibrillation in patients with hypertrophic cardiomyopathy. *Journal of the American College of Cardiology* 5, 393 (abstract)

Waxman HL, Sung RJ. (1980) Significance of fragmented ventricular electrograms observed using intracardiac recording techniques in man. *Circulation* 62, 1349

Wellens HJJ, Schuilenberg RM, Durrer D. (1972) Electrical stimulation of the heart in patients with ventricular tachycardia. *Circulation* 46, 216

Wellens HJJ, Lie KI, Durrer D. (1974) Further observations on ventricular tachycardia as studied by electrical stimulation of the heart: chronic recurrent ventricular tachycardia and ventricular tachycardia during acute myocardial infarction. *Circulation* 49, 647

Wellens HJJ, Duren D, Lie KI. (1976) Observations on the mechanisms of ventricular tachycardia in man. *Circulation* **54**, 237

Wellens HJJ, Bar FWHM, Lie KI. (1978) The value of the electrocardiogram in the differential diagnosis of tachycardia with a widened QRS complex. *American Journal of Medicine* **64**, 27

Wellens HJJ, Bar FW, Farre J, Ross DL, Weiner I, Vanagt EJ. (1980) Initiation and termination of ventricular tachycardia by supraventricular stimuli. *American Journal of Cardiology* **46**, 576

Wellens HJJ, Brugada P, Stevenson WG. (1985) Programmed electrical stimulation of the heart in patients with life-threatening ventricular arrhythmias. What is the significance of induced arrhythmias and what is the correct stimulation protocol? *Circulation* **72**, 1

Part IV

Therapies

11

Strategies

The investigation and treatment of patients with arrhythmias often requires many complex decisions at several stages, from the initial approach to diagnosis to the treatment which is finally chosen. Much of this (such as the selection of patients for further investigation, the type of investigation, etc.) is encompassed by well-formulated strategies within the clinical process, and a detailed description of all possible approaches to specific problems is not appropriate in this context. There are, however, some areas of investigation and treatment in which strategy is unclear or not appropriately applied. For the purposes of this chapter we have identified two such areas of clinical electrophysiology: (1) strategies during the clinical electrophysiological study; and (2) strategies for treatment.

Strategy during electrophysiological study

An electrophysiological study should be designed to suit the individual requirements of the patient. Factors which might influence this design include:

1. The nature of the problem.
2. Anatomical considerations such as the size of the patient and sites of access.
3. Events occurring during the study itself.

The problem

A patient undergoing study for investigation of suspected abnormalities of impulse generation or conduction (e.g. sinus node and AV conduction studies) is not likely to require the same rigorous study protocol as a patient being investigated for tachycardias. Thus, fewer catheters and sites of access will be needed. If appropriate, it may be possible to save time by performing the study at the same time as pacemaker implantation. There are, however, occasions when the diagnosis is in doubt, and it may be necessary to consider a full stimulation study to expose other possible causes of symptoms, such as re-entrant junctional tachycardias or ventricular tachycardia. Furthermore, in patients undergoing diagnostic studies (e.g. for syncope or palpitations) it is not sufficient to accept the first revealed abnormality as solely responsible for causing symptoms. Thus, if a markedly prolonged sinus node recovery time is discovered (see Chapter 4) the possibility of atrial or junctional tachycardia should not be automatically discounted.

Compared to bradycardias and conduction defects, investigation of recurrent paroxysmal tachycardias is usually more time consuming and the results of study are much more likely to have a bearing on final treatment. More electrodes are needed (for mapping and pacing, etc.) and often one or more repeat studies are undertaken to ascertain the effectiveness of treatment. Thus, some thought must be given to the number of catheters needed and the optimal insertion sites of these catheters. In patients likely to require serial drug studies, it is preferable to leave one catheter (sometimes more) *in situ* at the end of the study to enable recording and pacing to be undertaken over a period of several days. The subclavian vein is most suitable for this purpose as it is comfortable for the patient and may be kept clean and dry. The choice of electrode is also important in this respect. If it is likely that atrial and ventricular stimulation are needed for repeat studies, and appropriate catheter with atrial and ventricular electrodes (e.g. a hexapolar catheter) could be used. These factors should be considered when it is anticipated that further studies will be required.

Anatomical considerations

The size of the patient limits the number of electrodes which can safely be inserted. Thus, in children weighing under 10 kg it may be necessary to perform the entire study using one or two catheters. In such small children, however, the need for venous access should be carefully considered because it may be possible to obtain the desired information or therapeutic effect by transoesophageal techniques (see Chapter 2). For repeat studies, however, it is often easier to insert a subclavian electrode rather than attempt reinsertion of an oesophageal lead at each occasion. In patients with certain forms of congenital heart disease, the relationship of the electrodes to the conduction system is abnormal and different techniques are required to manipulate the catheters (Figs. 11.1 and 11.2).

Events during the study

An electrophysiological study should not be regarded as a rigid and inflexible event which follows a specified protocol in a stepwise manner. In different clinical settings there are different aims and the study should be tailored to the individual patient under consideration. Thus, in patients with junctional tachycardias the study will concentrate on abnormalities of the electrophysiology of AV junctional tissues. There are, however, many factors which may influence the course of the study, especially in patients investigated for tachycardias.

A standard protocol for study of a patient with junctional tachycardias might be as follows:

1. Anterograde conduction studies and provocation of tachycardia by extrastimulus testing during atrial pacing.
2. Retrograde conduction studies, etc., during ventricular pacing.
3. Study of the tachycardia (if induced).
4. Assessment of sinus node recovery times.
5. Initiation of atrial fibrillation (in patients with pre-excitation).
6. Administration of a drug and repeat of steps 1–4 as necessary.

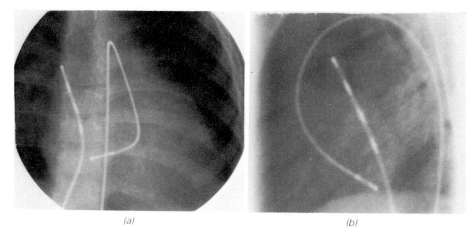

(a)   (b)

Fig. 11.1 (a) Posteroanterior and (b) lateral views showing position of electrode catheters for electrophysiological study of a 4½-year-old child who was suffering from rapid tachycardias after Mustard's operation for ventriculoarterial discordance (transposition of the great arteries). The quadripolar catheter was introduced in the right femoral vein and positioned in the systemic venous compartment of the atrium. The bipolar catheter was passed retrogradely from the right femoral artery to the systemic ventricle (morphologically right ventricle) and positioned retrogradely across the tricuspid valve to record the His potential. Recordings from a similar patient are shown in Fig. 11.2.

If tachycardia is induced at step 1, it may be necessary to modify this protocol to allow for detailed study of tachycardia (see below). In patients with a known (or suspected) tendency to atrial fibrillation in addition to tachycardia (e.g. patients with Wolff–Parkinson–White (WPW) syndrome) anterograde studies using atrial pacing and extrastimulus testing are more likely to cause atrial fibrillation which may interfere with the progress of the investigation. In this setting these studies are best deferred to later in the investigation after other important information has been acquired.

If tachycardia is initiated by extrastimulus testing or inadvertently during catheter manipulation, a decision must be made whether to study the arrhythmia or to terminate it and proceed with the predetermined protocol. If tachycardia appears infrequently or has not been observed or studied previously, it would be unfortunate to lose the opportunity of obtaining useful information by terminating tachycardia immediately. All clinical investigators recall occasions where this has been done and the identical tachycardia could not be initiated subsequently. If tachycardia is sustained, a 12-lead surface ECG should be recorded. Subsequently, information which does not depend on cardiac stimulation (which may terminate tachycardia) can be sought. If the catheters are in position, high speed recordings of intracardiac electrograms should be taken and, if relevant, detailed mapping studies can be performed. After the appropriate recordings of tachycardia have been made, the responses to atrial (bearing in mind the possibility of atrial fibrillation) and ventricular stimulation can be studied.

A retrogradely functioning anomalous VA pathway can be excluded by

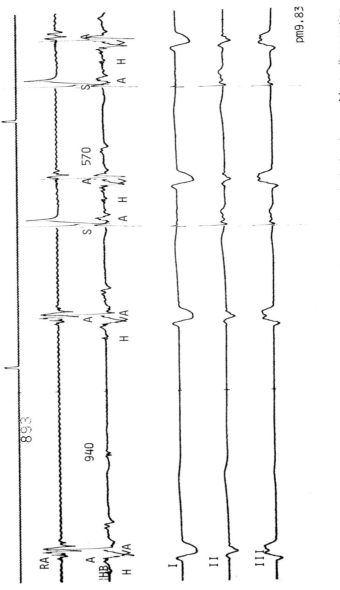

Fig. 11.2 Intracardiac recordings (obtained as shown in Fig. 11.1) from a patient who had undergone Mustard's operation. The strip begins with a junctional escape rhythm (cycle length 940 msec) with each QRS complex preceded by a His (H) potential. With the initiation of artial pacing (S), there is normal anterograde AV conduction. Paper speed 100 mm/sec. HB = His bundle region; RA = systemic venous atrium.

ventricular pacing. This can be performed at the outset before prolonged catheter manipulation. The presence of VA block during ventricular pacing despite inducible tachycardia excludes anomalous retrograde conduction during tachycardia. Definitive proof of anomalous retrograde conduction during tachycardia (obtained by atrial capture phenomena; see Chapter 9) should be obtained by ventricular stimulation during tachycardia. After these preliminary investigations, attention may be given to methods of terminating tachycardia by extrastimulation and rapid pacing. Conduction studies can be resumed when tachycardia has been terminated.

In patients undergoing study for sinoatrial disease and associated tachycardias, sinus node recovery time and sinoatrial conduction time may be more conveniently measured at the outset of the study to avoid the possible interference of tachycardia, especially atrial fibrillation.

Drugs are administered during an electrophysiological study either to assist in diagnosis or (more commonly) as part of efforts to establish treatment. If paroxysmal tachycardia is the clinical problem, the drug is usually given during sustained tachycardia (noting slowing and termination, etc.) or during sinus rhythm (if tachycardia is non-sustained or haemodynamically unstable) prior to repeat attempts to reinduce tachycardia (see Chapter 12). Occasionally, however, the order of events must be changed. For example, if atrial fibrillation is inadvertently initiated before the clinical tachycardia can be identified and studied the options are to abandon the study, to convert to sinus rhythm by external DC shock or to attempt pharmacological termination. If study of the tachycardia mechanism is important in the management decision (e.g. ablation or pacemaker treatment), pharmacological intervention is best avoided because initiation of the tachycardia may not be possible after the drug has been given. On the other hand, if the tachycardia has already been initiated and studied, an attempt at pharmacological termination of atrial fibrillation is reasonable because inducibility of other tachycardias can be restudied after drug administration. Junctional and atrial tachycardias can usually be restarted after DC cardioversion, although the electrophysiological effects of this procedure are not well documented.

It may be useful to frame a series of questions before embarking on a clinical study (Table 11.1). In the example of the WPW syndrome, many of the clinical questions may be answered by simple non-invasive tests (Table 11.2). The content and sequence of a comprehensive electrophysiological study of a patient

Table 11.1 WPW SYNDROME – QUESTIONS TO BE ANSWERED

Is pre-excitation present?

What type of pre-excitation is present?

How many pathways are present?

What are the functional properties of the pathways?

What tachycardias can be induced?

What is the involvement of the pathway(s) in the tachycardia(s)?

What is the effect of drugs on the pathway(s) and tachycardia(s)?

Table 11.2 NON-INVASIVE ASSESSMENT OF WPW SYNDROME

TEST	PURPOSE
12-lead ECG	Approximate location of anomalous pathway
Exercise ECG	Modification of pre-excitation and possible provocation of tachycardia
Holter (24 hour) ECG	Intermittency of pre-excitation and documentation of spontaneous tachycardia
Procainamide or ajmaline tests	To assess the approximate anterograde refractory period of anomalous pathway
Negative dromotropic agents/manoeuvres (verapamil, ATP, short-acting beta blockers, CSM, VM, etc.)	To reveal pre-excitation
Isoprenaline	To assess maximum conduction capacity of anomalous pathway during atrial fibrillation

ATP = adenosine triphosphate; CSM = carotid sinus massage; VM = Valsalva manoeuvre.

with the **WPW** syndrome is summarized in Table 11.3. The information provided by the non-invasive and invasive approaches should answer the questions enumerated in Table 11.1. It should be borne in mind, however, that a simple table or flow diagram is too rigid – a degree of flexibility is essential. A similar study plan for ventricular tachycardia is presented in Table 10.2.

In patients with serious or potentially serious symptoms (such as syncope or

Table 11.3 ELECTROPHYSIOLOGY STUDY SEQUENCE FOR WPW SYNDROME

Sinus rhythm

Pacing, at CL 600 msec and 400 msec, in the RV, then CS, then RA (?LV)

Assessment of refractory periods: single extrastimulus to the RV, CS and RA:
    At BCL 600 msec
    At BCL 400 msec

Induction of AVRT (if not already induced):
    Double extrastimulation at CL 600 msec, and 400 msec (RV, then CS, then RA)
    Burst pacing at incremental rates (up to 250 b.p.m.), (RV, then CS, then RA)
    Automatic manipulation – isoprenaline infusion, administration of atropine, etc.

Mapping of retrograde atrial sequence during tachycardia

Extrastimulation during tachycardia: RV then CS then RA (?LV)

Induction of atrial fibrillation: RA burst pacing (HRA preferable to RAA; avoid CS)

BCL = basic cycle length; CL = cycle length; CS = coronary sinus; HRA = high right atrium; LV = left ventricle; RA = right atrium; RAA = right atrial appendage; RV = right ventricle; AVRT = AV re-entrant tachycardia.

Table 11.4 COMPARISON OF STRATEGIES FOR ELECTROPHYSIOLOGICAL INVESTIGATION OF SUDDEN DEATH SYNDROME AND SYNCOPE

	Syncope	Sudden death syndrome
Before EPS	ECG, Holter, Echo Neurological evaluation Endocrine evaluation	ECG, Holter, Echo Exercise test Cardiac catheterization: Coronary arteriogram RV & LV angiogram ?Ventricular biopsy
At EPS	Sinus node function AV conduction studies Ventricular tachycardia provocation S1S2S3 – 1 site	Anomalous conduction tests AV conduction studies Ventricular tachycardia provocation S1S2S2S4 – 3 sites (including left ventricle)

sudden out-of-hospital cardiac arrest) it is essential to consider the overall strategy of investigation before proceeding to electrophysiological testing. For example, non-invasive investigations should be used to exclude other possible causes of the symptoms. This is well illustrated by comparing possible strategies of investigation in patients with unexplained syncope and in those who have suffered a sudden cardiac arrest outside hospital (Table 11.4). When using provocation testing to elicit ventricular arrhythmias in these patients, it should be recalled that the sensitivity and specificity of any given protocol are not known (see Chapter 10) and that non-specific responses to stimulation are probably not uncommon. In patients with potentially life-threatening arrhythmias, however, it may be prudent to use more aggressive stimulation protocols to elicit a response, even though it may be non-specific.

Strategies of therapy

The clinical decision of most importance in the treatment of bradycardias is whether or not a pacemaker should be implanted. In this respect the strategies for treatment of bradycardias are comparatively simple compared to those for tachycardias (see Table 11.5).

There are five basic strategies for the treatment of tachycardias:

1. Prevention of tachycardia.
2. Reduction in the ventricular response to continued tachycardia (amelioration of tachycardia).
3. Deliberate maintenance of tachycardia, the rate of which is controlled by another means.
4. Repeated termination of recurrent tachycardia.
5. Permanent abolition of tachycardia (cure?).

At present, the major therapeutic methods are:

1. Pharmacological.
2. Implantation of electrical devices.
3. Transvenous ablation or surgical ablation of the tachycardia substrate.

Table 11.5 THERAPY FOR TACHYCARDIA

ENDS	MEANS
Cure	Reassurance
Termination of paroxysm	Physical manoeuvres
Suppression	DC cardioversion/defibrillation
Amelioration	Drugs
	Surgery
	Catheter ablation
	Implantable devices:
	Pacemaker
	Cardioversion
	Defibrillator

Each strategy may be pursued with a particular therapeutic method. Some strategies are applied more effectively with a particular treatment (e.g. cure by surgery) and some treatments are not appropriate for a particular strategy (e.g. drug treatment aiming to effect a cure rather than prevent). Thus, for any given arrhythmia there is a hierarchy of therapeutic choices. In general, prevention is the usual approach and a trial of drugs is preferred prior to consideration of pacing or ablation. Many of the strategies are effectively applied only with the aid of information from the electrophysiological investigation.

Prevention

In patients with recurrent tachycardias the logical approach to treatment is prevention of recurrences. This strategy includes general measures such as correction of underlying, reversible abnormalities (e.g. structural defects and metabolic abnormalities) and removal of specific provocative factors (e.g. toxic drugs). If simple measures fail, antiarrhythmic drugs are considered.

Antiarrhythmic drugs for prevention

The choice of an antiarrhythmic drug to prevent or suppress tachycardia is determined by many factors, including the mechanism of tachycardia (e.g. re-entrant or automatic), location (e.g. atria or ventricles) and exacerbating influences (e.g. exertion). Theoretically, there are several possible approaches. If, for example, a tachycardia is always initiated by ventricular extrasystoles, prevention of sustained tachycardia can be achieved by abolition of the ventricular extrasystoles without regard to the mechanisms of tachycardia. Where the mechanism of tachycardia is different from the mechanism of the initiating event (e.g. AV re-entry, triggered by ventricular extrasystoles) it may be possible to modify each component of the clinical problem independently. Thus, drugs which alter the properties of a re-entrant circuit may prevent tachycardia without diminishing the frequency of potentially initiating events. However, because most antiarrhythmic drugs have several actions, such selective treatment is often impossible. It is also possible that although one particular action of a drug may be beneficial (e.g. suppression of ectopic beats) another may be deleterious (e.g. perpetuation of re-entry by slowing of conduction). The choice of strategy if drug prevention fails depends on the type of tachycardia. Some may be amenable to termination with drugs which can be administered by the patient, whereas others are more difficult to terminate and might be more conveniently and comfortably maintained with drugs (e.g. use of digoxin to convert paroxysmal to sustained atrial fibrillation) or pacing.

Pacemakers for prevention

The use of pacemakers to prevent the emergence of tachycardias associated with a slow heart rate is well known and is the simplest way in which pacing can be used to 'suppress' tachycardias. More complicated systems include dual site pacing and prestimulation to modify a potential re-entry circuit. These methods are often suitable for the short term but unreliable in the long term. They are discussed in more detail in Chapter 13.

Surgery for prevention

The place of surgery in the prevention of tachycardias (rather than their cure) is not clear. Coronary artery disease is the commonest surgically treated abnormality associated with symptomatic recurrent tachycardias. Revascularization of the myocardium does not, however, appear to have much effect (an unpredictable one at best) on these arrhythmias unless more specific surgical measures (see Chapter 14) are undertaken at the same time.

Amelioration of continuing tachycardia

This strategy is applicable to any tachycardia arising above the AV node. If the tachycardia cannot be prevented or terminated, symptomatic improvement can be achieved by reducing the ventricular response to tachycardia.

Amelioration by drugs

Agents which prolong AV nodal refractoriness are effective in reducing the ventricular response to atrial arrhythmias. The major groups of drugs used for this purpose are digitalis glycosides, beta blockers and some calcium antagonists. In patients with an anomalous AV pathway (see Chapter 6) this form of therapy will not work because these drugs have no significant effect on the anomalous pathway. In this setting, the drugs of choice are class 1 and class 3 drugs.

Amelioration by pacing

With so many effective antiarrhythmic drugs readily available, the use of pacing to ameliorate the ventricular response to continuing atrial tachycardia is rarely needed. When undertaken, it is usually as an emergency measure prior to more definitive treatment such as ablation. The pacing methods used are continuous atrial pacing (high rate pacing with second degree AV block reducing the ventricular rate), coupled atrial pacing (an atrial extrastimulus is coupled to each tachycardia beat so that the next beat is pre-empted but the extrastimulus blocks in the AV node), and paired atrial pacing (similar to coupled atrial pacing, but the atria are continuously overdriven and the extrastimulus is coupled to every paced beat). These techniques are cumbersome and largely obsolete. Ventricular pacing is occasionally effective in slowing the ventricular response to rapid atrial fibrillation (see Chapter 8).

Amelioration by ablation

The ventricles can be removed from the influence of continuing atrial tachycardias by ablation of AV conduction. This may be performed surgically or electrically (see Chapters 14 and 15). Not uncommonly, complete AV block is not obtained but the ventricular response rate is much reduced, presumably reflecting partial interference with the mechanism of AV nodal transmission.

Maintenance of tachycardia

In patients with frequently recurrent tachycardias which have not responded to prevention and are not suitable for termination, consideration should be given to maintaining the tachycardia and applying ameliorative strategies. A good example of this approach is in the treatment of paroxysmal atrial fibrillation or flutter where digoxin may be used to maintain the tachycardia (i.e. prevent paroxysmal changes of rhythm) and control the ventricular response. Rapid atrial pacing may be used to convert atrial flutter to atrial fibrillation, achieving the same result.

Termination of tachycardias

In many patients with tachycardias, especially those supported by junctional re-entrant mechanisms, recurrent attacks can be controlled by repeated termination. The utility and effectiveness of this strategy depend on many factors, including the type of tachycardia and the frequency of recurrences. Several therapeutic modes can be used: (1) physiological manoeuvres; (2) DC cardioversion; (3) drug termination; and (4) pacemaker termination.

Physiological manoeuvres

Many patients with junctional tachycardias have learned some manoeuvre which terminates the tachycardia. Most of these work by causing a surge of efferent vagal activity which slows AV nodal conduction and prolongs refractoriness. They include deep inspiration, the Valsalva manoeuvre (Fig. 11.3), the diving reflex, carotid sinus massage and eyeball pressure. The last is the least effective and the most uncomfortable. Ventricular tachycardias rarely respond to these procedures. Atrial tachycardias (including atrial fibrillation, atrial flutter and atrial tachycardia) do not usually terminate, although a beneficial effect is

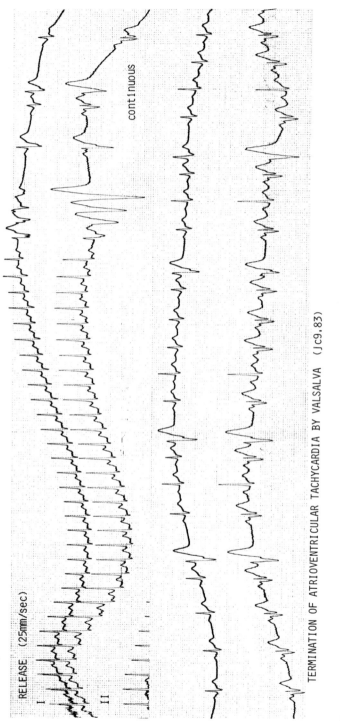

Fig. 11.3 Termination of atrioventricular tachycardia (left free wall anomalous pathway) by the Valsalva manoeuvre. Eight seconds after the release of the Valsalva manoeuvre, tachycardia is terminated in the anterograde limb. Immediately after termination, there is a short run of ventricular tachycardia, a phenomenon not uncommonly observed during the release phase. Ventricular ectopic beats were recorded for 30 seconds after the manoeuvre.

CONTROL

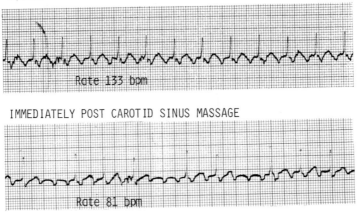

Fig. 11.4 Use of carotid sinus massage to slow the ventricular rate during atrial flutter. In the upper strip the atrial rate is 266 b.p.m. with 2:1 AV block. Immediately after carotid sinus massage, there is variable AV block due to prolonged AV nodal conduction time and refractoriness. The flutter waves are now clearly seen.

obtained by inducing increased AV block (Fig. 11.4). This effect may also clarify the diagnosis by revealing the underlying atrial rhythm disturbance.

Direct current cardioversion

This method is well tried and relatively safe for the termination of any paroxysmal tachycardia. It is most often used in an emergency for unstable ventricular tachycardias and for the elective cardioversion of atrial fibrillation or flutter. There is almost no need for this method in stable junctional tachycardias, which are more conveniently treated by drugs or pacing. Recently, this strategy has been applied to long-term treatment of refractory ventricular arrhythmias by implantation of an automatic defibrillator (see Chapter 13). The method is, however, not without dangers, and consideration should be given to other methods of termination if appropriate. An alternative to an automatic implanted device is the use of an automatic or 'semi-automatic' external defibrillator.

Drug termination

The understanding of tachycardias gained from intracardiac studies has provided a solid foundation for drug therapy. Drug termination of tachycardias should no longer be an empirical process, the success of which is determined by chance. The efficacy of this method depends on the type of arrhythmia and the drug used. Thus, junctional tachycardias are effectively terminated by agents which prolong AV nodal refractoriness, whereas atrial tachycardias are little affected by these drugs. This strategy is most useful for relatively infrequent attacks in patients who can attend a physician at the time of the attack. A major disadvantage of the method (especially with respect to ventricular tachycardia) is aggravation of the tachycardia. Drugs with very short half-lives are especially useful for the termination of tachycardia. In this respect lignocaine is valuable for termination of ventricular tachycardia, and recently available experimental agents such as adenosine (a purinergic agent), esmolol and flestolol (new ultrashort half-life beta-adrenergic blocking drugs) are useful for terminating junctional tachycardias.

Pacemaker termination

In patients with relatively infrequent tachycardias which are not controlled by drug treatment, or in whom drugs are not tolerated or accepted, termination of the arrhythmia can be achieved by pacing (see Chapter 13). This method is useful in an emergency (e.g. oesophageal pacing to terminate supraventricular tachycardia, see Chapter 2) and also to control symptoms outside of hospital. For this last application, specially built pacemakers are available. These units recognize tachycardia automatically and respond by stimulating the heart in a preset manner. This form of treatment avoids the uncertainty and discomfort of vagal manoeuvres and the inconvenience of frequent attendance at hospital for drug termination or cardioversion.

Permanent abolition of the tachycardia substrate

The physiological basis for tachycardia can be radically altered or destroyed by transvenous electrical ablation or surgical ablation at operation (e.g. ablation of an anomalous pathway or tachycardia focus). This strategy is the only one which offers the prospect of a 'cure' because the supposed tachycardia substrate is removed, or partly removed, rather than modified by drugs or pacing methods. The approach is based on accurate mapping techniques designed to localize the focus or circuit or an important component of it which is then destroyed. Surgical interruption of anomalous conduction is a most effective cure for tachycardias associated with the WPW syndrome. When applied to ventricular tachycardias, however, the method is less successful and cannot always be regarded as a cure in the same sense (recurrences are due to factors such

Table 11.6 TREATMENT OF WPW SYNDROME

Clinical presentation	Surgery	Medication	Device	No treatment
AF + short PRR	A	A	I	I
AVRT + short PRR	A	A	I	I
AVRT + long PRR	A	A	A	A
Asymptomatic + short PRR	A	A	I	A
Asymptomatic + long PRR	I	I	I	A

A = acceptable; I = generally inappropriate; short PRR = an interval of 250 msec or less between pre-excited QRS complexes; AF = atrial fibrillation; AVRT = re-entrant tachycardia.

as progressive disease, greater difficulty in localization, arrhythmogenic effects of surgery, etc.). These strategies are discussed in detail in Chapters 14 and 15.

In summary, it is clear that many options are available for the investigation and treatment of a particular tachycardia in an individual patient. The advantages of a chosen strategy and the therapeutic mode selected to apply it must be carefully weighed against the potential disadvantages and the advantages of many other possible forms of treatment. An example of the possible therapeutic approaches to the WPW syndrome is shown in Table 11.6.

12

Drug Studies

Prescription of treatment

Until the late 1970s the choice of an antiarrhythmic drug was largely empirical because it was based almost entirely on inadequate clinical experience. Furthermore, there was considerable misconception about the likely efficacy of such drugs and, apart from the well-known side effects seen with digoxin and to some extent with quinidine, it was hardly recognized that antiarrhythmic drugs might as readily provoke or aggravate arrhythmias as suppress them. However, it is now appreciated that the choice of antiarrhythmic therapy needs considerable care to ensure success and avoid tragedy. Nowhere is this more important than in the management of ventricular tachycardias, but some atrial and junctional tachyarrhythmias can also be better treated using electrophysiological techniques to derive the best prescription.

Atrial tachycardias

The method of serial drug testing (see below) can be used to evaluate which drugs will be most successful at preventing the artificial restimulation or spontaneous reinitiation of arrhythmias, such as atrial fibrillation or atrial flutter. In selected patients, potential adverse effects of these drugs, such as depression of AV conduction or worsening of sinus node function, may also be assessed before exposing the patient to out-of-hospital treatment. Conversely, some antiarrhythmics may so facilitate AV nodal conduction that atrial arrhythmias may conduct more rapidly to the ventricles, resulting in symptomatic and haemodynamic deterioration. Similarly, AV conduction of atrial arrhythmias over anomalous pathways can be most easily assessed by stimulating or simulating (by rapid atrial pacing) atrial arrhythmias after pretreatment with the drug (Table 12.1). Such studies have shown that class 1A, class 1C and class 3 antiarrhythmic agents may reduce the ventricular response by prolonging the refractoriness of the anomalous pathway (Fig. 12.1) whereas lignocaine, digoxin and verapamil may accelerate the ventricular response to atrial fibrillation in patients with Wolff–Parkinson–White (WPW) syndrome predominantly by reducing the anterograde refractoriness of the anomalous pathway. The mechanism of exacerbation caused by lignocaine (Barrett et al., 1980) and verapamil (Harper et al., 1982) is probably related to increased sympathetic tone secondary to the hypotensive effects of these drugs. Digoxin may shorten the refractoriness of the anomalous pathway or decrease the degree of anterograde concealed conduction into the pathway (Sellers et al., 1977).

Table 12.1 SLOWING OF VENTRICULAR RESPONSE TO ATRIAL FIBRILLATION

AVN (normal pathway)	WPW/LGL (anomalous pathway)
Digoxin	Procainamide
Verapamil	Quinidine
Beta blockade	Disopyramide
Amiodarone	Flecainide
	Amiodarone
Caution	**Caution**
Not disopyramide	Not digoxin
Not quinidine	Not verapamil
	Not lignocaine

Junctional tachycardia

The re-entrant basis and the substrate (circuit) of most junctional tachycardias have been well established. It may be possible, during tachycardia (by the introduction of single atrial or ventricular premature beats), to assess the conduction capacity (refractoriness) of several or all sections of the tachycardia circuit. Thus the weakest sector in the circuit (refractory period closest to the tachycardia cycle length) can be identified and the susceptibility to drugs of this and other parts of the circuit can be evaluated and balanced against any slowing of tachycardia circulation produced by the drug.

Junctional tachycardias may be initiated by atrial or ventricular premature beats, or by sinus tachycardia (see Chapter 9). Electrophysiological study allows assessment of these possibilities and subsequent appropriate drug therapy. Furthermore, differences in refractoriness critical to tachycardia initiation may be identified and treatment can be designed to minimize such differences (Fig. 12.2). For example, initiation of an orthodromic atrioventricular tachycardia by an atrial premature beat will occur only if the anterograde refractory period of the anomalous pathway is longer than that of the AV node. If this difference is found to be small, a drug which tends to lengthen AV nodal refractoriness (e.g. verapamil) is likely to be effective therapy, but treatment with a drug which shortens AV nodal refractoriness and increases anomalous pathway refractoriness (such as disopyramide) will probably be unsuccessful. Similar reasoning may suggest the use of a class 1 (Vaughan Williams' (VW) classification, see below) agent for prevention of a junctional tachycardia which is initiated by spontaneous ventricular premature beats (Fig. 12.2).

Ventricular tachycardia

The annual mortality of patients with chronic heart disease who have suffered a sustained ventricular arrhythmia (tachycardia or fibrillation not associated with an acute ischaemic event) approaches 40 per cent (see Chapter 10). Since death may be the consequence of failure to prescribe the 'best' therapy, successful management of this problem is essential. A variety of management strategies have been suggested; when the arrhythmias occur very frequently, or can be

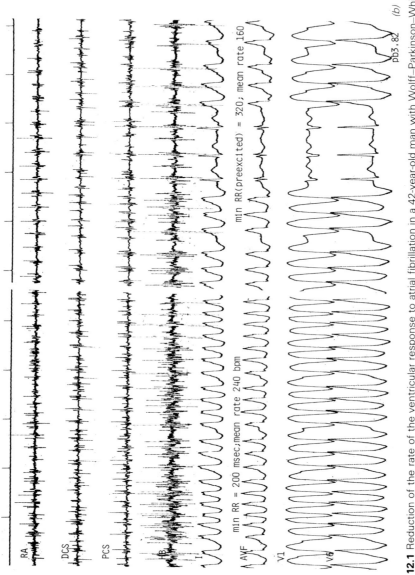

RA

DCS

PCS

HB

I

AVF   min RR = 200 msec;mean rate 240 bpm   min RR(preexcited) = 320; mean rate 160

V1

V6

pb3,82

(a)   (b)

Fig. 12.1 Reduction of the rate of the ventricular response to atrial fibrillation in a 42-year-old man with Wolff–Parkinson–White syndrome. (a) Rapid response (minimum pre-excited RR interval = 200 msec). (b) After intravenous flecainide (150 mg) the ventricular response was reduced (minimum pre-excited RR = 320 msec) and pre-excitation is intermittent. Note the slowing of the atrial electrograms after flecainide. Paper speed 25 mm/sec.

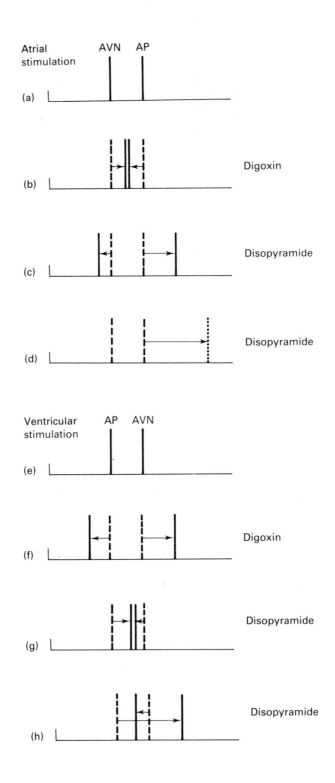

consistently provoked by exertion, long-term ambulatory ECG monitoring or exercise electrocardiography can be used to test the success of any treatment. Good results may be achieved provided that the published protocol is followed strictly. However, most ventricular tachycardias are not of this sort, but instead can be triggered by ventricular pacing (see Chapter 10). Such techniques may form a basis for the evaluation of medical management – the method is known as 'serial drug testing'. The ease and possibility of tachycardia provocation is determined before and after the administration of a sequence of drugs and drug combinations. Provided that a prescription which prevents tachycardia provocation is found, the long-term administration of such a regimen is likely to prove a successful therapy (Fig. 12.3). It is usual to test class 1 drugs (see below) first, followed by class 3 drugs or combinations of each class. When the intravenous administration of an antiarrhythmic results in suppression of the inducibility of tachycardia, the oral formulation should be similarly tested to ensure long-term efficacy.

Waxman et al. (1983) investigated the possibility of using the response to a single drug to predict responses to other drugs of a similar type. Some 86 per cent of sustained ventricular tachycardias suppressed by procainamide were also suppressed by other class 1 drugs or a beta blocker or combinations of these agents. In contrast, only 16 per cent of those tachycardias not suppressed by procainamide were suppressed by other regimens. Likewise, 64 per cent of drug regimens used in procainamide responders were also effective, whereas only 7 per cent were effective in non-responders. These preliminary studies suggest that the response to procainamide may predict the response to other selected agents and combinations of agents, thereby reducing the time needed for serial testing. These studies, however, require confirmation with other agents and in large numbers of patients. The specific value of procainamide (compared to other drugs) in this context is not proven.

Unfortunately, there is no agreement on the selection of protocols to be used for the serial drug studies in patients with ventricular tachycardia. The assessment of drug efficacy in this context has been seriously hampered by difficulties in the interpretation of results of numerous studies using different

---

Fig. 12.2 The theoretical effects of digoxin and disopyramide on the tachycardia initiation windows with (a–d) atrial and (e–h) ventricular extrastimulation. (a) The anterograde effective refractory periods (ERP) of the AV node (AVN) and the anomalous pathway (AP). The ERP of the AP exceeds that of the AV node and orthodromic tachycardia is induced by block in the AP. (b) Digoxin prolongs the AV nodal ERP and may shorten the ERP of the AP, thus narrowing the tachycardia zone. (c) The opposite effect induced by disopyramide. The atropine-like effect may outweigh the direct action of the drug on the AV node and the tachycardia zone is widened. Usually, however, disopyramide only prolongs the ERP of the AP (d). (e) The retrograde ERP of the normal (VA) pathway and the anomalous pathway (AP). The ERP of the VA pathway exceeds that of the AP and tachycardia is initiated by a ventricular extrastimulus which blocks in the normal VA pathway., Digoxin may widen the initiation zone as indicated in (f) by prolonging the VA pathway ERP and reducing the AP retrograde ERP. Disopyramide has the opposite effect (g) by prolonging the ERP of the AP and reducing the normal VA pathway ERP. Marked prolongation of the retrograde ERP of the AP such that it exceeds that of the VAP may abolish the tachycardia zone altogether (h) unless antidromic tachycardia is initiated by retrograde block in the AP but conduction in the normal VA pathway and continued anterograde AV re-entry over the AP.

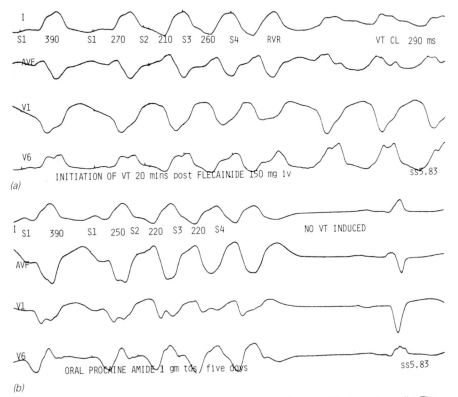

I
S1   390   S1   270   S2   210   S3   260   S4   RVR   VT CL   290 ms

AVF

V1

V6
      INITIATION OF VT 20 mins post FLECAINIDE 150 mg iv   ss5.83
(a)

I
S1   390   S1   250 S2   220   S3   220   S4   NO VT INDUCED

AVF

V1

V6
      ORAL PROCAINE AMIDE 1 gm tds / five days   ss5.83
(b)

Fig. 12.3 Serial drug testing in a patient with recurrent sustained ventricular tachycardia. The control tachycardia cycle length was 220 msec. After intravenous flecainide tachycardia was still inducible by right ventricular pacing (S1S1) and triple extrastimuli (S2S3S4) although the cycle length was increased to 290 msec (a). After oral procainamide (b) triple extrastimuli failed to induce tachycardia. The patient did well for 6 months with no symptoms, when he suddenly collapsed and died. Paper speed 100 mm/sec.

protocols. One such protocol for serial testing is shown in Table 12.2. (DiMarco et al., 1980). Another, devised by Wellens et al. (1985), is described in Chapter 10.

There is little information about the predictive value of administering the drug during induced ventricular tachycardia. Clearly, this is possible only if the tachycardia is haemodynamically stable. Most agents used for the treatment of ventricular tachycardias tend to depress myocardial 'contractility' and may cause profound hypotension during tachycardia in patients with important left ventricular disease. This approach should therefore be used cautiously. In selected patients, however, administration of the drug during tachycardia may provide useful information. Preliminary information using flecainide suggests that termination of induced tachycardia may be a more useful predictor of long-term effectiveness than suppression of tachycardia induction after oral or intravenous drug administration (Ward et al., 1986).

The precise schedule of drug testing must depend on certain important clinical

Table 12.2 GRADES OF PROVOCATION FOR SERIAL DRUG TESTING IN VENTRICULAR TACHYCARDIA (DiMarco et al., 1980)

I	Extrastimulus testing during sinus rhythm or atrial pacing
II	Single extrastimulus after ventricular drive pacing
III	Double extrastimulus after ventricular drive pacing
IV	Ventricular burst pacing

factors. In particular, previous drug history, current therapy with amiodarone, the status of left ventricular function and the type of ventricular tachycardia are relevant to the choice of drug(s) to be tested. A specific scheme of serial drug testing is set out below:

1. A class 1B (VW) drug (e.g. mexiletine).
2. A class 1A (VW) drug (e.g. disopyramide).
3. A class 1C (VW) drug (e.g. flecainide).
4. A class 3 (VW) drug (e.g. sotalol).
5. Another class 3 (VW) drug (e.g. amiodarone).
6. Class 1 and class 3 (VW) combinations.

Such a schedule would be appropriate for a patient with recently diagnosed tachycardia without significantly impaired left ventricular function and no prior therapy. In the presence of severe left ventricular disease steps 2, 3 and 4 may be hazardous because of further depression of 'contractility', and are best omitted.

There is limited information about the efficacy of drug combinations assessed by programmed electrical stimulation (Kim et al., 1985a; Greenspan et al., 1986). Clearly, it is not possible to assess multiple combinations and permutations of a large number of drugs, so some means of predicting which combinations are likely to be effective are needed. A combination of two agents which have a partial antiarrhythmic effect when used alone (e.g. slowing of induced tachycardia, suppression of ventricular ectopy) seems more likely to be effective than combinations which include an inactive drug (Matos et al., 1984). Further carefully designed studies of drug combinations are needed to clarify this potentially important aspect of antiarrhythmic therapy, especially in relation to ventricular arrhythmias.

There are limitations to this method of assessment. In particular, there is a proportion of ventricular tachycardias (about 10 per cent of sustained, monomorphic tachycardia due to ischaemic heart disease, 25 per cent of idiopathic tachycardia and almost 70 per cent of exercise-induced tachycardia) which cannot be consistently provoked by electrical stimulation. Whilst the predictive accuracy of a fully positive response (tachycardia cannot be initiated) is high, the value of a negative study (the same tachycardia is still inducible) or of an equivocal result (a non-sustained tachycardia or one of shorter duration, a slower (Fig. 12.4) tachycardia or tachycardia which can be provoked only by more 'vigorous' stimulation) is less certain. What constitutes 'effective' drug treatment in patients in whom ventricular tachycardia remains inducible, is unanswered. Platia and Reid (1985) showed that induction of non-sustained

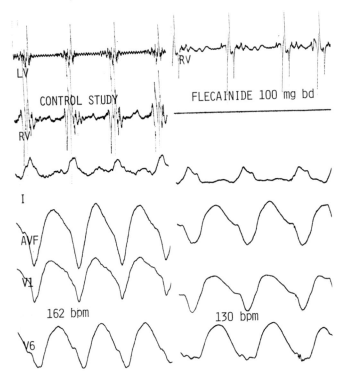

LV

RV

CONTROL STUDY

FLECAINIDE 100 mg bd

RV

I

AVF

V1

162 bpm

130 bpm

V6

Fig. 12.4 Slowing of ventricular tachycardia on drug treatment. The control tachycardia rate is 160 b.p.m. Although oral antiarrhythmic treatment failed to suppress initiation of tachycardia, the induced tachycardia was considerably slowed and better tolerated. This patient had no recurrences on long-term therapy. Paper speed 50 mm/sec. LV = left ventricle; RV= right ventricle.

tachycardia of five or more beats is an indication of inadequate treatment. On the other hand, Swerdlow et al. (1983b) concluded that suppression of sustained tachycardia with antiarrhythmic therapy was significantly more likely to be effective in patients with inducible tachycardias of less than 15 complexes' duration than in patients with sustained arrhythmias. Data concerning the significance of slowing of tachycardia rate are not available. Overall, drug testing identifies effective drug treatment in about 25–45 per cent of patients with monomorphic sustained ventricular tachycardia.

Several investigators have attempted to define variables which can be used to predict the outcome of serial electrophysiological drug testing. Unfortunately, no single factor distinguishes 'successes' (those in whom drug suppression was possible) and 'failures' (those in whom drug suppression was not possible). Among multivariate determinants of success (Spielman et al., 1983; Swerdlow et al., 1983c) are female sex, fewer episodes of arrhythmia and fewer coronary arteries affected by severe lesions, young age (<45 years) and limited left ventricular damage (hypokinesia only and ejection fraction >50 per cent). Factors contributing to failure include left ventricular aneurysm, Q waves and tachycardia induction with a single stimulus (see also Chapter 10). By extrapolation, it seems that patients at most risk of death (poor LV function, more residual coronary stenoses, etc.) are less likely to benefit from serial drug testing.

There is continued debate about the applicability of this form of testing for certain drugs, particularly amiodarone. The available evidence suggests that inducibility of tachycardia on amiodarone therapy does not predict failure of long-term treatment. If tachycardia is rendered non-inducible by treatment, however, spontaneous recurrences are unlikely. Furthermore, many investigators believe that serial testing is applicable after longer periods of treatment with amiodarone.

Another disadvantage of this technique is the financial cost and emotional strain of the repeated tachycardia stimulation necessary for multiple drug testing. Some protocols demand repeated insertion of electrodes for such studies. A protocol which requires stimulation at a single site (e.g. the Wellens' protocol, see Chapter 10) has considerable advantages in this respect. A single catheter may be left *in situ* via a neck vein and no manipulation of the catheter is necessary during the restudy. A potential disadvantage of this approach has been pointed out by Duff et al. (1986). These authors have shown, using an indwelling electrode, that changes in the response to ventricular extrastimulation can occur passively with time, resulting in loss of the ability to induce tachycardia where it existed at the baseline study. This phenomenon may mimic an antiarrhythmic drug effect. It may be caused by local tissue reactions to the indwelling electrode. The authors advise electrode replacement for serial testing. Variations in autonomic tone, however, could also account for these findings.

Finally, widespread and proper use of this technique demands the provision of specialist facilities and highly trained personnel.

Assessment of proarrhythmic effects (arrhythmogenic potential)

Drugs which modify properties of cardiac conduction and refractoriness must certainly be capable of either building or breaking potential tachycardia substrates. Thus a drug given for the purpose of preventing a tachycardia may paradoxically sustain the arrhythmia or render it more easily inducible. Alternatively, the treatment may provoke a quite different arrhythmia (either a bradycardia or tachycardia). Results such as these are described as 'proarrhythmic'.

It may be very difficult to distinguish these proarrhythmic effects from natural variation, but apparent deterioration in response to electrophysiological testing must be taken very seriously. Proarrhythmic effects are usually manifest as:

1. Acceleration of tachycardia.
2. Conversion of non-sustained to sustained tachycardia.
3. Conversion of monomorphic to multimorphic tachycardia.
4. Degeneration to ventricular fibrillation.
5. Resistance to termination by pacing or defibrillation.
6. Emergence of new types of tachycardia (Fig. 12.5).
7. Development of sinus node dysfunction, AV block or intraventricular block.

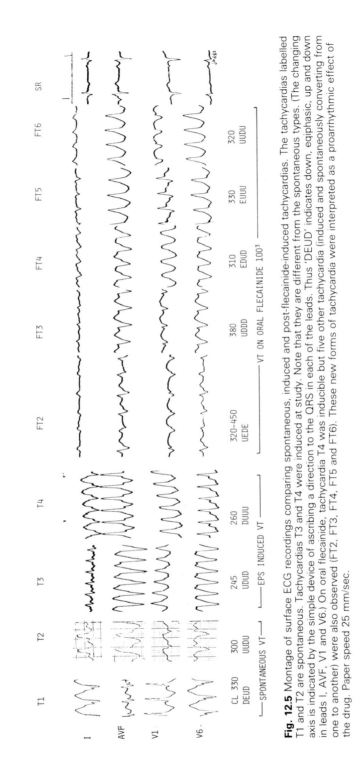

Fig. 12.5 Montage of surface ECG recordings comparing spontaneous, induced and post-flecainide-induced tachycardias. The tachycardias labelled T1 and T2 are spontaneous. Tachycardias T3 and T4 were induced at study. Note that they are different from the spontaneous types. (The changing axis is indicated by the simple device of ascribing a direction to the QRS in each of the leads. Thus 'DEUD' indicates down, eqiphasic, up and down in leads I, AVF, V1 and V6.) On oral flecainide, tachycardia T4 was inducible but five other tachycardia (induced and spontaneously converting from one to another) were also observed (FT2, FT3, FT4, FT5 and FT6). These new forms of tachycardia were interpreted as a proarrhythmic effect of the drug. Paper speed 25 mm/sec.

It is also important to consider and test the possibility that patients presenting with arrhythmias may be suffering largely because of current 'antiarrhythmic' drug therapy. Such a thesis (Ruskin et al., 1983) has been shown to be correct in a small proportion of those who sustain out-of-hospital cardiac arrest or recurrent ventricular tachycardia.

Use of drugs during an electrophysiological study

Tissue characterisation

In Chapter 3 cardiac conduction tissue is differentiated into so-called decremental and non-decremental types. Conduction in decremental tissue, such as the AV node, is largely due to the 'slow' action potentials typically produced by transmembrane calcium ion flux (and, to a limited extent, slow sodium ion flux). Such ionic movements are impeded by 'calcium antagonists' such as verapamil and by purinergic drugs such as adenosine. Adenosine also increases potassium ion flux and may be antiadrenergic. Because both drugs are quite specific, and adenosine has an extremely short half-life, they can be used to assess whether conduction is occurring through the AV node or via another pathway. For example, depression of retrograde conduction through the normal AV nodal pathway may reveal eccentric retrograde atrial activation via an anomalous pathway. It should be noted that some rare types of anomalous pathway share the same type of response to these drugs (Perrot et al., 1984).

Fast, sodium ion-dependent action potentials are not affected by adenosine or by calcium antagonists. On the other hand, ajmaline (a rauwolfia derivative) and other drugs such as the class 1C (VW) agents (see below) do impair this type of conduction. Theoretically, anomalous pathway conduction can be distinguished from AV nodal conduction by the depressive effect of ajmaline on anomalous pathway conduction. Unfortunately, ajmaline is not very specific and conduction pathways respond even less specifically. In particular, retrograde conduction via putative para- or intranodal pathways is partially sensitive to both verapamil and ajmaline.

Since ajmaline has a very short half-life, it is most successful for this type of testing and it is usually used before verapamil or after adenosine is given. The intravenous dose of verapamil is 0.1 mg/kg body weight over 5–10 minutes; that of ajmaline is 1 mg/kg body weight (or a total dose of 50 mg) over 3–10 minutes and adenosine is given in a dose of 0.25 mg/kg body weight as quickly as possible. Adenosine triphosphate (10–20 mg) or Striadyne (30 mg) may be used instead of adenosine. (Striadyne is a mixture of the mono-, di- and triphosphates of adenosine.) Table 12.3 summarizes the properties and effects of drugs which may be of use at an electrophysiological study.

Pharmacological stress tests

His–Purkinje system

Drugs have been used to 'stress' the His–Purkinje system in two ways, both of which are used to reveal latent abnormalities of conduction. The administration

Table 12.3 ELECTROPHYSIOLOGICAL EFFECTS OF DRUGS GIVEN AT ELECTROPHYSIOLOGICAL STUDY

Drug	Time of Administration	SCL	AERP	AH	WP	AV ERP	HV	V ERP	AP ERP	INDICATIONS FOR USE AT EPS
Verapamil (0.1 mg/kg)	5 min	0/+	0	++	--	++	0	0	0/-	Terminate AVRT/AVNRT Reveal AP conduction Impair decremental conduction
Adenosine (37.7 µg/kg)	Rapid	++	-	+++	---	+++	0	NA	+/-	Block AV node conduction Reveal AP conduction
Propranolol (0.1–0.2 mg/kg)	1 min	++	0	++	--	++	0	0	0	Sympathetic (partial autonomic) blockade Suppress torsade de pointes
Ajmaline (0.5–1 mg/kg)	5 min	+/-	+	+	0/-	+	++	+	++	Block AP conduction Stress HP conduction
Disopyramide (2 mg/kg up to 150 mg)	10 min	0/-	+	+/0	+	-	0/+	+	++	Terminate AF Block AP conduction
Flecainide (2 mg/kg up to 150 mg)	10 min	0/+	0/+	+	-	+	++	0/+	++	Terminate AF Block AP conduction
Procainamide (10 mg/kg)	5 min	0/-	++	0	+	-	+	+	++	Block AP conduction Stress HP conduction
Lignocaine (1.0–1.5 mg/kg)	Rapid	0	0	0	0	0/+	0	0	0/-	Terminate VT Suppress VEA Local anaesthetic
Atropine (0.02–0.04 mg/kg)	Rapid	--	0	--	++	--	0	0	0	Cholinergic (partial autonomic) blockade Provoke AVNRT/AVRT
Isoprenaline 1–5 µg/min	Continuous infusion	--	0/-	--	++	--	0	0/-	-	Provoke AVNRT/AVRT Stimulate AP conduction Provoke VT Provoke torsade de pointes

0 = no effect; - = small reduction; - - = moderate reduction; - - - = large reduction; + = small increase; + + = moderate increase; + + + = large increase; +/- = small but variable effect.

AERP = atrial effective refractory period; AH = atrio–His interval; APERP = anomalous pathway effective refractory period; AVERP = atrioventricular nodal effective refractory period; HV = His–ventricular interval; SCL = sinus cycle length; VERP = ventricular effective refractory period; WP = Wenckebach period.

AF = atrial fibrillation; AP = anomalous pathway; AVNRT = atrioventricular nodal re-entrant tachycardia; AVRT = atrioventricular re-entrant tachycardia; HP = His–Purkinje system; NA = not available; VEA = ventricular ectopic activity; VT = ventricular tachycardia.

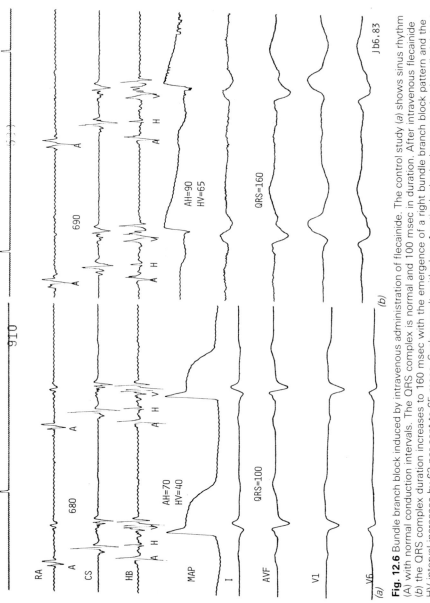

Fig. 12.6 Bundle branch block induced by intravenous administration of flecainide. The control study (a) shows sinus rhythm (A) with normal conduction intervals. The QRS complex is normal and 100 msec in duration. After intravenous flecainide (b) the QRS complex duration increases to 160 msec with the emergence of a right bundle branch block pattern and the HV interval increases by 63 per cent to 65 msec. Such a result, with class 1 antiarrhythmic drugs, may imply a diminished intraventricular conduction 'reserve'. Paper speed 100 mm/sec. CS = coronary sinus; HB = His bundle region; MAP = monophasic action potential; RA = right atrium.

of atropine will result in a reduction of the functional refractoriness of the AV node and allow the His–Purkinje tissue to be exposed to closely coupled stimulation. Alternatively, drugs such as ajmaline, procainamide, disopyramide or flecainide which impair conduction in the His–Purkinje system may, by marginally increasing its refractoriness, reveal reduced conduction reserve. In their simplest form (e.g. prolongation of the HV interval to beyond 90 msec or an increase of 100 per cent following the injection of ajmaline, 1 mg/kg body weight) such tests are neither specific nor sensitive but elaborate versions such as the 'disopyramide test' may prove clinically useful.

In the disopyramide test (Bergfeldt et al., 1985), disopyramide phosphate, 2 mg/kg body weight, is infused over 5 minutes. In patients with bifascicular block a positive test is:

1. Induction of second or third degree HV block during sinus rhythm.
2. A similar result during atrial pacing.
3. A similar result after abruptly terminating a period of ventricular pacing.
4. A 50 per cent increase in the HV interval.

A positive disopyramide test has been claimed to have a predictive value of 80 per cent for subsequent development of AV block. Flecainide has also been advocated for use as a pharmacological provocation but its depressant effect on conduction not uncommonly causes bundle branch delay or block in patients with normal intraventricular conduction (Fig. 12.6).

Anomalous pathways

The 'conduction capacity' of an anomalous pathway may also be assessed using pharmacological tests. Ajmaline and procainamide may block anterograde conduction in a direct AV anomalous pathway (disappearance of the delta wave) when the anterograde effective refractory period in the control state is greater than 270 msec (Fig. 12.7). Pathways with shorter refractory periods will not be completely blocked after acute intravenous administration of one of these drugs. Such tests are not completely reliable because both false positives and false negatives occur.

For these tests the following doses are used:

1. Procainamide: 10 mg/kg body weight i.v. over 5 minutes.
2. Ajmaline: 1 mg/kg body weight (maximum 50 mg) i.v. over 5 minutes.

In each test electrocardiographic observation is continued for 20 minutes after the end of the infusion.

Facilitation of tachycardia induction

Tachycardias which should otherwise have been easily provoked by electrical stimulation may be rendered non-inducible by spontaneous variations of autonomic tone (Fig. 12.8). For example, reduced sympathetic or increased parasympathetic stimulation may result in increased refractoriness of part of the circuit and so prevent junctional re-entry over atrioventricular or intra-AV nodal routes. The intravenous administration of atropine (in 0.03 mg increments up

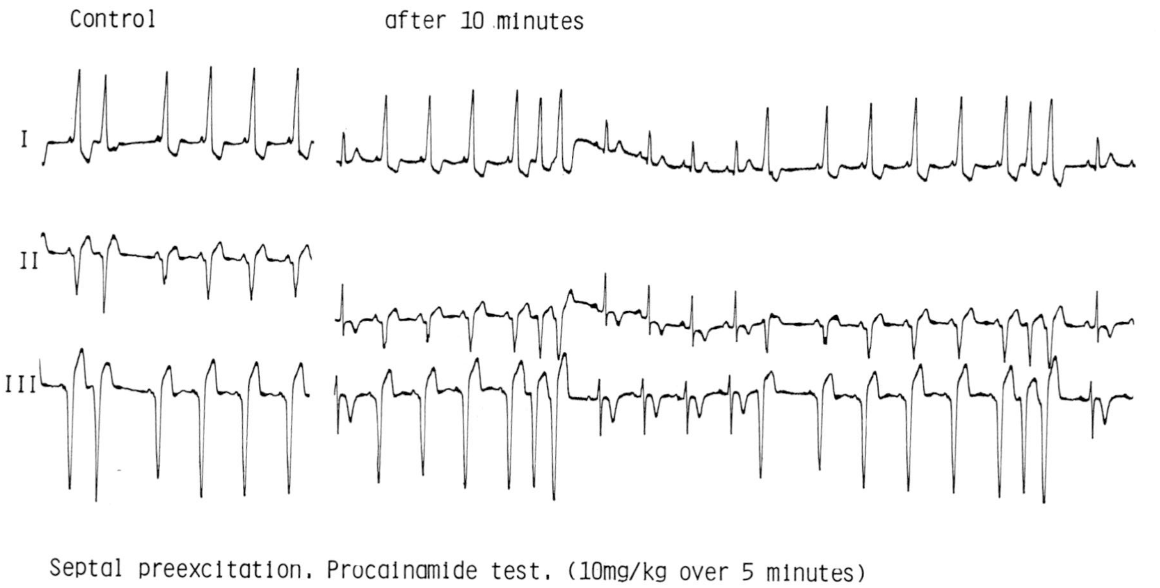

Control after 10 minutes

I

II

III

Septal preexcitation. Procainamide test. (10mg/kg over 5 minutes)

Fig. 12.7 The procainamide test for anomalous AV conduction. The baseline recordings show septal pre-excitation. Ten minutes after an infusion of procainamide the delta wave disappears, revealing normal AV conduction (with inferior T wave changes secondary to long-standing pre-excitation). These results suggest that the refractory period of the anomalous pathway is long. Paper speed 25 mm/sec.

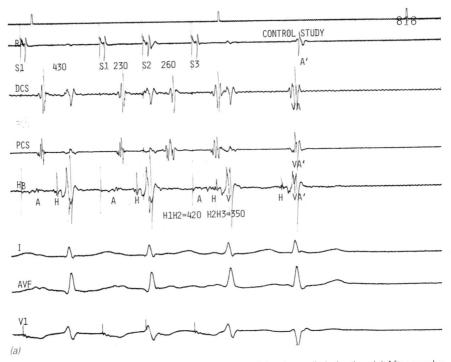

(a)

Fig. 12.8 Effect of isoprenaline and atropine on AV nodal tachycardia induction. (*a*) After regular atrial pacing at a cycle length of 430 msec (S1S1), double atrial premature stimulation (S2S3) results in a single atrial echo beat (A') (dual AH pathways were demonstrated). The atrial activation sequence was normal and inscribed simultaneously with the QRS. (*b*) During isoprenaline infusion (to enhance anterograde conduction), double atrial extrastimuli resulted in two cycles of tachycardia which terminated with block in the retrograde limb. (*c*) After intravenous atropine alone (not shown), a similar effect was seen. Sustained tachycardia (cycle length 245 msec) was initiated only after isoprenaline was reintroduced. The exact mechanisms involved in this example are not clear. Improvement of anterograde conduction by isoprenaline may not have been accompanied by shortening of retrograde refractoriness with consequent VA block. When atropine was administered with isoprenaline retrograde refractoriness was reduced sufficiently to allow re-entry. Paper speed 100 mm/sec. DCS = distal coronary sinus; HB = His bundle region; PCS = proximal coronary sinus; RA = right atrium.

to 1.2 mg) or isoprenaline (2 μg/min) may reverse these effects and allow stimulation of the tachycardia. It is preferable to use isoprenaline first because its elimination half-life is shorter than that of atropine. When tachycardia initiation is thwarted by excessively long refractoriness of an anomalous pathway, isoprenaline will generally be more effective than atropine. On the other hand, but not so invariably, atropine will more readily allow re-entry which was blocked by AV nodal refractoriness. Successful provocation of junctional tachycardias following the administration of these drugs probably indicates that such tachycardias occur spontaneously.

The intravenous infusion of catecholamines, particularly isoprenaline, has also been employed as an adjuvant for provocation of ventricular tachycardia. This has been claimed to be effective for the induction of those ventricular

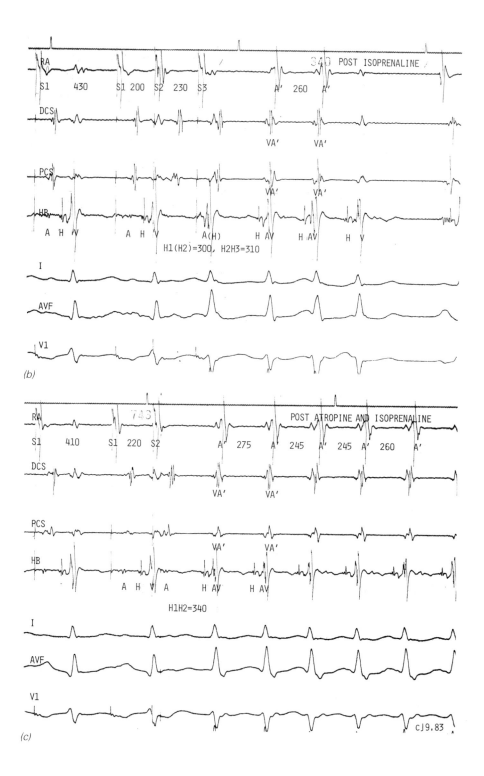

(b)

(c)

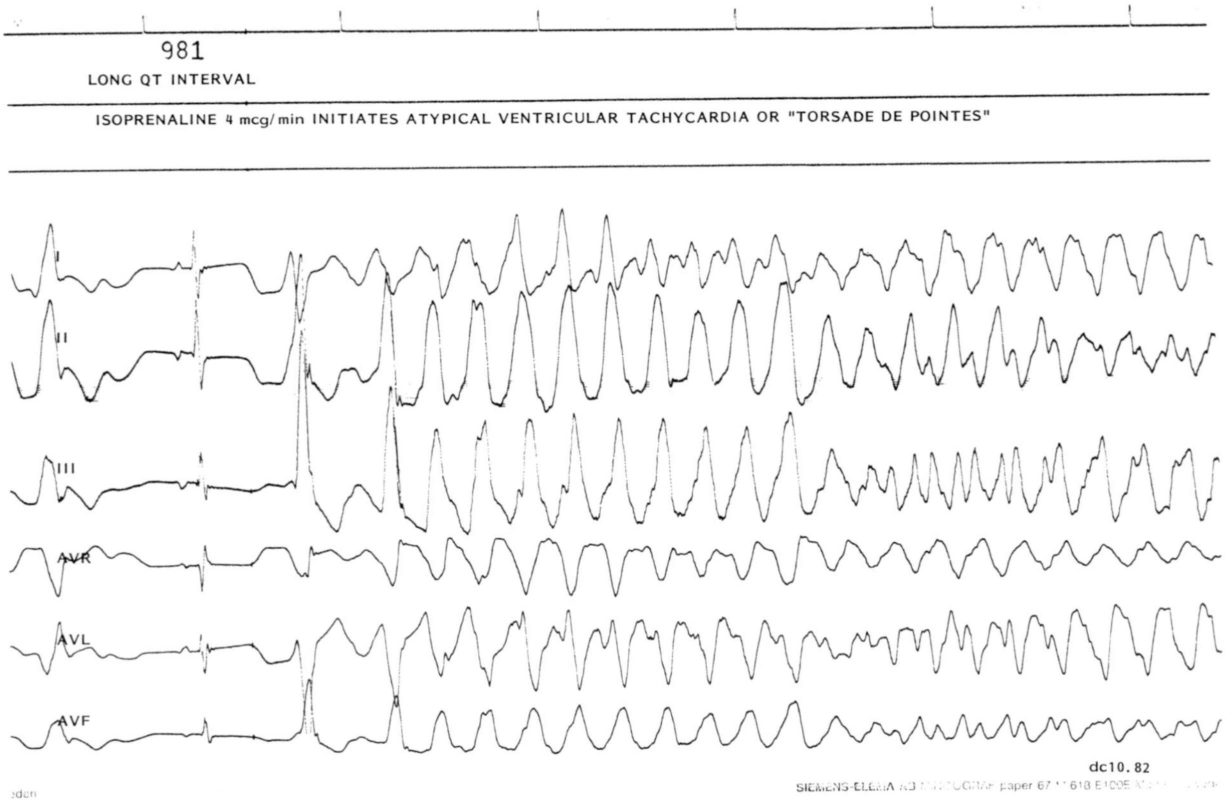

981

LONG QT INTERVAL

ISOPRENALINE 4 mcg/min INITIATES ATYPICAL VENTRICULAR TACHYCARDIA OR "TORSADE DE POINTES"

dc10. 82

Fig. 12.9 Induction of torsade de pointes by isoprenaline infusion in a 3-year-old child with congenital prolongation of the QT interval and associated nerve deafness (his brother aged 1 year was similarly affected). The patient had suffered several sudden attacks of collapse. Isoprenaline was used as a provocation test. The infusion caused marked variability of the morphology of T waves and in the duration of the ST interval prior to initiation of torsade de pointes. Note the cyclical changes in axis and the marked QRS phase difference in the different leads. The arrhythmia was promptly suppressed by propranolol. Paper speed 50 mm/sec.

tachycardias which are provoked by exercise. The role of isoprenaline for inducing other forms of ventricular tachycardia is very uncertain. Nevertheless, provided that the induced tachycardia resembles the tachycardia which occurs spontaneously (clinical tachycardia), it is appropriate to use this form of provocation (see Chapter 10). There is possibly a special role for the use of isoprenaline as a stimulant of torsade de pointes associated with congenital long QT syndrome (Fig. 12.9).

Assessment of intrinsic function by autonomic blockade

The sinus and AV nodes are richly innervated and their function may be enhanced or depressed by changes in autonomic tone. Therefore, tests of their electrophysiological responses are not complete until the influence of the autonomic nervous system has been evaluated in such a way that the 'intrinsic' nodal function and the sensitivity of the node to autonomic tone have been assessed. First, it is important to measure the response to 'physiological' forms of autonomic manipulation, such as carotid sinus massage or the Valsalva manoeuvre. Then, in the case of the sinus node (see Chapter 4), and sometimes the AV node, it is usual to repeat conventional tests after autonomic blockade with atropine (0.04 mg/kg) and propranolol (0.2 mg/kg). Of course these doses are not sufficient to effect complete autonomic blockade. Other pharmacological blocking drugs, such as alpha blockers, are not usually employed. Tests of intrinsic function are theoretically attractive but they are not usually clinically useful.

Treatment of arrhythmias complicating electrophysiological studies

During the course of an electrophysiological study, arrhythmias may be provoked (mechanically or by electrical stimulation) which are not reversible by simple stimulation techniques. In some cases, pharmacological therapy must be considered. However, it should be realized that most drugs have a long elimination half-life relative to the duration of an electrophysiological study and will therefore disturb the remainder of the study. For this reason DC cardioversion, although possibly troublesome to arrange, is usually preferred. Should antiarrhythmic drug therapy be chosen, the effects of the administration should be carefully monitored and recorded. Such a course is particularly relevant in the management of recurrent unwanted provocations of atrial fibrillation and sometimes atrial flutter or tachycardia. In these cases disopyramide (2 mg/kg body weight, over 10 minutes) or flecainide (2 mg/kg body weight, over 10 minutes) is usually administered intravenously.

Electrophysiological characteristics of antiarrhythmic drugs

Classification of antiarrhythmic drugs

The electrophysiological effects of antiarrhythmic drugs on the monocellular action potential of His–Purkinje tissue have been used as the basis for several

Table 12.4 VAUGHAN WILLIAMS' CLASSIFICATION

	Effect on action potential	Examples
Class 1	Reduction of rate of rise of phase 0:	
	+ prolongation	A. Quinidine, disopyramide, procainamide
	+ shortening	B. Lignocaine, tocainide, mexiletine, phenytoin, penticainide
	+ no effect on duration	C. Flecainide, propafenone, encainide, ajmaline, aprindine, lorcainide, recainam, cercainide
Class 2	Reduction of rate of rise of phase 4	Beta blockers and other antisympathetic agents
Class 3	Prolongation	Sotalol, amiodarone, bretylium, meobentine, clofilium
Class 4	Depression of phase 2–3	Verapamil, diltiazem
Class 5	Reduction of rate of rise of phase 4	Alinidine

classifications of such drugs, the best known and most enduring of which is widely referred to as the Vaughan Williams classification (Table 12.4). The exact criteria for this scheme have been changed on several occasions and the current form is illustrated in the Table. This classification is of limited clinical value, perhaps because most of the electrophysiological data on which it is based is derived from healthy, isolated animal tissue. The recently added class 1C is an exception because, at least when first suggested, drugs in this category were distinguished by their slowing effect on human His–Purkinje conduction.

Touboul et al. (1979) have suggested a classification based entirely on results from human clinical electrophysiology (Table 12.5). In this scheme drugs are divided into those which impair AV nodal conduction (type A) and those which affect His–Purkinje properties (type B). The latter group is subdivided into those which predominantly slow conduction (type B1) and those which do not affect conduction but do affect infranodal refractoriness (type B2). Antiarrhythmics

Table 12.5 TOUBOUL'S CLASSIFICATION OF ANTIARRHYRHMIC DRUGS

Group A	Impair AV nodal conduction (prolong AH time) e.g. digitalis, beta blockers, verapamil
Group B	1. Impair infranodal conduction (prolong HV time) e.g. quinidine, procainamide, disopyramide 2. Potentially improve infranodal conduction (reduce HP ERP) e.g. lignocaine, mexiletine
Group C	Impair both intra- and infra-AV nodal conduction (prolong AH and HV times) e.g. flecainide, encainide, propafenone, lorcainide

ERP = effective refractory period; HP = His–Purkinje system.

which affect conduction both above and below the AV node are known as type C.

The assessment of new drugs

Protocols

The assessment of any new antiarrhythmic drug must include an evaluation of its *in vivo* electrophysiological effects on human cardiac tissue (Fig. 12.10). This information is derived at the time of clinical electrophysiological testing.

For the purpose of the electrophysiological characterization of the new drug, the following parameters are usually measured in patients with normal, or near normal, physiology:

1. Sinus node function.
2. Anterograde conduction intervals.
3. Atrial, AV nodal and ventricular refractory periods.
4. Retrograde refractory periods.
5. Retrograde conduction intervals.

Because antiarrhythmic drugs may have a major effect on the heart rate, measurements should be made not only during sinus rhythm but also at several (at least two) identical rates before and after drug administration.

The following electrophysiological effects of antiarrhythmic drugs should also be studied:

1. Anomalous pathways, particularly in WPW syndrome.
2. Abnormal His–Purkinje tissue (bifascicular block).
3. Pathological tachycardias (termination and reinducibility).

In addition to the data derived from conventional studies, it is also appropriate to obtain information about the effect of drugs on other electrophysiological parameters such as monophasic action potentials, defibrillation thresholds (at open heart surgery), pacemaker thresholds (at pacemaker implantation) and late potentials (surface averaged ECG).

Use of implanted pacemakers or oesophageal pacemakers

Repeated volunteer studies in individual patients can be undertaken by re-inserting intracardiac electrodes. For the comfort and safety of the patient, 'non-invasive' methods such as oesophageal pacing are preferred. However, even these may prove rather uncomfortable. A better model for repeat studies is a patient implanted with a sophisticated pacemaker incorporating electrophysiological stimulation protocols. Pacemakers, particularly those designed to interrupt tachycardia (so-called 'implantable electrophysiology laboratories'), are increasingly being equipped with this facility. Before considering a patient for study of an antiarrhythmic drug, it must be remembered that the drug could render the pacemaker ineffective by increasing the pacing threshold or by slowing the rate of tissue depolarization to such an extent that pacemaker sensing is lost.

Drug: Dose: oral/i.v.	Patient's name:			Diagnosis:	
OBSERVATIONS IN MILLISECONDS	**BEFORE DRUG**			**AFTER DRUG**	
Basic sinus cycle length (mean of 10 cycles)					
Sinus node recovery time — SNRT (max.)					
Sinus node recovery time — CSNRT (max.)					
Sino-atrial conduction time — $A_1 - A_1$					
Sino-atrial conduction time — $A_3 - A_4$					
Sino-atrial conduction time — SACT INDEX					
	SR	**PACED**		**SR**	**PACED**
Sinus cycle length (single beat)/paced cycle length					
P—A interval/S—A interval					
HRA—LA interval/S—LA interval (DCS)					
A—H interval					
H—V interval					
QRS duration					
QRS morphology					
QT interval					
QT_c interval ($QT/\sqrt{RR}$ (in secs))					
Atrial effective R.P.					
A—V node effective R.P.					
A—V node functional R.P.					
A—V Wenckebach cycle length					
Accessory pathway anterograde effective R.P.					
Ventricular effective R.P.					
Retrograde V—A (nodal) effective R.P.					
V—A Wenckebach cycle length					
Accessory pathway retrograde effective R.P.					
Tachycardia C.L./Type					
? Termination of tachycardia (Yes/No)					
Investigator:				Date:	

Fig. 12.10 A specimen form used for comprehensive logging of data collected during an electrophysiological assessment of an investigational antiarrhythmic agent.

Drug administration

The electrophysiological effects of both an acute intravenous bolus and a maintenance infusion of antiarrhythmic drug should be assessed. Subsequently the effect of orally administered drug must be evaluated in order to account for the accumulation of active metabolites. If the kinetics of the drug allow, a repeat study performed within a few days can usually be accomplished using temporary pacing catheters which have been left *in situ*. However, it may be necessary to repeat the study after several weeks, in which case the methods for repeat study discussed above should be considered.

Usually, electrophysiological assessments of antiarrhythmic drugs are performed in patients who have not taken any other antiarrhythmic medication for at least five elimination half-lives prior to the study. The trend to combine antiarrhythmic medication suggests that detailed electrophysiological tests should be made on drug combinations. This is particularly true of combinations with amiodarone which has such a long half-life that therapeutic combination is inevitable. Similarly the electrophysiological consequences of co-administration with commonly prescribed cardioactive drugs such as digoxin, beta blockers and calcium antagonists must be determined.

Although antiarrhythmic drugs may have marked electrophysiological effects in the resting state, many of these effects may be neutralized or reversed by exercise or isoprenaline infusion. It is now conventional to assess this effect. Usually this is performed by three evaluations:

1. Control.
2. After antiarrhythmic drug.
3. After antiarrhythmic drug and isoprenaline.

Surprisingly, the effect of isoprenaline on control electrophysiological measurements is not usually assessed. Such measurements would improve the interpretation of the data.

References and further reading

Akhtar M, Damato AN, Batsford WP, Caracta AR, Ruskin JN, Weisfogel JN, Lau SH. (1975) Induction of atrioventricular nodal reentrant tachycardia after atropine. *American Journal of Cardiology* **36**, 286

Barrett PA, Laks MM, Mandel WJ, Yamaguchi I. (1980) The electrophysiologic effects of intravenous lidocaine in the Wolff–Parkinson–White syndrome. *American Heart Journal* **100**, 23

Bauernfeind RA, Wyndham CR, Dhingra R, Swiryn SP, Palileo E, Strasberg B, Rosen KM. (1980) Serial drug testing of multiple drugs in patients with atrioventricular nodal reentrant paroxysmal tachycardia. *Circulation* **62**, 1341

Benedini G, Cuccia C, Bognese R, Affatato A, Gallo G, Renaldini E, Visioli O. (1984) Value of purinic compounds in assessing sinus node dysfunction in man: a new diagnostic method. *European Heart Journal* **5**, 394

Bergfeldt L, Rosenqvist M, Vallin H, Edhag O. (1985) Disopyramide induced second and third degree atrioventricular block in patients with bifascicular block: an acute stress test to predict atrioventricular block progression. *British Heart Journal* **53**, 328

Bigger JT, Reiffel JA. (1983) Holter versus electrophysiologic studies in the management of malignant ventricular arrhythmias. *American Journal of Cardiology* **51**, 1464

Breithardt G, Seipel L, Abendroth RR, Loogen F. (1980) Serial electrophysiological testing of antiarrhythmic drug efficacy in patients with recurrent ventricular tachycardia. *European Heart Journal* 1, 11

Breithardt G, Borgreffe M, Seipel L. (1984) Selection of optimal drug treatment of ventricular tachycardia by programmed electrical stimulation of the heart. *Annals of the New York Academy of Sciences* 427, 429

Brugada P, Dassen WR, Braat S, Gorgels AP, Wellens HJJ. (1983) Value of the ajmaline–procainamide test to predict the effect of long-term oral amiodarone on the anterograde effective refractory period of the accessory pathway in the Wolff–Parkinson–White syndrome. *American Journal of Cardiology* 52, 70

Brugada P, Wellens HJJ. (1985) Effects of oral amiodarone on rate-dependent changes in refractoriness in patients with Wolff–Parkinson–White syndrome. *American Journal of Cardiology* 56, 863

Brugada P, Facchini M, Wellens HJJ. (1986) Effects of isoproterenol and amiodarone and the role of exercise in initiation of circus movement tachycardia in the accessory atrioventricular pathway. *American Journal of Cardiology* 57, 146

Buxton AE, Josephson ME. (1986) Role of electrophysiologic studies in identifying arrhythmogenic properties of antiarrhythmic drugs. *Circulation* 73, suppl. II, 67

Cavalli A, Maggioni A, Tusa M, Volpi A. (1985) Two false negative responses to the ajmaline test in the Wolff–Parkinson–White syndrome. *Pacing and Clinical Electrophysiology* 8, 832

Cheesman M, Ward DE. (1985) Exacerbation of ventricular tachycardia by tocainide. *Clinical Cardiology* 8, 47

Chiale PA, Pryzbylski J, Laino RA, Halpern MS, Nau GJ, Sanchez GJ, Lazzari JO, Elizari MV, Rosenbaum M. (1982) Usefulness of the ajmaline test in patients with bundle branch block. *American Journal of Cardiology* 49, 21

Critelli G, Grassi G, Perticone F, Coltorti F, Monda F, Condorelli M. (1983) Transesophageal pacing for prognostic evaluation of preexication syndrome and assessment of protective therapy. *American Journal of Cardiology* 51, 513

DiMarco J, Gara H, Ruskin J. (1980) Partial suppression of induced ventricular arrhythmias during serial electrophysiologic testing. *Circulation* 62, suppl. II, 261

DiMarco JP, Sellers TD, Lerman BB, Greenberg ML, Bern RM. Belardinelli L. (1985) Diagnostic and therapeutic use of adenosine in patients with supraventricular tachyarrhythmias. *Journal of the American College of Cardiology* 6, 417

Doherty JU, Josephson ME. (1983) Role of electrophysiologic testing in the therapy of ventricular arrythmias. *Pacing and Clinical Electrophysiology* 6, 1071

Duff HJ, Mitchell LB, Wyse DG. (1986) Programmed electrical stimulation studies for ventricular tachycardia induction in humans. II. Comparison of indwelling electrode catheter and daily catheter replacement. *Journal of the American College of Cardiology* 8, 576

Fisher JD, Cohen HL, Mehra R, Altschuler H, Escher DJW, Furman S. (1977) Cardiac pacing and pacemakers. II. Serial electrophysiologic–pharmacologic testing for control of recurrent tachyarrhythmias. *American Heart Journal* 93, 658

Greenspan AM, Spielman SR, Horowitz LN. (1986) Combination antiarrhythmic drug therapy for ventricular tachyarrythmias. *Pacing and Clinical Electrophysiology* 9, 565

Gulamhusein S, Ko P, Carruthers SG, Klein GJ. (1982) Acceleration of the ventricular response during atrial fibrillation in the Wolff–Parkinson–White syndrome after verapamil. *Circulation* 65, 348

Hamer AW, Finerman WB, Peter T, Mandel WJ. (1981) Disparity between the clinical and electrophysiologic effects of amiodarone in the treatment of recurrent ventricular tachyarrythmias. *American Heart Journal* 6, 992

Hamer A, Peter T, Mandel W. (1983) Atrioventricular nodal reentry: intravenous verapamil as a method of defining multiple electrophysiologic types. *American Heart*

Journal **105**, 629

Harper RW, Whitford E, Middlebook K, Federman J, Anderson S, Pitt A. (1982) Effects of verapamil on the electrophysiologic properties of the accessory pathway in patients with the Wolff–Parkinson–White syndrome. *American Journal of Cardiology* **50**, 1323

Heger JJ, Prystowsky EN, Jackman WM, Naccarelli GV, Warfel KA. Rinkenberger RL, Zipes DP. (1981) Amiodarone. Clinical efficacy and electrophysiology during long-term therapy for recurrent ventricular tachycardia and ventricular fibrillation. *New England Journal of Medicine* **305**, 539

Horowitz LN, Josephson ME, Spielman SR, Michelson EL, Greenspan AM. (1978) Recurrent ventricular tachycardia. 3. Role of the electrophysiologic study in selection of antiarrhythmic regimens. *Circulation* **58**, 986

Horowitz LN, Josephson ME, Kastor JA. (1980) Intracardiac electrophysiologic studies as a method for the optimization of drug therapy in chronic ventricular arrhythmia. *Progress in Cardiovascular Diseases* **23**, 81

Horowitz LN, Greenspan AM, Spielman SR, Webb CR, Morganroth J, Rotmensch H, Sokoloff NM, Rae AP, Segal BL, Kay HR. (1985) Usefulness of electrophysiologic testing in evaluation of amiodarone therapy for sustained ventricular tachyarrhythmias associated with coronary heart disease. *American Journal of Cardiology* **55**, 367

Josephson ME. (1978) Paroxysmal supraventricular tachycardia: an electrophysiological approach. *American Journal of Cardiology* **41**, 1123

Kim SG, Seiden SW, Matos JA, Waspe LE, Fisher JD. (1985a) Combination of procainamide and quinidine for better tolerance and additive effects for ventricular arrhythmias. *American Journal of Cardiology* **56**, 84

Kim SG, Seiden SW, Matos JA, Waspe LE, Fisher JD. (1985b) Discordance between ambulatory monitoring and programmed electrical stimulation in assessing efficacy of class IA antiarrhythmic agents in patients with ventricular tachycardia. *Journal of the American College of Cardiology* **6**, 539

Levy S, Hilaire J, Albin H, Corbelli J-L, Burtey J-P, Bricaud H, Gerard R. (1986) A new method for evaluating the effect of antiarrhythmic drugs on atrioventricular nodal conduction. *British Heart Journal* **55**, 569

McKenna WJ, Rowland E, Davies J, Krikler D. (1980) Failure to predict development of atrioventricular block with electrophysiological testing supplemented by ajmaline. *Pacing and Clinical Electrophysiology* **3**, 666

Mason JW, Winkle RA. (1978) Electrode-catheter arrhythmia induction in the selection and assessment of antiarrhythmic drug therapy for recurrent ventricular tachycardia. *Circulation* **58**, 971

Mason JW, Swerdlow CD, Winkle RA, Griffin JC, Ross DL, Keefe DL, Clusin WT. (1982) Programmed ventricular stimulation in predicting vulnerability to ventricular arrhythmias and their response to antiarrhythmic therapy. *American Heart Journal* **103**, 633

Matos JA, Wiener D, Siegel S, Fisher JD, Kim SG, Waspe LE. (1984) Treatment of refractory ventricular tachycardia with antiarrhythmic drug combinations. *Pacing and Clinical Electrophysiology* **7**, 461 (abstract)

Morady F, Sledge C, Shen E, Sung RJ, Gonzales R, Scheinman MM. (1983) Electrophysiologic testing in the management of patients with the Wolff–Parkinson–White syndrome and atrial fibrillation. *American Journal of Cardiology* **51**, 1623

Morady F, DiCarlo LA, Krol RB, Baerman JM, de Buitleir M. (1986) Acute and chronic effects of amiodarone on ventricular refractoriness, intraventricular conduction and ventricular tachycardia induction. *Journal of the American College of Cardiology* **7**, 148

Mueller RA. (1986) Flecainide: a new antiarrhythmic drug. *Clinical Cardiology* **9**, 1

Nathan AW, Hellestrand KJ. (1984) Flecainide acetate. A review. *Clinical Progress in Pacing and Electrophysiology* **2**, 43

Oseran DS, Gang ES, Rosenthal ME, Mandel WJ, Peter T. (1985) Electropharmacologic testing in sustained ventricular tachycardia associated with coronary heart disease: value of the response to intravenous procainamide in predicting the response to oral procainamide and oral quinidine treatment. *American Journal of Cardiology* **56**, 883

Perrot B, Clozel JP, Faivre G. (1984) Effect of adenosine triphosphate on the accessory pathways. *European Heart Journal* **5**, 382

Platia EV, Reid PR. (1984) Comparison of programmed electrical stimulation and ambulatory electrocardiographic (Holter) monitoring in the management of ventricular tachycardia and ventricular fibrillation. *Journal of the American College of Cardiology* **4**, 493

Platia EV, Reid PR. (1985) Non-sustained ventricular tachycardia during programmed ventricular stimulation: criteria for a positive test. *American Journal of Cardiology* **56**, 79

Podrid PJ, Schoeneberger A, Lown B, Lampert S, Matos J, Porterfield J, Raeder E, Corrigan E. (1983) Use of nonsustained ventricular tachycardia as a guide to antiarrhythmic drug therapy in patients with malignant ventricular arrhythmia. *American Heart Journal* **105**, 181

Poser RF, Podrid PJ, Lombardi F, Lown B. (1985) Aggravation of arrhythmia induced with antiarrhythmic drugs during electrophysiologic testing. *American Heart Journal* **110**, 9

Puech P, Sassine A, Munoz A, Masse C, Zettelmaier F, Leenhardt A, Yoshimura H. Electrophysiologic effects of purines: clinical applications. In: *Cardiac Electrophysiology and Arrhythmias* p. 443. Ed. by D Zipes, J Jalife. Grune & Stratton: Orlando, Fla

Rae AP, Greenspan AM, Spielman SR, Sokoloff NM, Webb CR, Kay HR, Horowitz LN. (1985) Antiarrhythmic drug efficacy for ventricular tachycarrythmias associated with coronary artery disease as assessed by electrophysiologic studies. *American Journal of Cardiology* **55**, 1494

Reddy CP, Gettes LS. (1979) Use of isoproterenol as an aid to electric induction of chronic recurrent ventricular tachycardia. *American Journal of Cardiology* **44**, 705

Reddy CP, McAllister RG. (1984) Effect of verapamil on retrograde conduction in atrioventricular nodal reentrant tachycardia. *American Journal of Cardiology* **54**, 535

Rinkenberger RL, Prystowsky EN, Jackman WM, Naccarelli GV, Heger JJ, Zipes DP. (1982) Drug conversion of nonsustained ventricular tachycardia to sustained ventricular tachycardia during serial electrophysiologic studies: identification of drugs that exacerbate tachycardia and potential mechanisms. *American Heart Journal* **103**, 177

Ruskin JN, McGovern B, Garan H, DiMarco JP, Kelly E. (1983) Antiarrhythmic drugs: a possible cause of out-of-hospital cardiac arrest. *New England Journal of Medicine* **309**, 1302

Schoenfeld MH, Ruskin JN, Garan H. (1984) Role of electrophysiologic studies in the treatment of tachycardias. In: *Tachycardias*, p. 551. Ed. by B Surawicz, CP Reddy, EN Prystowsky. Martinus Nijhoff: Boston, Mass

Sellers TD, Bashore TM, Gallagher JJ. (1977) Digitalis in the pre-excitation syndrome: analysis during atrial fibrillation. *Circulation* **56**, 260

Spielman SR, Schwartz JS, McCarthy DM, Horowitz LN, Greenspan AM, Sadowski LM, Josephson ME, Waxman HL. (1983) Predictors of the success or failure of medical therapy in patients with chronic recurrent sustained ventricular tachycardia: a discriminant analysis. *Journal of the American College of Cardiology* **1**, 401

Spurrell RAJ, Krikler DM, Sowton E. (1974) Concealed bypasses of the atrioventricular node in patients with paroxysmal supraventricular tachycardia revealed by intracardiac stimulation and verapamil. *American Journal of Cardiology* **33**, 590

Spurrell RAJ, Thorburn CW, Camm AJ, Sowton E, Deuchar DC. (1975) Effects of disopyramide on electrophysiological properties of specialised conduction system in man and on accessory atrioventricular pathway in Wolff–Parkinson–White syndrome. *British Heart Journal* **37**, 861

Swerdlow CD, Blum J, Winkle RA, Griffin JC, Ross DL, Mason JW. (1982) Decreased incidence of antiarrhythmic drug efficacy at electrophysiologic study associated with the use of a third extrastimulus. *American Heart Journal* **104**, 1004

Swerdlow CD, Winkle RA, Mason JW. (1983a) Determinants of survival in patients with chronic recurrent ventricular tachycardia. *New England Journal of Medicine* **308**, 1436

Swerdlow CD, Winkle RA, Mason JW. (1983b) Prognostic significance of the number of induced ventricular complexes during assessment of therapy for ventricular tachyarrhythmias. *Circulation* **68**, 400

Swerdlow CD, Gong G, Echt DS, Winkle RA, Griffin JC, Ross DL, Mason JW. (1983c) Clinical factors predicting successful electrophysiologic–pharmacologic study in patients with ventricular tachycardia. *Journal of the American College of Cardiology* **1**, 409

Tajima T, Muramatsu T, Kanaka S, Yanagishita Y, Ide M, Dohi Y. (1986) Intravenous adenosine triphosphate disodium: its efficacy and electrophysiologic effects on patients with paroxysmal supraventricular tachycardias. *Pacing and Clinical Electrophysiology* **9**, 401

Tonkin AM, Heddle WF, Tornos P. (1978) Intermittent atrioventricular block: procainamide adminstration as a provocative test. *Australian and New Zealand Journal of Medicine* **8**, 594

Torres V, Flowers D, Somberg JC. (1985) The arrhythmogenicity of antiarrhythmic agents. *American Heart Journal* **109**, 1090

Touboul P, Attalah G, Gressade A, Michelson G, Chatelain MT, Delahaye JP. (1979) Affets electrophysiologique des agents antiarrhythmiques chez l'homme. Tentative de classification. *Archives des Maladies du Coeur* **72**, 72

Vaughan Williams EM. (1970) Classification of antiarrhythmic drugs. In: *Symposium on Cardiac Arrhythmias*, p. 449. Ed. by E Sandoe, E Flensted-Jensen KH Olsen. Astra Pharmaceuticals: Sodertalje, Sweden

Vaughan Williams EM. (1984) A classification of antiarrhythmic actions reassessed after a decade of new drugs. *Journal of Clinical Pharmacology* **24**, 129

Velebit V, Podrid P, Lown B, Cohen BH, Graboys TB. (1982) Aggravation and provocation of ventricular arrhythmias by antiarrhythmic drugs. *Circulation* **65**, 886

Veltri EP, Reid PR, Platia EV, Griffith LSC. (1985) Results of late programmed electrical stimulation and long-term electrophysiologic effects of amiodarone therapy in patients with refractory ventricular tachycardia. *American Journal of Cardiology* **55**, 375

Walsh KA, Denes P. (1985) Tocainide. A review. *Clinical Progress in Electrophysiology and Pacing* **3**, 163

Ward DE, Bennett DH, Camm AJ. (1984) Mechanisms of junctional tachycardia showing ventricular preexcitation. *British Heart Journal* **52**, 369

Ward DE, Cheesman M, Dancy M. (1986) Effect of intravenous and oral flecainide on ventricular tachycardia. *International Journal of Cardiology* **10**, 251

Waxman HL, Buxton AE, Sadowski LM, Josephson ME. (1983) The response to procainamide during electrophysiologic study for sustained ventricular tachycarrhythmias predicts the response to other medications. *Circulation* **67**, 30

Waxman HL, Buxton AE, Marchlinski FE, Josephson ME. (1984) Pharmacologic therapy of sustained ventricular tachyarrhythmias. In: *Tachycardias: mechanisms, diagnosis and treatment*, p. 399. Ed. by ME Josephson, HJJ Wellens, Lea & Febiger: Philadelphia, Pa

Wellens HJJ, Durrer D. (1974) Effect of procainamide, quinidine and ajmaline in the Wolff–Parkinson–White syndrome. *Circulation* 50, 114

Wellens HJJ, Lie KI, Bar FW, Wesdorp JC, Dohmen HJ, Duren DR, Durrer D. (1976) Effect of amiodarine in the Wolff–Parkinson–White syndrome. *American Journal of Cardiology* 38, 189

Wellens HJJ, Bar FWHM, Lie KI, Durren DR, Dohmen HJ. (1977) Effect of procainamide, propranolol and verapamil on mechanism of tachycardia in patients with chronic recurrent ventricular tachycardia. *American Journal of Cardiology* 40, 579

Wellens HJJ, Bar FW, Gorgels AP, Vanagt EJ. (1980a) Use of ajmaline in patients with Wolff–Parkinson–White syndrome to disclose a short refractory period of the accessory pathway. *American Journal of Cardiology* 45, 130

Wellens HJJ, Bar FW, Dassen WRM, Brugada P, Vanagt EJ, Farre J. (1980b) Effect of drugs in the Wolff–Parkinson–White syndrome. Importance of initial length of effective refractory period of the accessory pathway. *American Journal of Cardiology* 46, 665

Wellens HJJ, Braat S, Brugada P, Gorgels AP, Bar FW. (1982) Use of procainamide in patients with Wolff–Parkinson–White syndrome to disclose a short refractory period of the accessory pathway. *American Journal of Cardiology* 50, 1087

Wellens HJJ, Brugada P, Abdollah H. (1984) Drug therapy of patients with arrhythmias associated with bypass tracts. *Annals of the New York Academy of Sciences* 432, 272

Wellens HJJ, Brugada P, Stevenson WG. (1985) Programmed electrical stimulation of the heart in patients with life-threatening ventricular arrhythmias: what is the significance of induced arrhythmias and what is the correct stimulation protocol? *Circulation* 72, 1

Wu D, Amat-y-Leon F, Simpson RJ, Latif P, Wyndham CR, Denes P, Rosen KM. (1977) Electrophysiological studies with multiple drugs in patients with atrioventricular reentrant tachycardias utilizing an extranodal pathway. *Circulation* 56, 727

Zipes DP, Prystowsky EN, Heger JJ. (1982) Electrophysiologic testing of antiarrhythmic agents. *American Heart Journal* 103, 610

13

Use of Pacing Methods to Treat Tachycardias

Since the 1960s pacing techniques have been applied to the control of a variety of tachycardias. The first use of pacing was to suppress the emergence of dangerous ventricular arrhythmias by continuous ventricular pacing to prevent the slow heart rates which may predispose to these arrhythmias. This method was extended to controlling similar arrhythmias by pacing at a rate slightly faster than the normal sinus rate, so-called 'overdrive suppression'. Since the discovery of clinical re-entrant mechanisms, pacing has been mostly used to terminate paroxysms of tachycardia rather than to prevent their initiation. The various applications of pacing to the control of tachycardias are listed in Table 13.1. Conventional pacing energies (25 microjoules (μJ) which is enough to 'capture' the heart) and, more recently, higher energies (25 J which is enough to defibrillate the heart) have been used for terminating tachycardias.

Tachycardia-prevention pacing

Rate control

Slow ventricular rates associated with complete AV block may predispose to the emergence of malignant ventricular arrhythmias. Similarly, sinus bradycardia in

Table 13.1 PACEMAKERS FOR THE PREVENTION OR TERMINATION OF TACHYCARDIA

PREVENTION

Physiological overdrive

Pre-excitation pacing (two channels)

Pre-emptive pacing (single channel)

TERMINATION

Single beat:	1. Underdrive:	(a) single channel
		(b) two channels
	2. Critical timing:	(a) simple scan
		(b) intelligent scan
Multiple beat:	1. Simple burst	
	2. Adaptive burst	
	3. Rate-related burst	

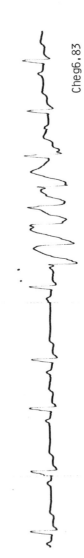

VENTRICULAR PACING AT 100 bpm

Cheg6.83

1 minute post switch-off. Repetitive ventricular activity.

Fig. 13.1 The effect of ventricular overdrive pacing on recurrent ventricular tachycardia and fibrillation. These recordings are from a 75-year-old woman who had recurrent episodes of ventricular fibrillation triggered by polymorphic ventricular tachycardias which were unresponsive to drug therapy. Overdrive ventricular pacing completely suppressed the tachycardias. When the pacemaker was switched off (lower trace), non-sustained polymorphic tachycardia appeared within minutes. Paper speed 25 mm/sec.

the setting of sinoatrial disease may allow atrial tachycardias (and sometimes ventricular tachycardias) to develop. Restoring the heart rate to normal increases the uniformity of cellular repolarization, reduces the tendency for spontaneous diastolic ectopic automaticity, changes the direction of myocardial activation and produces complex biochemical effects (including liberation of endogenous acetylcholine, accumulation of extracellular potassium and electrogenic extrusion of sodium ions; Vassalle, 1977). All of these electrophysiological effects may act to reduce the propensity to tachycardias or ectopic impulse formation.

Pacing the heart at rates in excess of the normal intrinsic sinus rate (80–140 b.p.m.) has similar beneficial effects. This is called physiological overdrive suppression, and may be used in settings where bradycardia is not an obvious precipitating factor. A classic application of the method is in the control of arrhythmias associated with QT prolongation. In this circumstance, atrial pacing is preferred to ventricular pacing, provided that AV conduction is intact. Another example of the value of overdrive pacing is in the acute control of ventricular arrhythmias when many antiarrhythmic drugs have been given (Fig. 13.1).

At present, the use of these techniques is empirical because there is no method of predicting their effect. Electrophysiological studies have not been applied to their assessment. Thus a trial of therapy must be conducted to allow retrospective evaluation.

Altered activation sequence

Pacing the myocardium directly (e.g. right ventricular pacing) necessarily alters the cardiac activation sequence, which itself may have an antiarrhythmic effect. This principle has been applied to the control of refractory junctional tachycardias, particularly those associated with a direct anomalous AV pathway.

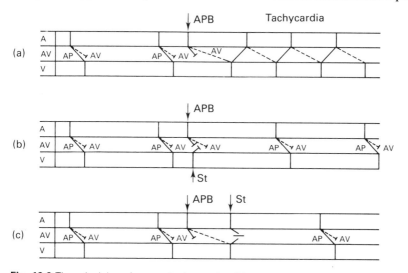

Fig. 13.2 The principles of pre-excitation pacing (b) and pre-emptive pacing (c) in preventing the initiation of atrioventricular tachycardia by an atrial stimulus (APB) as indicated in (a). AP = anomalous pathway; St = stimulus.

Such tachycardias are almost always dependent on AV conduction delay for their initiation (see Chapter 9). When delayed activation of the ventricles is prevented by ventricular pacing shortly after atrial depolarization, tachycardia is not initiated. This has been called 'pre-excitation pacing' (Figs. 13.2 and 13.3). An alternative approach is to pre-empt critical circuit delay by atrial pacing after an atrial event or by ventricular pacing after a ventricular event (Kuck et al., 1984). This has been called 'pre-emptive pacing' (Fig. 13.2 and 13.4). In the short term both techniques are effective, but pre-emptive pacing may induce arrhythmias (e.g. atrial fibrillation when pacing the atria) because of closely coupled

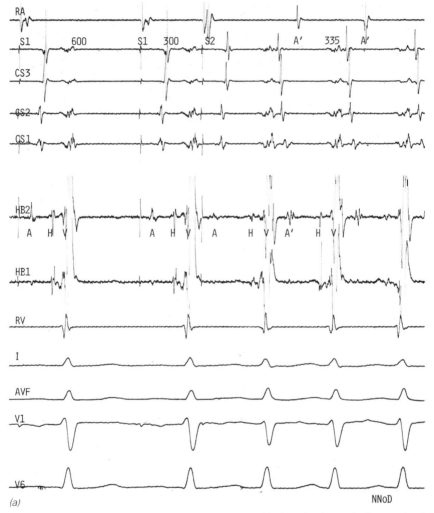

(a)   NNoD

Fig. 13.3 The use of pre-excitation pacing to prevent initiation of atrioventricular re-entrant tachycardia. (*a*) After regular atrial pacing (S1S1) at a cycle length of 600 msec, an atrial premature stimulus (S2) at 300 msec initiates atrioventricular tachycardia. (*b*) After a similar sequence

extrastimulation. In the long term both techniques are often unsuccessful because of the multiplicity of mechanisms of spontaneous tachycardia initiation, many of which are not countered by this type of pacing. These techniques are usually dependent on pacing in response to a sensed event ('triggered pacing'), but pacing at two sites ('dual site stimulation') may achieve similar results.

In an occasional instance of refractory junctional tachycardia, preventative pacing may (for various reasons) be the only option. In such cases, a detailed electrophysiological assessment is essential prior to implantation of a permanent device (usually a standard dual chamber pacemaker with a programmable short

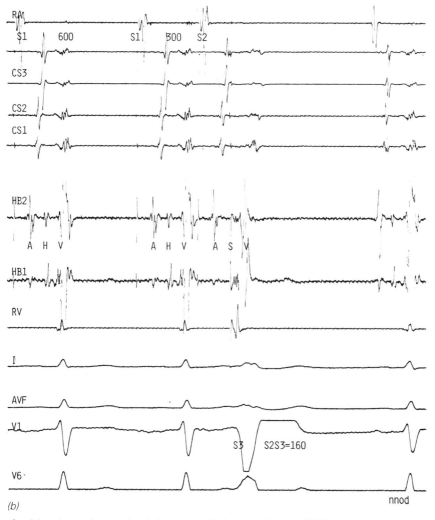

(b)

of atrial pacing and extrastimulation, a ventricular extrastimulus (S3) is coupled at 160 msec after S2, and initiation of tachycardia is prevented. Paper speed 100 mm/sec. CS 1–4 = 'unipolar' coronary sinus; HB 1, 2 = His bundle region; RA = right atrium; RV = right ventricle.

AV delay, short atrial refractory period and high tracking rate). In particular, the assessment must include evaluation of modes of initiation of tachycardia. The potential proarrhythmic effects of the pacemaker (e.g. unwanted initiation of the tachycardia) must be investigated during the study.

Dual site stimulation or triggered pacing may modify the substrate for ventricular tachycardias. Thus, right ventricular outflow tract pacing triggered by a sensed event at the right ventricular apex may prevent emergence of a tachycardia which is dependent for its initiation on critical right bundle branch

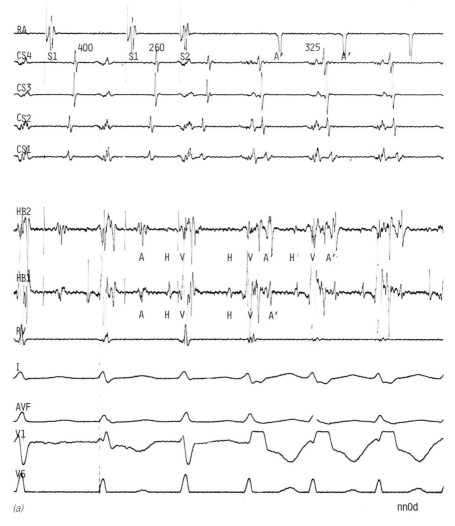

(a)   nn0d

Fig. 13.4 The use of pre-emptive pacing to prevent the initiation of atrioventricular re-entrant tachycardia. (*a*) After regular atrial drive (S1S1) at 400 msec, an extrastimulus (S2) atrioventricular re-entrant tachycardia is initiated. (*b*) After a similar sequence, tachycardia initiation is prevented

delay. In practice, it is difficult to determine the critical timing and electrode positions needed to achieve the effect.

Inhibition pacing

It has recently been shown that subthreshold stimulation of the ventricular myocardium may prevent capture by a following suprathreshold impulse. This phenomenon has been called 'inhibition'. It has been suggested that this effect

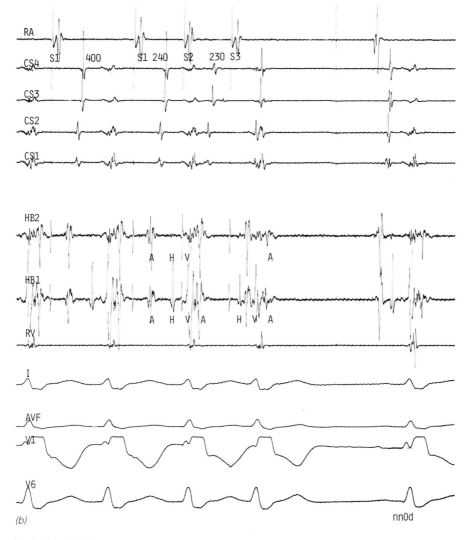

(b)

by the introduction another atrial extrastimulus (S3) coupled to S2 at an interval of 230 msec. Paper speed 100 mm/sec. CS 1–4 = 'unipolar' coronary sinus; HB 1, 2 = His bundle region; RA = right atrium; RV = right ventricle.

may be used to prevent tachycardia, but it is likely that electrode positioning will be extremely critical (Prystowsky and Zipes, 1983).

Tachycardia-termination pacing

General principles

Re-entrant tachycardias can typically be terminated by stimulation. The electrophysiological basis for this effect is well understood. In classical re-entrant excitation (fixed pathway) there is an 'excitable gap' between the advancing head of the circulating wavefront and its receding refractory tail. If this were not so, the advancing head would collide with the receding tail and tachycardia would terminate. Thus if the excitable gap is 'plugged' by an artificially stimulated wavefront, tachycardia can no longer continue (Fig. 13.5). When tachycardia is the result of re-entry around refractory tissue (so-called 'leading circle' mechanism), artificial stimulation probably terminates re-entry by progressive invasion and capture of the entire circuit. Triggered automaticity in cells can also be halted by premature or rapid pacing. It is not known whether this mechanism is important in human tachycardias (see Chapter 7).

Conditions and modes of pacing

Depolarization of the excitable gap requires critical timing of stimulation in relation to the circulating wavefront (see Chapter 7). Attempts to stimulate (with a single stimulus) the myocardium artificially during tachycardia may result in one of several possible responses (Fig. 13.5):

1. Failure to capture the myocardium (refractory zone).
2. Collision of the stimulated wavefront with the wavefront spreading from the tachycardia circuit (collision zone).
3. Invasion of the tachycardia circuit, resulting in resetting the position of the circulating wavefront (reset zone).
4. Invasion of the tachycardia circuit, resulting in complete depolarization and abolition of the excitable gap (termination zone).

The closer stimulation is to the circuit, the smaller the zone of collision and the larger the zones of reset and termination. The collision zone is non-existent if stimulation is actually on-circuit. The termination zone diminishes in duration and may disappear when the site of stimulation is remote from the circuit. In this case, two or more stimuli may be necessary to 'rephase' the tissue intervening between the pacing site and the circuit, thus allowing activation of the excitable gap. The use of multiple beats is known as 'burst overdrive' pacing and single or double beats are referred to as 'extrastimulus' pacing. The termination zone is intrinsically variable because of physiological influences such as changes in autonomic tone. Because of this it is necessary to scan the cycle by adjusting the coupling of single or double premature extrastimuli. Such critical timing becomes less important when more stimuli are used (burst pacing). Similarly, the site of stimulation must be close to the re-entrant circuit for only one or two extrastimuli, whereas with burst pacing the stimulation site is less critical.

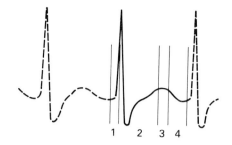

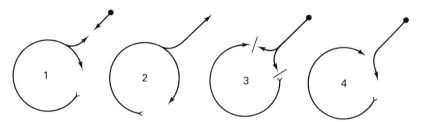

Fig. 13.5 The possible responses to a premature stimulus during tachycardia. An early stimulus (1) encounters the tachycardia wavefront emerging from the circuit (zone of collision). A later stimulus (2) may find surrounding tissue or the circuit itself totally refractory and will not propagate (zone of refractoriness). A little later (3), stimulation may result in penetration of the circuit with abolition of the excitable gap (zone of termination). A late stimulus (4) may enter the circuit ahead of the circulating tachycardia impulse and follow the circuit, resulting in reset of the tachycardia cycle (zone of reset).

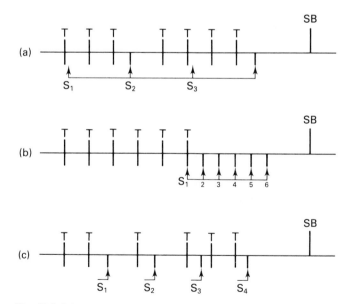

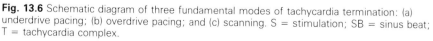

Fig. 13.6 Schematic diagram of three fundamental modes of tachycardia termination: (a) underdrive pacing; (b) overdrive pacing; and (c) scanning. S = stimulation; SB = sinus beat; T = tachycardia complex.

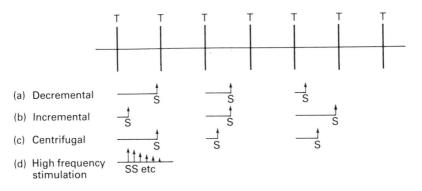

Fig. 13.7 Schematic diagram of four methods of effecting a scan of the tachycardia cycle. The decremental scan (a) operates by progressive reduction of the coupling interval between the tachycardia complex (T) and the stimulus (S). An incremental scan (b) operates in reverse. A centrifugal scan (c) is a type of 'search' (or optimization) procedure in which the termination zone is found by scanning back and forth around a median point. Using high frequency stimulation (d), a single cycle is rapidly scanned.

In clinical practice tachycardias may be terminated by single or multiple beat methods. The critical timing of single beat termination can be achieved by using fixed, constant rate pacing (underdrive, Fig. 13.6) during tachycardia such that stimulation during the termination zone eventually occurs by change (assuming that the rates of pacing and tachycardia are not harmonically related). Another system is systematic 'scanning' (Figs. 13.6 and 13.7) of the cycle either manually or automatically. The versatility of multiple beat methods (burst pacing) is increased by automatically linking the burst characteristics to the tachycardia (rate-related pacing) and, if termination is not effected, changing these characteristics before a further attempt is made (adaptive pacing, Fig. 13.8). The simplicity of the underdrive and simple burst modes makes them most suitable for temporary application (e.g. in the coronary care unit). The more sophisticated termination algorithms are safer and more likely to succeed. They are therefore incorporated into fully implantable and automatic systems.

Arrhythmias amenable to pacing termination

Prevention by pacemaker is applicable to tachycardias which are incessant or frequently recurrent (repetitive). It has been most successfully applied to junctional tachycardias associated with anomalous conduction. Tachycardia termination is inappropriate when tachycardia returns immediately after termination. Thus, incessant or repetitive temporal patterns are not suitable for this form of therapy. The termination method is most suitable for paroxysmal episodes which are relatively infrequent.

Tachycardia features which favour pacemaker termination include:

1. Slower rates.
2. Regularity of rate.
3. Monomorphic ECG pattern.

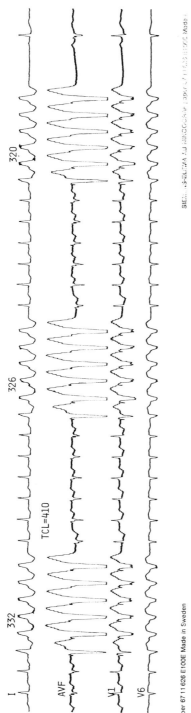

Fig. 13.8 The use of adaptive burst ('concertina') pacing to terminate tachycardia. The tachycardia cycle length (TCL) is 410 msec. The initial coupling interval of the pacemaker is set at 338 msec (not shown). If the burst of six beats is ineffective, tachycardia is again detected, and another burst delivered at a coupling interval shortened by 6 msec. The cycle length of the burst is also reduced by 6 msec. This process continues until tachycardia is terminated or until the minimum coupling interval is reached. Paper speed 25 mm/sec.

4. Haemodynamic stability.
5. No tendency to accelerate or degenerate during stimulation.
6. Easy, consistent termination by a given pacing sequence.

Atrial fibrillation is not amenable to termination by pacing techniques (see Chapter 8). Atrial flutter can be terminated by rapid atrial pacing usually at rates 50–100 b.p.m. faster than the flutter rate. A single stimulus is rarely effective. Atrial tachycardia, if re-entrant, will respond to single atrial premature beats or rapid pacing depending on the rate of tachycardia.

All junctional re-entrant tachycardias are amenable to pacing termination by rapid atrial pacing or premature stimulation. Ventricular extrastimulation is more efficacious but more dangerous (see below) than atrial stimulation (see Chapter 9). Automatic junctional tachycardias and idiojunctional escape or accelerated rhythms do not terminate in response to pacing.

Chronic recurrent sustained monomorphic ventricular tachycardia (see Chapter 10) can be terminated by pacing but there is some risk of inducing unwanted arrhythmias. Ventricular tachycardias in excess of 250 b.p.m. or with multiple morphologies will not readily terminate. Atypical ventricular tachycardia, ventricular flutter and ventricular fibrillation are not amenable to this technique.

The safety and efficacy of various pacing modalities and sites in relation to ventricular and supraventricular arrhythmias are detailed in Table 13.2.

Potential dangers of pacing termination methods

Unwanted tachycardias may be provoked by extrastimulus or burst pacing (Table 13.3.) For example, atrial pacing can induce atrial flutter or fibrillation, and ventricular pacing may induce ventricular tachycardia or fibrillation or accelerate ventricular tachycardia. For these reasons, termination pacing is preferably confined to atrial pacing. Ventricular tachycardia does not usually respond to atrial burst pacing (because the AV node prevents high ventricular rates or close ventricular coupling intervals) and will respond only to ventricular pacing. Pacing termination of ventricular tachycardias is relatively dangerous.

Table 13.2 SAFETY AND EFFICACY OF PACEMAKER TERMINATION OF TACHYCARDIA

Paced chamber	Tachycardia	Single beat		Multiple beat	
		Efficacy	Safety	Efficacy	Safety
Atrium	SVT	+/−	+	++	+
	VT	−	NA	−	NA
Ventricle	SVT	+	+/−	+	−
	VT	+/−	+/−	+	−

SVT = supraventricular tachycardia; VT = ventricular tachycardia.

++ = very effective/safe; + = moderately effective/safe; − = ineffective/unsafe; NA = not applicable.

Table 13.3 MAJOR FACTORS IN THE PROVOCATION OF 'DETRIMENTAL' ARRHYTHMIAS

Pacing modalities	Prematurity
	Rate
	Duration
	Energy
	Polarity
Tachycardia	Rate
	Stability
Patient	Ischaemia
	Electrolyte abnormality
	Personality
	Stress
	Medication (e.g. digoxin)
	Ventricular function

This should be performed only in hospital with a defibrillator available. The use of automatic implantable devices should be limited to highly selected patients or to patients 'protected' by an implanted defibrillator.

Factors which predispose to the induction of serious unwanted arrhythmias include:

1. Rapid tachycardia rates.
2. Rapid pacing rates.
3. Closely coupled extrastimulation.
4. High stimulus intensity (more than twice diastolic threshold).
5. Ventricular stimulation.
6. Acute myocardial ischaemia.
7. Myocardial disease (old infarction, cardiomyopathy).
8. Drug intoxication (especially with antiarrhythmic drugs, digoxin).
9. Metabolic disturbances (especially electrolyte abnormalities).
10. Stimulation during catecholamine excess (e.g. exercise, isoprenaline infusion).

After the termination of tachycardia there may be a significant bradycardia or asystolic pause. Bradycardia standby pacing must therefore be available (as part of the external or implantable pacing system) whenever tachycardia is to be terminated by pacing methods. Occasionally, however, bradycardia support pacing may reinitiate the tachycardia by one of several mechanisms (e.g. retrograde VA conduction).

During burst pacing, hypotension or haemodynamic distress may develop, especially if the burst is rapid or prolonged or if the ventricles are paced. This is an important consideration when burst pacing is frequently repeated by an automatic implanted device.

False recognition of sinus tachycardia as pathological tachycardia will cause an automatic system to pace inappropriately. Pacing during the sinus tachycardia produced by exercise may be particularly prone to induce unwanted arrhythmias. This potential malfunction of an automatic device is less likely when criteria additional to rate are used to trigger the pacemaker. Such criteria include:

1. Sudden change of rate (absolute interval change or 'delta' heart rate.
2. The stability (lack of variation in beat to beat cycle length) of the high heart rate.
3. The duration of the tachycardia.
4. Differences between timing of two electrograms (e.g. AV relationships during tachycardia.
5. Electrogram characteristics (e.g. amplitude, shape, etc.).

These criteria may be used on a hierarchical basis as indicated in Table 13.4.

Permanent pacing for tachycardia termination

Indications

Any patient with paroxysmal regular tachycardia which is responsive to pacing is a potential candidate for this treatment. Most patients have had unsuccessful drug treatment (failed treatment, side effects, poor patient compliance, patient unsuitable for drug therapy as in pregnancy, patient preference) and have had repeated hospital visits for acute termination of the arrhythmia. At present it is not considered as a first line of treatment.

Patient assessment

Detailed electrophysiological studies must be undertaken to determine the mechanism of tachycardia, the location of the tachycardia source and the efficacy and safety of various modes of pacemaker termination. A versatile stimulator which can reproduce the pacing responses of implantable devices must be available. The likelihood of confusion of sinus and pathological tachycardias must be explored by exercise testing and ambulatory ECG monitoring. The psychological suitability of the patient for permanent pacing ('bioprosthesis neurosis', scar, etc.) must be considered and, if necessary, formally assessed. Detailed testing at the time of electrophysiological study can be minimized by using versatile, fully programmable systems which can be tested and adjusted accordingly after implantation.

Table 13.4 TACHYCARDIA RECOGNITION

Criterion	Diagnosis
Rate	Tachycardia
Rate of change of rate	Sudden tachycardia
Activation sequence	Abnormal tachycardia
Electrogram morphology	Abnormal tachycardia

Tachycardia-termination pacemakers

There are several fully implantable automatic devices specially designed and constructed for tachycardia termination. Most are highly programmable (recognition and response algorithms, 'Holter' functions, telemetry and conventional pacing parameters can be programmed by an external programmer), small and lightweight and are single-chamber (channel) systems. Versatile programmability allows fine adjustment after implantation such that prolonged implantation procedures are not necessary.

Implantable systems

Cybertach 60 (Intermedics)   The Cybertach 60 (Griffin et al., 1980) automatic implantable pacemaker was introduced following the success of patient-activated rapid atrial pacing systems. In response to the development of a rapid heart rate, a preprogrammed but fixed burst of asynchronous pacing was delivered. This unit proved successful in a high proportion of cases but had several important drawbacks:

1. Diagnosis of pathological tachycardia relied on heart rate analysis with only two heart rates available to distinguish pathological tachycardia from sinus tachycardia.
2. Asynchronous pacing was used, which is likely to induce unwanted arrhythmias.
3. There was only one non-adaptive and non-responsive reaction to tachycardia – the pacemaker repeated futile attempts to terminate tachycardia.

Subsequent versions of implantable pacemaker were designed to correct these limitations.

Pasar 4151 (Telectronics)   The PASAR (programmable automatic scanning arrhythmia reversion) 4151 was the first device to incorporate the scanning principle (Spurrell et al., 1982). The pacemaker was a first generation, implantable, bipolar system designed exclusively for tachycardia termination. Bradycardia support pacing was not provided in this pacemaker, to ensure that the device was not used in patients who predominantly required relief from bradycardia. The unit automatically detected the occurrence of tachycardia and terminated the arrhythmia by delivering one or two critically timed extrastimuli. Tachycardia was confirmed when four successive cycles occurred at a rate faster than the programmed tachycardia detection rate (eight rates available). If tachycardia did not terminate in response to the extrastimuli, the coupling interval between the tachycardia complex and the first extrastimulus was progressively reduced (decremental scan) by approximately 6 msec. The coupling interval between the first and second extrastimuli was not automatically varied but was programmable. Successful coupling intervals were retained (memory function) for subsequent reuse if tachycardia recurred.

Pasar 4151 was recommended for the treatment of supraventricular tachycardia and 122 were implanted for this purpose (in 70 instances for atrioventricular tachycardia and 42 cases for intra-AV nodal tachycardia).

However, the electrode was most often placed in the ventricle (61 per cent). The average age of the patients was 46 years (range: 8–78 years) and 57 per cent were female. In the majority of cases the pacemaker was consistently effective in terminating spontaneous attacks of tachycardia but in approximately half continuing antiarrhythmic drug therapy was necessary. There were some technical failures and sensing difficulties with this pulse generator. When the second generation device (Pasar 4171 – see below) became available the original was no longer investigated.

Of particular concern was the report of four sudden deaths in patients fitted with this pacemaker. Two of these deaths occurred in female patients with Wolff–Parkinson–White (WPW) syndrome paced from the ventricles with two extrastimuli. It was possible that pacing had directly stimulated ventricular tachycardia or fibrillation, but in each case the anterograde refractoriness of the anomalous pathway was short and it is also possible that ventricular stimulation produced atrial fibrillation (by retrograde conduction) which in turn resulted in ventricular fibrillation (by anterograde conduction over the anomalous pathway). The other two patients who died suddenly had structural heart disease and the pacemaker might not have played a significant role. However, in one instance a Holter ECG monitor was being recorded at the time of death. The mode of death was ventricular fibrillation and the pacemaker was active at the initiation of this arrhythmia but the significance of this is still not clear. Nevertheless, from this experience it has been suggested that:

1. Double ventricular stimulation should not be used to treat supraventricular tachycardia.
2. Patients with WPW syndrome and a short anterograde refractory period of the anomalous pathway should not be treated with tachycardia interruption pacing.
3. Patients with structural heart disease should be treated with caution.

Tachylog (Siemens)   This pacemaker includes a variety of conventional and novel modalities for tachycardia conversion. In addition to straightforward burst pacing and precisely coupled extrastimuli, geometrical centrifugal scanning and responsive scanning are also available. Geometrical centrifugal scanning to alternate incremental and decremental movement of the extrastimulus dividing tachycardia diastole into geometric intervals. Responsive scanning is a method of actively searching for the tachycardia termination zones. It relies on the termination zone being bracketed by the zone of refractoriness (to the left) and the zone of reset (to the right). A stimulus delivered too early in the cycle does not affect the timing of subsequent tachycardia but a stimulus which is too late resets the tachycardia timing. Based on an analysis of tachycardia timing the termination zone is rapidly discovered.

With Tachylog, diagnosis of tachycardia requires not only a high heart rate but also a sudden change of rate at the onset of tachycardia. Both features are programmable.

Results are available from 25 patients (Sowton, 1984) with supraventricular tachycardia (16 patients) or ventricular tachycardia (9 patients). The results with ventricular tachycardia were very variable – 4 with severe coronary artery disease and poor left ventricular function died. Patients with supraventricular tachycardia did well over a follow-up period of 5–19 months. However, 2 patients with WPW syndrome underwent division of the anomalous pathway because of the development of atrial fibrillation with a rapid ventricular response, and 3 other patients needed additional antiarrhythmic drug treatment.

Pasar 4171 (Telectronics) Studies of two major determinants (pacing cycle length and duration of pacing) of the ability of pacing to terminate paroxysmal supraventricular tachycardia had demonstrated that, as the number of beats within a burst of pacing was increased, the longest coupling interval needed to terminate the tachycardia also increased. Similarly, it was shown that, at least at atrial level, the provocation of unwanted arrhythmias was less with longer coupling intervals and longer bursts. With these principles in mind the Pasar 4171 was designed and built. This unit is similar to Pasar 4151 but up to seven extrastimuli can be delivered. When more than two extrastimuli are selected their minimum coupling interval is restricted. This pacemaker also incorporates optional bradycardia support pacing at a single rate of 60 b.p.m.

The burst (multiple extrastimuli) mode of this pacemaker involved the concept of scanning. The coupling interval between the burst and the tachycardia (shifting burst) and the interval between successive beats within the burst (concertina bursts) may be progressively decremented if tachycardia does not terminate. The concertina scanning mode has proved so effective and safe that this pacemaker is now widely approved for the treatment of supraventricular tachycardia.

In a small personal series of 8 patients (4 atrioventricular tachycardia and 4 intra-AV nodal tachycardia) satisfactory long-term control has been achieved in all over a follow-up period of 31–36 (mean 34) months. In only 1 patient was concomitant antiarrhythmic drug therapy necessary. Sinus tachycardia inappropriately triggered the tachycardia conversion response in 3 patients.

The initial world-wide evaluation of Pasar 4171 involved 78 patients (47 female) aged 17–78 (average 47) years. Fifty patients suffered from intra-AV nodal re-entrant tachycardia and the remainder had atrioventricular tachycardia associated with WPW syndrome. In 95 per cent atrial electrodes were used. Over a total follow-up period of 1134 patient-months there were only 17 instances of failure to terminate tachycardia. A noteworthy feature of this series was the reduction of antiarrhythmic drug usage after implantation of the device. Before the implantation, 77 patients received antiarrhythmic drugs but afterwards only 30 patients needed concomitant drug therapy.

Intertach 262-12 (Intermedics) This latest tachycardia conversion pacemaker (Fig. 13.9) incorporates a wide range of tachycardia detection and interruption modalities, in addition to full multiprogrammable bradycardia support pacing. Tachycardia reversion capabilities include scans (incremental and decremental) and bursts (constant rate, rate-related and adaptive). Tachycardia detection algorithms consist of high heart rate, rate of change of heart rate at the onset of tachycardia, stability of the high rate and duration of the tachycardia. The high heart rate criterion is programmable but obligatory, whilst the other three variables are optional in various combinations.

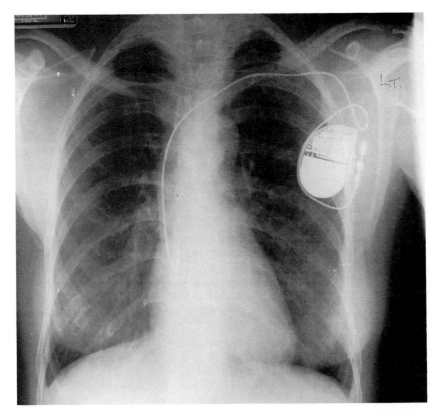

Fig. 13.9 Chest radiograph showing bipolar electrode lodged in the right atrial appendage and connected to an Intertach 262–12 (Intermedics) pacemaker.

Personal experience suggests that this device is safe and effective. Of the 13 patients fitted with the pacemaker, the tachycardia interruption modality has been activated in 12 (concertina, rate related in 11). In one instance the tachycardia was easily managed with antiarrhythmic drugs plus bradycardia support pacing. The 12 patients with active tachycardia interruption pacing have intra-AV nodal (9 patients) or atrioventricular (3 patients) tachycardia. All have been virtually asymptomatic and only 1 case has required concomitant drug therapy. The tachycardia interruption response has been triggered by sinus tachycardia on seven documented instances in 5 patients. Judicious programming has reduced but not eradicated this problem.

Implantation

The device is implanted in the same manner as a conventional pacemaker, with the following differences:

1. The electrode must be positioned at a site which allows repeated reliable and safe termination of tachycardia as determined by electrophysiological study.

2. The pacing threshold must be determined accurately during sinus rhythm and during tachycardia.
3. Ensure that the electrograms recorded from the pacing lead are adequate for reliable sensing during both tachycardia and sinus rhythm.

Postimplantation adjustments

The pacemaker should be programmed to recognize pathological tachycardia and distinguish this from sinus rhythm of any rate. The assessments should be made with the patient recumbent, upon standing and during exercise. Ambulatory ECG tape monitoring is necessary to ensure that no inappropriate pacing occurs. A standard pacemaker check is carried out prior to discharge.

Follow-up assessments

When possible, the pacemaker should first be interrogated to document its recent history (e.g. number of tachycardias detected, pacing responses and successes, etc.). A clinical record of the patient's symptoms should be made. The standard system checks are repeated. The pacemaker is adjusted accordingly.

Tachycardia termination by high energy techniques

Internal cardioversion

This system differs from conventional tachycardia termination in that higher energies (0.05–2 J) are used and the stimulus is delivered synchronously with the

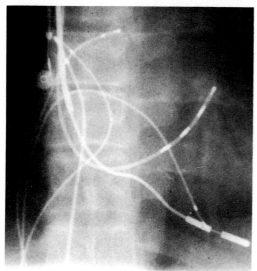

Fig. 13.10 The cardioverter catheter positioned at the right ventricular apex during an electrophysiological study. The shock is delivered between the apical electrodes (connected to form a single pole) and similar electrodes positioned at the junction between the superior vena cava and the right atrium.

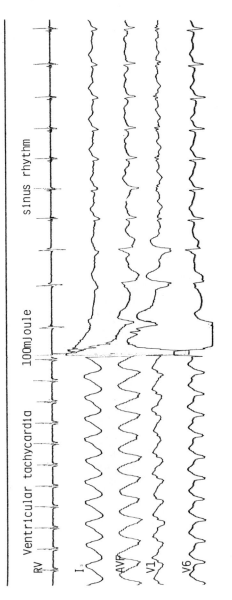

Fig. 13.11 Use of an external cardioverter (see Fig. 2.9) to terminate ventricular tachycardia. A synchronized discharge of 100 mJ results in prompt reversion to sinus rhythm. Paper speed 25 mm/sec.

tachycardia complex (QRS or electrogram). Specifically constructed, large surface area electrodes are required for use with the cardioverter device (Fig. 13.10). It has been almost exclusively applied to the termination of ventricular tachycardia by ventricular stimulation (Fig. 13.11). The stimulus energy depolarizes sufficient myocardium to terminate tachycardia. This method of tachycardia termination is useful for the treatment of recurrent tachycardias, especially in the coronary care unit or the cardiac catheterization laboratory. It is also particularly useful during electrophysiological study of ventricular tachycardias.

There are several drawbacks to the method:

1. The stimulus causes pain in conscious patients.
2. The timing of the stimulus is critical to the safety and success of the method but synchronization is difficult during ventricular tachycardias.
3. The stimulus may cause acceleration of ventricular tachycardia or initiate ventricular fibrillation (Fig. 13.12).
4. Atrial arrhythmias may be provoked (atrial fibrillation (Fig. 13.13) or atrial flutter).
5. It may be unsuccessful in as many as 50 per cent of patients.

Automatic implantable cardioverter/defibrillator (AICD)

This device has been perfected over the last 20 years. It is designed to detect and terminate malignant ventricular arrhythmias by delivering a discharge of 25–30 J (synchronized in the presence of distinct electrograms in as many cases of

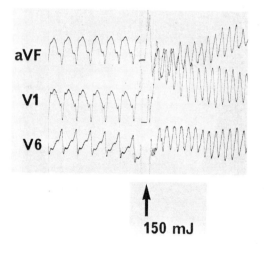

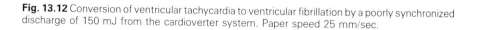

Fig. 13.12 Conversion of ventricular tachycardia to ventricular fibrillation by a poorly synchronized discharge of 150 mJ from the cardioverter system. Paper speed 25 mm/sec.

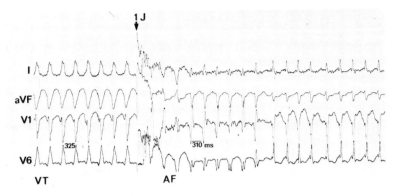

Fig. 13.13 Initiation of atrial fibrillation (AF) in response to internal cardioversion of ventricular tachycardia (VT). Paper speed 25 mm/sec.

ventricular tachycardia). The system currently available (CPI/Intec) comprises a generator (weight 290 g, volume 250 ml) powered by lithium iodide cells sufficient to deliver about 100 discharges. The shocks are delivered via two epicardial patch electrodes (Fig. 13.14) or by one patch electrode and an intravascular spring-coil electrode (right atrium–superior vena cava). In patients not requiring cardiac surgery for other reasons, the preferred method of

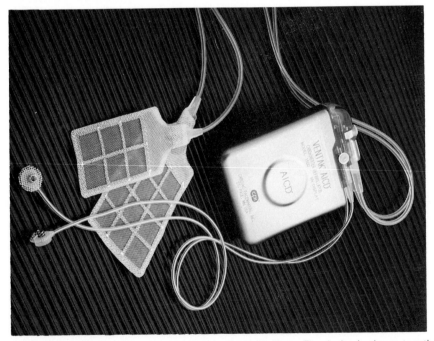

Fig. 13.14 The automatic implantable cardioverter/defibrillator. The device is shown together with a 10 cm^2 and 20 cm^2 patch electrode and two epicardial sensing electrodes. (Photograph kindly supplied by Mr S. Nisam.)

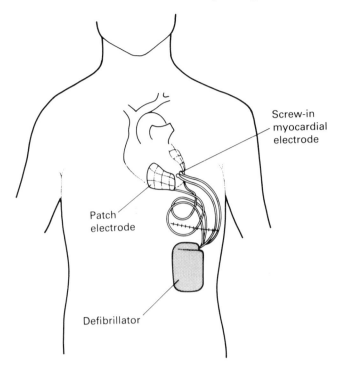

Fig. 13.15 The left subcostal approach for placement of two epicardial patch electrodes and two screw-in myocardial sensing leads.

implantation is the epicardial approach (Fig. 13.15). Electrograms are sensed from right ventricular bipolar electrodes or epicardial screw electrodes. Ventricular fibrillation is detected when there is no distinct isoelectric baseline (the algorithm is called a 'probability density function') or by absolute rate, and ventricular tachycardia is detected by rate criteria alone.

The precise indications for the use of this device have not been determined. It seems clear that any patient with recurrent serious ventricular arrhythmias which are life-threatening should be considered if other therapies are ineffective. Other indications (see also Table 13.5) which have been suggested include:

1. Patients with sustained ventricular tachycardia irrespective of the 'apparent' effectiveness of drug treatment.
2. Cases of out-of-hospital cardiac arrest not associated with an acute myocardial infarction.
3. Patients with severely impaired left ventricular function after myocardial infarction.
4. Patients with 'electrical instability' after myocardial infarction (see Chapter 10).
5. Patients with atypical ventricular tachycardias associated with prolonged repolarization (long QT syndromes).

Table 13.5 INDICATIONS FOR DEFIBRILLATOR IMPLANTATION

Definite	Recurrent, documented (or clinically certain), life-threatening ventricular tachyarrhythmias (ventricular fibrillation or hypotensive/ syncopal ventricular tachycardia):
	Not due to a transient cause (e.g. within 2 weeks of acute myocardial infarction)
	Not due to a reversible cause (e.g. drug toxicity or electrolyte imbalance)
	Not responsive to conventional therapy
Probable	A single episode of documented life-threatening ventricular tachyarrhythmia
	Recurrent, undocumented episodes of life-threatening ventricular tachyarrhythmias in a patient with inducible ventricular tachyarrhythmia
	Life-threatening ventricular tachyarrhythmias which cannot be evaluated for possible therapy by conventional means
Possible	As supplementary therapy to:
	Specific arrhythmia surgery
	Tachycardia interruption pacing
	Imperfect antiarrhythmic drug therapy

Table 13.6 CONTRAINDICATIONS TO DEFIBRILLATOR IMPLANTATION

Presence of concurrent terminal ($\leqslant$6 months) disease

Psychological unsuitability

Recurrent unsuppressible, non-sustained ventricular tachyarrhythmias

Recurrent uncontrollable supraventicular tachycardias

Virtually incessant, or very frequently recurrent ventricular tachycardias

Whilst awaiting definitive antiarrhythmic therapy (e.g. cardiac transplantation, potentially curative cardiac surgery, etc.)

Arrhythmias which are not suitable for treatment (see also Table 13.6) with this device include:

1. Frequently repetitive ventricular arrhythmias.
2. Associated short self-terminating bursts of ventricular arrhythmia which may trigger the device unnecessarily (Fig. 13.16).
3. Associated supraventricular arrhythmias causing inappropriate triggering.
4. Arrhythmias which are unlikely to recur (e.g. in association with the acute phase of myocardial infarction.
5. Arrhythmias in patients with a reduced life expectancy from other causes (e.g. malignancy).

For patients with ventricular tachycardia the electrophysiological assessment includes provocation of the arrhythmia in the laboratory. Testing patients with

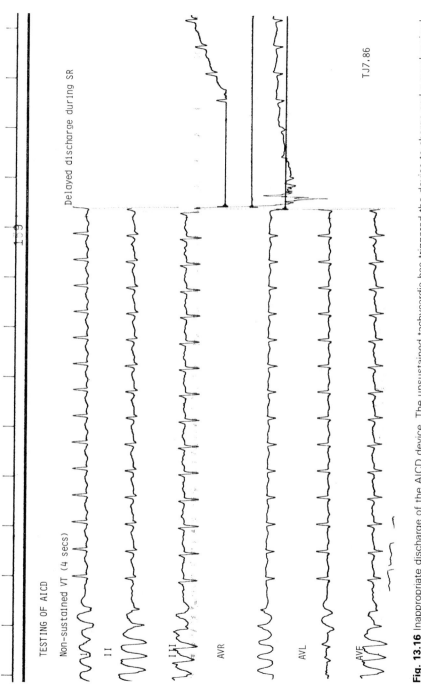

Fig. 13.16 Inappropriate discharge of the AICD device. The unsustained tachycardia has triggered the device to charge and a synchronized shock is given during sinus rhythm. Paper speed 25 mm/sec.

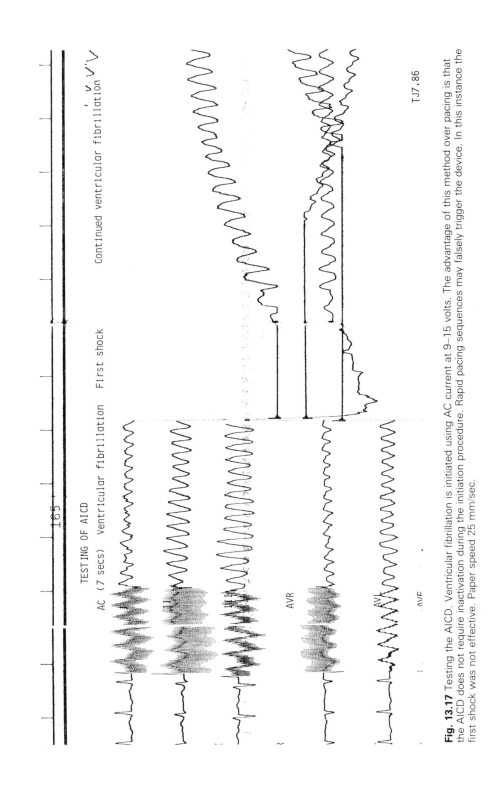

Fig. 13.17 Testing the AICD. Ventricular fibrillation is initiated using AC current at 9–15 volts. The advantage of this method over pacing is that the AICD does not require inactivation during the initiation procedure. Rapid pacing sequences may falsely trigger the device. In this instance the first shock was not effective. Paper speed 25 mm/sec.

recurrent ventricular fibrillation is performed at the time of implantation when the arrhythmia is induced by low energy AC stimulation (Fig. 13.17). This method has the advantage that the AICD need not be inactivated during the induction procedure (ventricular pacing may trigger the device). The defibrillation threshold is measured using a specially constructed device (external cardioverter/defibrillator – ECD).

Ambulatory monitoring, exercise testing and repeat electrophysiological testing, including the induction of ventricular fibrillation, are essential after implantation. No general anaesthetic is used during the testing procedure so that the patient may experience the sensation of the discharge. Ventricular arrhythmias are induced using alternating current transmitted to the heart using a bipolar electrode. It is important to ensure that the arrhythmias are sustained because, once the device is inactivated, it will discharge regardless of spontaneous termination (see Fig. 13.15). The postimplantation assessment documents the safety and efficacy of the device prior to the patient's discharge from hospital.

The AICD is activated by placing a magnet over the device for 30 seconds. A continuous tone is emitted during this period. This is followed by a random sequence of bleeps lasting a few seconds before the conversion to synchronous bleeping with the QRS complex which indicates that the AICD is activated. Inactivation of the AICD is achieved by holding the magnet in position for 30 seconds until a continuous tone is heard. If the magnet is removed before this period, a magnet test will result. The results of this test are displayed using the AIDCHECK which is used to monitor the performance of the AICD. A sensing probe is held over the AICD during the magnet test. The monitor displays the total number of discharges given and the current charge time of the capacitors. This latter measurement serves as a battery end-of-life indicator. Factors related to capacitor deformation require this check procedure to be repeated twice, and the second reading taken as the test result.

Several versions of this device have now been implanted on an experimental basis in over 1300 patients. Major modifications in the specification of the AICD

Table 13.7 MODALITIES FOR TERMINATION OF VENTRICULAR TACHYCARDIA

Modality	Efficacy			Safety	Pain	Prompt action
	VT	Fast VT	VF			
Single beat pacemaker	+	+/−	−	+	None	Yes
Multiple beat pacemaker	+ +	+	−	+/−	None	Yes
Internal cardioversion	+ +	+	+/−	+	+ +	Yes
Implantable defibrillator	+ +	+ +	+ +	+ +	+ +	No

VF = ventricular fibrillation; VT = ventricular tachycardia.
+ + = very effective/safe; + = moderately effective/safe; − = ineffective/unsafe.

are expected in the near future. These include extensive programmability, pacing modalities and data-logging functions. Each method of tachycardia termination has its particular merits and problems (Table 13.7). In future, tachycardia termination by pacing, by cardioversion and by defibrillation are likely to be incorporated within a single device which will automatically select the most appropriate response for a particular arrythmia.

It appears that expected mortality in this group of patients has been significantly reduced. There are, however, several disadvantages to the technique, some of which are technical and can be corrected in future models. The painful stimulus seems to be well tolerated by the majority of these patients.

References and further reading

Akhtar M, Gilbert CJ, Al-Nouri M, Schmidt DH. (1979) Electrophysiologic mechanisms for modification and abolition of atrioventricular junctional tachycardia with simultaneous and sequential atrial and ventricular pacing. *Circulation* **60**, 1443

Barold SS, Linhart JW, Samet P, Lister JW. (1969) Supraventricular tachycardia initiated and terminated by a single electrical stimulus. *American Journal of Cardiology* **24**, 37

Batchelder JE, Zipes DP. (1975) Treatment of tachyarrhythmias by pacing. *Archives of Internal Medicine* **135**, 1115

Bennett MA, Pentecost BL. (1970) Suppression of refractory ventricular tachycardia by transvenous rapid cardiac pacing and antiarrhythmic drugs. *American Heart Journal* **79**, 44

Bertholet M, Demoulin JC, Waleffe A, Kulbertus H. (1985) Programmable extrastimulus pacing for long-term management of supraventricular and ventricular tachycardias: clinical experience in 16 patients. *American Heart Journal* **110**, 582

Bertholet M, Demoulin JC, Waleffe A, Kulbertus H. (1985) Programmable extrastimuls pacing for long-term management of supraventricular and ventricular tachycardias: clinical experience in 16 patients. *American Heart Journal* **110**, 582

Camm AJ, Ward DE, Washington HG, Spurrell RAJ. (1979) Intravenous disopyramide phosphate and ventricular overdrive pacing in the termination of paroxysmal ventricular tachycardia. *Pacing and Clinical Electrophysiology* **2**, 395

Camm AJ, Ward DE. (1983) *Pacing for Tachycardia Control*. Telectronics: Sydney, Aus.

Chapman PD, Troup P. (1986) The automatic implantable cardioverter-defibrillator: evaluating suspected inappropriate shocks. *Journal of the American College of Cardiology* **7**, 1075

Cohen LS, Buccino RA, Morrow AG, Braunwald E. (1967) Recurrent ventricular tachycardia and fibrillation treated with a combination of beta-adrenergic blockade and electrical pacing. *Annals of Internal Medicine* **66**, 945

Cooper T, MacLean WAH, Waldo AL. (1978) Overdrive pacing for supraventricular tachycardias: a review of theoretical implications and therapeutic techniques. *Pacing and Clinical Electrophysiology* **1**, 196

Curry PVL, Rowland E, Krikler D. (1979) Dual-demand pacing for refractory atrioventricular reentry tachycardias. *Pacing and Clinical Electrophysiology* **2**, 137

Davies DW, Nathan AW, Camm AJ. (1985) Antitachycardia prophylaxis: DDD defeated. *Clinical Progress in Electrophysiology and Pacing* **3**, 224

DeFrancis NA, Giordano RP. (1968) Permanent epicardial atrial pacing in the treatment of refractory ventricular tachycardia. *American Journal of Cardiology* **22**, 742

den Dulk K, Bertholet M, Brugada P, Bar FE, Demoulin J, Waleffe A, Bakels N, Lindemans F, Bourgeois I, Kulbertus H, Wellens HJJ. (1984) Clinical experience with implantable devices for control of tachyarrhythmias. *Pacing and Clinical Electrophysiology* **7**, 548

Dreifus LS, Arriaga J, Watanabe Y, Downing D, Haiat R, Morse D. (1971) Recurrent Wolff–Parkinson–White tachycardia in an infant. Successful treatment by a radio-frequency pacemaker. *American Journal of Cardiology* **28**, 586

Echt D. (1984) Potential hazards of implanted devices for the electrical control of tachyarrhythmias. *Pacing and Clinical Electrophysiology* **7**, 580

Echt DS, Armstrong K, Schmidt P, Oyer PE, Stinson EB, Winkle RA. (1985) Clinical experience, complications, and survival in 70 patients with the automatic implantable cardioverter/defibrillator. *Circulation* **71**, 289

Fisher JD, Mehra R, Furman S. (1978) Termination of ventricular tachycardia with bursts of rapid ventricular pacing. *American Journal of Cardiology* **41**, 94

Fisher JD, Matos JA, Kim SG. (1982a) The sparkling joules of internal cardiac stimulation: cardioversion, defibrillation and ablation. *American Heart Journal* **104**, 177

Fisher JD, Kim SG, Furman S, Matos JA. (1982b) Role of implantable pacemakers in control of recurrent ventricular tachycardia. *American Journal of Cardiology* **49**, 194

Fisher JD, Matos JA, Ostrow E. (1983a) Comparative effectiveness of pacing techniques for termination of well-tolerated sustained ventricular tachycardia. *Pacing and Clinical Electrophysiology* **6**, 915

Fisher JD, Lawrence KA, Waspe LE, Matos JA. (1983b) Mechanisms for success and failure of pacing for termination of ventricular tachycardia: clinical and hypothetical considerations. *Pacing and Clinical Electrophysiology* **6**, 1094

Friedberg CK, Lyon LJ, Donoso E. (1970) Suppression of refractory recurrent ventricular tachycardia by transvenous rapid cardiac pacing and antiarrhythmic drugs. *American Heart Journal* **79**, 44

Gardener MJ, Waxman HL, Buxton AE, Cain ME, Josephson ME. (1982) Termination of ventricular tachycardia. Evaluation of a new method. *American Journal of Cardiology* **50**, 1338

Griffin JC, Mason JW, Calfee RV. (1980) Clinical use of an implantable automatic tachycardia terminating pacemaker. *American Heart Journal* **100**, 1093

Haft JI, Kosowsky BD, Lau SH, Stein E, Damato AN. (1967) Termination of atrial flutter by rapid electrical pacing of the atrium. *American Journal of Cardiology* **20**, 239

Haft JI. (1974) Treatment of arrhythmias by intracardiac electrical stimulation. *Progress in Cardiovascular Diseases* **16**, 539

Hartzler GO. (1979) Treatment of recurrent ventricular tachycardia by patient-activated radiofrequency ventricular stimulation. *Mayo Clinic Proceedings* **54**, 75

Hartzler GO, Holmes DR, Osborn MJ. (1981) Patient activated transvenous cardiac stimulation for the treatment of supraventricular and ventricular tachycardia. *American Journal of Cardiology* **47**, 903

Herre JM, Griffin JC, Nielson AP, Mann DE, Luck JC, Magro SA, Scheunemeyer T, Wyndham CRC. (1985) Permanent triggered antitachycardia pacemakers in the management of recurrent sustained ventricular tachycardia. *Journal of the American College of Cardiology* **6**, 206

Hornbaker HJ, Humphries JO, Ross RS. (1969) Permanent pacing in the absence of heart block. An approach to the management of intractable arrhythmias. *Circulation* **39**, 189

Hunt NC, Cobb FR, Waxman MB, Zeft HJ, Peter RH, Morris JJ. (1968) Conversion of supraventricular tachycardias with atrial stimulation. Evidence for re-entry mechanisms. *Circulation* **38**, 1060

Jackman W, Zipes DP. (1982) Low-energy synchronous cardioversion of ventricular tachycardia using a catheter electrode in a canine model of subacute myocardial infarction. *Circulation* **66**, 187

Kappenberger L, Sowton E. (1981) Programmed stimulation for long-term treatment and non-invasive investigation of recurrent tachycardia. *Lancet* **i**, 909

Kastor JA, DeSanctis RW, Harthorne JW, Schwartz GH. (1967) Transvenous atrial pacing in the treatment of refractory ventricular irritability. *Annals of Internal Medicine* **66**, 939

Krikler D, Curry PVL, Buffet J. (1976) Dual-demand pacing for reciprocating atrioventricular tachycardia. *British Medical Journal* **1**, 1114

Kuck KH, Kunze KP, Schluter M, Bliefeld W. (1984) Tachycardia prevention by programmed stimulation. *American Journal of Cardiology* **54**, 550

Lew HT, March HW. (1967) Control of recurrent ventricular fibrillation by transvenous pacing in the absence of heart block. *American Heart Journal* **73**, 794

Lister JW, Cohen LS, Bernstein WH, Samet P. (1968) Treatment of supraventricular tachycardias by rapid atrial stimulation. *Circulation* **38**, 1044

Lister JW, Gosselin AJ, Nathan DA, Barold SS. (1973) Rapid atrial stimulation in the treatment of supraventricular tachycardia. *Chest* **63**, 995

McCallister BD, McGoon DC, Connolly DC. (1966) Paroxysmal ventricular tachycardia and fibrillation without complete heart block. Report of a case treated with a permanent internal cardiac pacemaker. *American Journal of Cardiology* **18**, 898

Mandel WJ, Laks MM, Yamaguchi I, Fields J, Berkovits B. (1976) Recurrent reciprocating tachycardias in the Wolff–Parkinson–White syndrome. Control by the use of a scanning pacemaker. *Chest* **69**, 769

Massumi RA, Kistin AD, Tawakkol AA. (1967) Termination of reciprocating tachycardia by atrial stimulation. *Circulation* **36**, 637

Mirowski M, Mower MM, Staewen WS, Denniston RH, Mendeloff AI. (1972) The development of the transvenous automatic defibrillator. *Archives of Internal Medicine* **129**, 773

Mirowski M, Reid PR, Watkins L, Weisfeldt ML, Mower MM. (1981) Clinical treatment of life-threatening ventricular tachyarrhythmias with the automatic implantable defibrillator. *American Heart Journal* **102**, 265

Mirowski M, Reid PR, Winkle RA, Mower MM, Watkins L, Stinson EB, Kallman C, Weisfeldt M. (1983) Mortality in patients with implanted automatic defibrillators. *Annals of Internal Medicine* **98**, 585

Mirowski M. (1985) The automatic implantable cardioverter-defibrillator: an overview. *Journal of the American College of Cardiology* **6**, 461

Moss AJ, Rivers RJ, Griffith LSC, Carmel JA, Millard EB. (1968) Transvenous left atrial pacing for control of recurrent ventricular fibrillation. *New England Journal of Medicine* **278**, 928

Nathan AN, Bexton RS, Spurrell RAJ, Camm AJ. (1984) Internal transvenous low-energy cardioversion for the treatment of cardiac arrhythmias. *British Heart Journal* **52**, 377

O'Keeffe DB, Curry PVL, Sowton E. (1981) Treatment of paroxysmal nodal tachycardia by dual demand pacemaker in the coronary sinus. *British Heart Journal* **45**, 105

Osborn MJ, Holmes DR. (1985) Antitachycardia pacing. *Clinical Progress in Electrophysiology and Pacing* **3**, 239

Prystowsky EN, Zipes DP. (1983) Inhibition in the human heart. *Circulation* **68**, 707

Reddy CP, Todd EP, Kuo CS, DeMaria AN. (1984) Treatment of ventricular tachycardia using an automatic scanning extrastimulus pacemaker. *Journal of the American College of Cardiology* **3**, 225

Reid PR, Mirowski M, Mower MM, Platia EV, Griffith LSC, Watkins L, Bach SM, Imran M, Thomas A. (1983) Clinical evaluation of the internal automatic cardioverter-defibrillator in survivors of sudden cardiac death. *American Journal of Cardiology* **51**, 1608

Ruskin JN, Gara H, Poulin F, Harthorne JW. (1980) Permanent radiofrequency ventricular pacing for management of drug-resistant ventricular tachycardia. *American Journal of Cardiology* **46**, 317

Ryan GF, Easley RM, Zaroff LI, Goldstein S. (1968) Paradoxical use of a demand pacemaker in treatment of supraventricular tachycardia due to Wolff–Parkinson–White syndrome. Observation on termination of reciprocal rhythm. *Circulation* **38**, 1037

Sowton E, Leatham A, Carson P. (1964) The suppression of arrhythmias by artificial pacemaking. *Lancet* **2**, 1098

Sowton E, Balcon R, Preston T, Leaver D, Yacoub M. (1969) Long-term control of intractable supraventricular tachycardia by ventricular pacing. *British Heart Journal* **31**, 700

Sowton E, O'Keeffe DB, Curry PVL. (1980a) Use of multiprogrammable pacemaker in the dual demand mode: influence of pacing rate on termination of tachycardias. *European Heart Journal* **1**, 165

Sowton E, O'Keeffe DB, Curry PVL. (1980b) Use of a multiprogrammable pacemaker in the dual demand mode: influence of pacing rate on termination of tachycardias. *European Heart Journal* **1**, 165

Sowton E. (1984) Clinical results with the Tachylog antitachycardia pacemaker. *Pacing and Clinical Electrophysiology* **7**, 1313

Spurrell RAJ, Sowton E. (1976) Pacing techniques in the management of supraventricular tachycardias. *Journal of Electrocardiology* **8**, 287

Spurrell RAJ. (1982) Use of cardiac pacemakers in the management of tachycardias. *Cardiovascular Reviews and Reports* **3**, 123

Spurrell RAJ, Nathan AN, Bexton RS, Hellestrand KJ, Nappholz T, Camm AJ. (1982) Implantable automatic scanning pacemaker for termination of supraventricular tachycardia. *American Journal of Cardiology* **49**, 753

Sung RJ, Styperek JL, Castellanos A. (1980) Complete abolition of the reentrant supraventricular zone using a new modality of cardiac pacing with simultaneous atrioventricular stimulation. *American Journal of Cardiology* **45**, 72

Vassalle M. (1977) The relationship between cardiac pacemakers. Overdrive suppression. *Circulation Research* **41**, 269

Vergara GS, Hildner FJ, Schoenfeld CB, Javier RP, Cohen LS, Samet P. (1972) Conversion of supraventricular tachycardias with rapid atrial pacing. *Circulation* **46**, 788

Waldecker B, Brugada P, den Dulk K, Zehender M, Wellens HJJ. (1985) Arrhythmias induced during termination of supraventricular tachycardia. *American Journal of Cardiology* **55**, 412

Waldo AL, Kongrad E, Kupersmith J, Levine R, Bowman FO, Hoffman BF. (1976a) Ventricular paired pacing to control rapid ventricular heart rate following open heart surgery. *Circulation* **53**, 176

Waldo AL, MacLean WAH, Karp RB, Kouchoukos NT, James TN. (1976b) Continuous rapid atrial pacing to control recurrent or sustained supraventricular tachycardias following open heart surgery. *Circulation* **54**, 245

Ward DE, Camm AJ, Spurrell RAJ. (1979) The response of regular reentrant supraventricular tachycardia to right heart stimulation. *Pacing and Clinical Electrophysiology* **2**, 586

Ward DE, Camm AJ, Gainsborough J, Spurrell RAJ. (1980) Autodecremental pacing – a microprocessor based modality for the termination of paroxysmal tachycardias. *Pacing and Clinical Electrophysiology* **3**, 178

Ward DE, Rigby M, Dawson P, Collins M, Shinebourne EA. (1884) Rapid ventricular pacing to control resistant neonatal atrioventricular reentrant tachycardias. *Pediatric Cardiology* **5**, 45

Wellens HJJ. (1978) Value and limitations of programmed electrical stimulation of the heart in the study and treatment of tachycardias. *Circulation* **57**, 845

Wellens HJJ, Bar FW, Gorgels AP, Muncharaz JF. (1978) Electrical treatment of arrhythmias with an emphasis on the tachycardias. *American Journal of Cardiology* **41**, 1025

Winkle RA. (1983) The implantable defibrillator in ventricular arrhythmias. *Hospital Practice* **18**, 149

Zeft HJ, McGowan RL. (1969) Termination of paroxysmal junctional tachycardia by right ventricular stimulation. *Circulation* **40**, 919

Zeft HJ, Cobb FR, Waxman MB, Hunt NC, Morris JJ. (1969) Right atrial stimulation in the treatment of atrial flutter. *Annals of Internal Medicine* **70**, 447

Zipes DP, Wallace AG, Sealy W, Floyd WI. (1969) Artificial and atrial and ventricular pacing in the treatment of arrhythmias. *Annals of Internal Medicine* **70**, 885

Zipes DP, Jackman WM, Heger JJ, Chilson DA, Browne KF, Nacarrelli GV, Rahilly GT, Prystowsky EN. (1982) Clinical transvenous cardioversion of recurrent life-threatening ventricular tachyarrhythmias: low energy synchronized cardioversion of ventricular tachycardia and termination of ventricular fibrillation in patients using a catheter electrode. *American Heart Journal* **103**, 789

14

Operative Electrophysiological Studies and Surgical Treatment of Tachycardias

Surgical treatment of tachycardias (Table 14.1) is considered in any patient with severely symptomatic tachycardias in whom other forms of therapy have failed, are not suitable or are unacceptable for any reason – drug side effects, the patient's preference (e.g. patient may not wish to continue drug treatment for life), failed pacing treatment, etc. There are four basic applications of surgical treatment. The precise strategy of surgery differs with each category (Fig. 14.1).

1. Treatment of atrial tachycardias (atrial fibrillation, flutter and tachycardia) and junctional tachycardias (AV nodal re-entrant tachycardia, AV re-entrant tachycardia). The aim is to remove the ventricles from the influence of tachycardia by ablation of the AV node–His bundle. This strategy may be regarded as ameliorative.

2. Treatment of tachycardias associated with the presence of an anomalous AV connection (rapid atrial fibrillation with ventricular pre-excitation, AV re-entrant tachycardias). In this setting the strategy is to prevent conduction in the anomalous pathway, thereby preventing the expression of the symptomatic arrhythmia (i.e. re-entrant excitation cannot occur because the circuit is broken and rapid responses to atrial fibrillation with ventricular pre-excitation are prevented by abolition of anterograde anomalous conduction. This approach can be regarded as a cure.

Table 14.1 SPECIFIC SURGERY FOR ARRHYTHMIAS

| Method | Arrhythmia | | |
	Atrial	WPW	Ventricular
Exclusion	Left atrial isolation Right atrial (sinus) isolation His bundle division	NA	Encircling ventriculotomy Right ventricular isolation
Incision	Atriotomy	Division of AP or His bundle	Ventriculotomy
Excision	Atrial appendectomy	NA	Endocardial resection Aneurysmectomy Mitral valve replacement

AP = anomalous pathway; NA = not applicable.

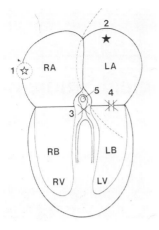

Fig. 14.1 Operative strategies for surgical treatment of supraventricular tachycardia. Atrial foci may be ablated (1) or isolated (2) from the rest of the atria. If this is not feasible, these foci may be prevented from driving the ventricles by His bundle ablation (3). This method is also applicable to AV nodal tachycardias. Atrioventricular re-entrant tachycardias can be approached by ablation of the His bundle (3) or the anomalous pathway (4). Recently, it has been possible to ablate selectively part of the AV node (5) in patients with dual pathways such that fast anterograde conduction persists but slow pathway conduction is abolished.

3. Treatment of certain types of atrial tachycardia by direct ablation or excision. This approach may be regarded as curative rather than ameliorative.
4. Treatment of recurrent ventricular tachycardias associated with a localized substrate (e.g. recurrent sustained monomorphic ventricular tachycardia associated with old myocardial infarction). The strategy is to ablate or in some way modify the substrate for tachycardia, such that re-entrant excitation responsible for the clinical arrhythmia is prevented. This strategy cannot be regarded as a cure in the sense that the substrate is permanently destroyed.

Principles of operative electrophysiology

Effective surgical treatment of a tachycardia is dependent on two requirements: (1) accurate localization of the area or specific structure to be ablated. This can be achieved by 'operative mapping'; and (2) effective ablation of the area or structure supporting the tachycardia.

Operative mapping

The basic mapping procedure involves sampling of electrograms from strategically selected sites in the region of interest. This type of mapping is referred to as 'electrogram mapping' and is the fundamental method of operative electrophysiology for any of the indications described above. Clearly, the technique is modified according to the particular clinical setting but there are general principles common to all applications of the method.

When the heart is exposed, several fixed electrodes are sutured to the atria and

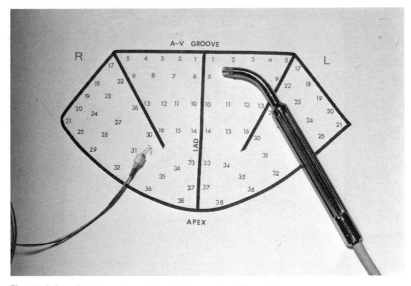

Fig. 14.2 A stylized mapping grid with electrodes. The grid is superimposed on a representation of the unfolded ventricular surface (LAD = left anterior descending artery). A bipolar hook electrode (lower left) is used to obtain atrial and ventricular reference electrograms. The mapping probe (upper right) has three platinum electrodes at its tip.

ventricles. These act as recording reference electrodes and may also be used to stimulate tachycardias by the standard methods. Electrograms are sampled from various points over the epicardial or endocardial surface or both (depending on the clinical problem) using a purpose-built hand-held roving electrode probe (Fig. 14.2) containing three electrodes at its tip. Bipolar electrograms are recorded and filtered and amplified as described in Chapter 2. Each electrogram from the roving pole is timed against a reference and related to the sample position by a predetermined stylized grid (Fig. 14.2). Data points obtained from these techniques can be used to construct a simple activation map (Fig. 14.3). From the clinical point of view this rarely is necessary since the main objective of the procedure is to localize a specific area (e.g. the His bundle or the earliest point of activation). On-line computing facilities using multiplexing can generate activation maps at the time of surgery. Another device which may reduce the Multipolar endocardial balloon electrodes are also under investigation (de Bakker et al., 1983).

Surgical ablation

Methods of surgical ablation have included direct incision, microdissection, diathermy, ligature, excision, circumferential incision, cryothermal ablation and many more. The method used is determined by the nature of the operation. Thus, for AV nodal ablation, cryotherapy or microdissection are both currently used. For ventricular tachycardia a wide variety of procedures are available. The choice of method may be determined by the exact nature of the problem or as

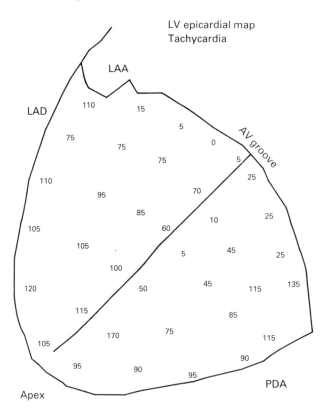

Fig. 14.3 Simple activation map of ventricular tachycardia in a 60-year-old woman with a left ventricular scar and recurrent refractory ventricular tachycardias. The local activation times are superimposed on this stylized grid of the left ventricular surface. The shortest interval between the reference electrode and the local activation time is situated just anterior to the obtuse margin of the left ventricle. The junction between healthy and fibrous tissue was paper thin at this point and cryothermal mapping confirmed this as the origin of tachycardia. LAA = left atrial appendage; LAD = left anterior descending artery; PDA = posterior descending artery.

a matter of preference. The cryothermal method is applicable to all types of tachycardia surgery. Ablation is achieved by using a cryothermal system capable of freezing to about −60°C. A special probe applies cooling to the appropriate area (Fig. 14.4). In certain settings the temperature is initially reduced to about −10°C during the appropriate rhythm. Thus, if cooling during tachycardia results in termination of that tachycardia, this is taken as confirmatory evidence of the accurate localization of the tachycardia substrate (or part of it) and the correct location of the probe. This is called 'cryothermal mapping' (Camm et al., 1980). Further cooling to −60°C for 2 minutes causes a spherical zone of damage about 1 cm in diameter, resulting in permanent ablation. Other advantages of the method include haemostasis and preservation of fibroblastic healing processes. The long-term effect of cryotherapy on nearby coronary arteries is not known.

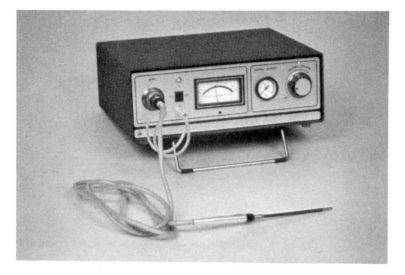

Fig. 14.4 The cryothermal apparatus used for cryoablation at the time of surgery. The probe shown in the foreground is of the straight variety commonly used for His bundle cryoablation. Curved probes are available for less easily accessible areas.

Surgical ablation of the AV node–His bundle

This method has now been superseded by electrical ablation of the AV node–His bundle (see Chapter 15). Nevertheless, there are likely to be occasions when electrical ablation fails and a surgical approach may have to be considered. The main indication for surgical ablation of the AV node–His bundle is therefore failed electrical ablation. The principle of surgical AV node ablation is identical to that of electrical ablation. The region of the AV node–his bundle is identified using a specially constructed tripolar mapping probe. The region of the AV junction is explored using this probe until a distinct His spike is recorded. This potential is usually found at the apex of the triangle of Koch (Fig. 14.5). The operation is performed during full cardiopulmonary bypass.

Ablation of the AV node–His bundle is undertaken by cryotherapy. If AV block is induced (Fig. 14.6), indicating that the probe is correctly located (Fig. 14.7), the temperature is reduced to −60°C for 2 minutes. This results in permanent complete AV block in 80 per cent of patients, and in the remainder there is significant modification of AV nodal function preventing a high rate of AV nodal responses.

In patients with AV nodal tachycardias, a new approach has recently been developed by Ross et al. (1985). Tissue overlying the AV node–His bundle is carefully dissected away from its inferior attachments. This has resulted in abolition of inducible AV nodal re-entrant tachycardia without damage to normal AV conduction, and, in particular, with preservation of the AV nodal dual pathway features so commonly seen in these patients. Further information about the results of this method is awaited.

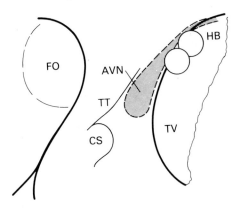

Fig. 14.5 The His bundle region as approached from the right atrium at surgery. The AV node (AVN) and penetrating bundle of His (HB) lie at the apex of Koch's triangle which is bounded by the tricuspid valve annulus (TV), the tendon of Todaro (TT) and the ostium of the coronary sinus (CS). FO = fossa ovalis. (See also Figs. 14.6 and 14.7).

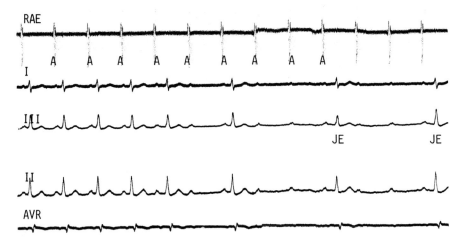

Fig. 14.6 The effect of cooling in the apex of the triangle of Koch. This patient was undergoing surgical AV nodal–His bundle ablation for refractory AV nodal tachycardias. Application of the cryoprobe and cooling to −10°C resulted in immediate complete AV block. Paper speed 25 mm/sec. RAE = right atrial reference electrogram.

Surgical ablation of anomalous direct AV connections

The main indications for this operation are refractory AV re-entrant tachycardias and rapid atrial fibrillation due to AV conduction over the anomalous pathway itself (see Chapters 6 and 9). Ablation of the anomalous pathway will prevent both types of arrhythmia, offering a cure. Central to the success of the procedure is accurate localization of the anomalous pathway. A fairly accurate idea of its location will have been gained at preoperative electrophysiological studies, a

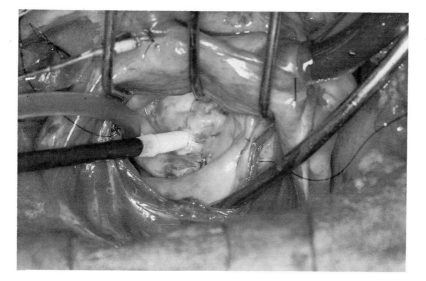

Fig. 14.7 View of the right atrium at surgery. The cryoprobe is shown applied to the endocardium at the apex of the triangle of Koch.

necessary prerequisite in all patients referred for operative treatment of this condition.

All direct anomalous AV pathways are located in the AV groove. Electrogram mapping of the epicardium and the endocardium in the region of the AV groove are the standard methods used to localize the anomalous pathway. Epicardial mapping of the ventricular surface during anterograde conduction in the anomalous pathway (atrial pacing or sinus rhythm with ventricular pre-excitation or during antidromic tachycardia) identifies the earliest point of ventricular activation as a result of conduction over the anomalous pathway. This information is of indirect value in that surgery is not performed at the ventricular insertion of the anomalous pathway. Nevertheless, the atrial insertion is usually at or near to a corresponding point on the atrial side of the AV groove.

The atrial activation pattern during ventricular pacing is determined by the degree of fusion between the normal retrograde AV nodal wavefront and the retrograde anomalous wavefront. Detailed mapping can separate the two wavefronts. It is, however, preferable to map the atria during orthodromic tachycardia when retrograde conduction is exclusively via the anomalous pathway. Endocardial activation reveals earliest activation around the valve rings and this accurately localizes the atrial insertion of the anomalous pathway (Fig. 14.8). Endocardial surgery (incision or ablation) could then be performed in this region. Atrial epicardial mapping provides accurate localization for epicardial ablation methods. Note that if no tachycardia can be induced, it is still possible to locate the anomalous pathway by mapping during atrial and ventricular pacing. Occasionally, the anomalous pathway is dormant at operation. This emphasizes the value of detailed preoperative mapping.

Surgical ablation of the anomalous pathway has been achieved using a variety

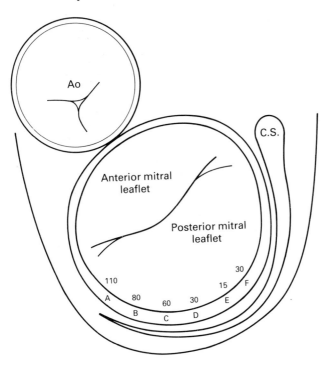

Fig. 14.8 Localization of the atrial insertion of an anomalous pathway. The atrial endocardium is mapped during atrioventricular re-entrant tachycardia using the roving probe (see Fig. 14.2). The shortest interval between the ventricular reference and the probe electrogram during tachycardia is 15 msec, indicating that the insertion of the anomalous pathway is in the territory of point E on the free wall of the atrium. CS = coronary sinus.

of methods (Fig. 14.9). The classic method devised by Sealy and colleagues (1974) has been endocardial atrial incision at the atrial margin of the AV ring, with or without cryothermal ablation at the earliest point of atrial activation. This approach requires full cardiopulmonary bypass. Cryothermal mapping (freezing to − 10°C for 30 seconds) can be used to confirm the location of the anomalous pathway by cooling during tachycardia, causing termination of the tachycardia in the retrograde limb. Alternatively, the probe may be applied during sinus

Fig. 14.9 Four methods of achieving surgical ablation of an anomalous pathway. Each diagram shows a cross-section at the mitral annulus. (*a*) Endocardial incision and dissection: in this method the mitral leaflet is lifted away from its insertion and the subannuluar tissue dissected through to the epicardial fat adjacent the AV groove. (*b*) Endocardial cryothermal injury: in this technique the cryoprobe is applied to the atrial endocardial aspect of the mitral ring. (*c*) Closed heart dissection: the fat pad is dissected away from the AV groove down to the annulus itself, thereby interrupting anomalous pathways running in the epicardial fat. Additional damage can be achieved using the cryothermal method. (*d*) Epicardial electrical discharges: this novel method is based on the principle of endocardial ablation (see Chapter 15). Localized discharges delivered through an epicardial plate abolish anomalous conduction.

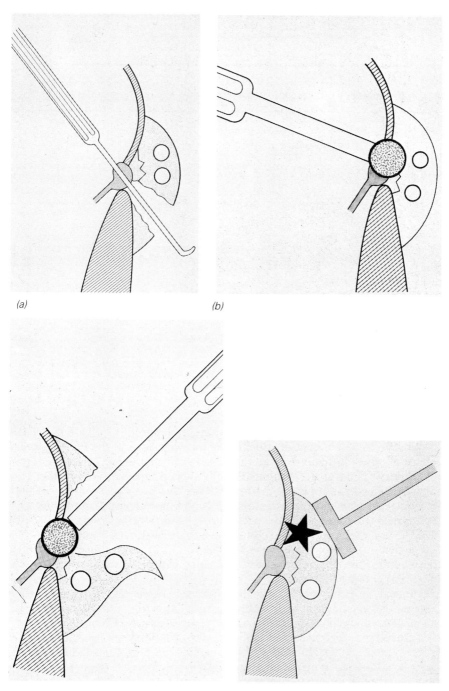

(a)

(b)

(c)

(d)

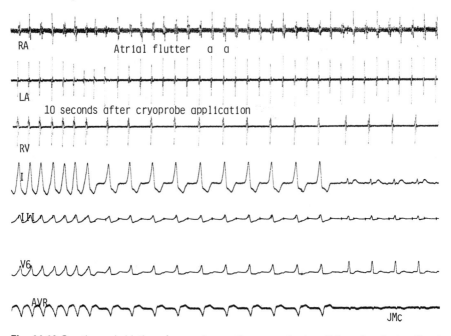

Fig. 14.10 Cryothermal ablation of anomalous pathway conduction. This patient had suffered from frequent episodes of tachycardia and atrial fibrillation with a rapid ventricular response due to conduction over a right septal pathway. The recording shows atrial flutter (a) with 1:1 anomalous AV conduction. Ten seconds after cooling to $-10°C$, the 1:1 ratio changes to 2:1 conduction and finally pre-excitation disappears altogether. Paper speed 25 mm/sec. LA = left atrial reference electrogram; RA = right atrial reference electrogram; RV = right ventricular reference electrogram.

rhythm or atrial pacing with ventricular pre-excitation (Fig. 14.10). This method is effective in 95 per cent of patients. Pathways located in the posterior-septal region are most difficult to locate and ablate, often requiring careful dissection of the crux. Camm et al. (1980) successfully ablated anomalous conduction using cryosurgery without opening the heart. Recently, Klein and colleagues (1984) have reported an improved method of closed-heart epicardial ablation. The epicardial fat in the region of the AV groove is dissected away from the AV groove and the cryoprobe applied directly to the epicardial surface of the atrial wall in the region of the anomalous pathway. The results of this technique, which has been applied to right, left free wall and septal pathways, are encouraging with near 100 per cent success to date.

Surgical dissection of the posteroseptal region has also been successfully applied to ablation of tachycardias associated with atypical posteroseptal anomalous conduction (so-called long RP' tachycardias, see Chapter 9).

Transvenous electrical ablation of anomalous conduction is feasible in selected patients (see Chapter 15). Recently, this method has been applied directly to the surface of the heart at operation. An electrode with a large surface area is applied to the appropriate area, and epicardial shocks of 100–300 j are delivered, resulting in abolition of anomalous conduction. Cardiopulmonary bypass is not needed for this method. Further information is required before it can be more widely used.

Surgical ablation or exclusion of atrial tachycardia foci

Atrial tachycardias may be automatic or re-entrant in type. In either case, the origin of tachycardia may be confined to a small area of atrial myocardium which can be localized by electrogram mapping techniques. The focus can then be excised, isolated by an encircling incision or ablated by cryothermal injury. Transvenous electrical ablation has also been applied to this type of tachycardia (see Chapter 15).

Surgical ablation or exclusion of ventricular tachycardias

Although surgical methods of treating ventricular tachycardias have been applied without using operative electrophysiological methods (simple coronary grafting, 'blind' aneurysmectomy, etc.), the available evidence suggests that, with appropriate patient selection, the results of operative treatment are greatly improved by specific electrophysiologically guided procedures. Thus the aim of mapping is to locate the area of earliest ventricular activation, because this is closely associated with the origin of the tachycardia whatever the mechanism. When operative methods were first applied to the treatment of ventricular tachycardias, the emphasis was on epicardial electrogram mapping. It is now appreciated, however, that most ventricular tachycardias arise from the endocardium or subendocardium. Electrophysiological and surgical procedures are therefore directed at this region, especially in relation to the left ventricle. Many tachycardias are localized to a small area of endocardium (microre-entrant) but recent studies have suggested that macrore-entry may be more common than has been recognized (Mason et al., 1985).

Mapping procedures

Localization of the origin of tachycardia requires detailed activation mapping. Some idea of the source of tachycardia can be obtained by analysis of the surface ECG and patients will have undergone endocardial activation mapping at electrophysiological study prior to surgery. To construct an activation map of the ventricular endocardium, about 50–100 points must be sampled which may take several minutes, even in skilled hands. Tachycardia may not be haemodynamically stable, preventing detailed mapping. Degeneration to unstable rhythms such as polymorphic tachycardia (changing activation patterns) also prevents mapping. Tachycardia may be non-sustained. Attempts to reduce mapping times have included multiple electrode arrays (on a balloon, on a patch, on an epicardial sock) and computing facilities (real-time analysis, multiplexing, isochrone maps etc.). Earliest endocardial activation during tachycardia may be up to 80 msec before the onset of the surface QRS complex.

The technique of electrogram activation mapping is complemented by cryothermal mapping (Camm et al., 1980). The general method is described above. The principle of cryothermal mapping of ventricular tachycardia has been to identify the earliest point of endocardial activation during ventricular tachycardia and apply cooling to −10°C for 15–30 seconds to this area, observing the effect on tachycardia. Termination of tachycardia indicates that the probe is at, or close to, the point of origin. Thus, ventricular tachycardias caused by microre-entry or focal mechanisms of any sort can be accurately localized by this method. Recent activation studies of ventricular tachycardias have suggested that macrore-entry may be the underlying mechanism in a small proportion of instances (Mason et al., 1985). Corroborative evidence for this has been provided by cryothermal termination of tachycardia at a site activated late after the onset of the QRS. This suggests that cooling blocked conduction in a relatively large circuit. The application of cryothermal mapping may provide useful information about the mechanism, as well as the location, of the tachycardia.

If tachycardia cannot be induced at surgery, localization by activation searching for the 'earliest point of activation' is not possible. In this case, other methods of localization can be used. As described in Chapter 10, fractionated and delayed endocardial electrograms are often recorded during sinus rhythm from the region of origin of tachycardia. These signals can be used at surgery as a rough guide to the source of tachycardia, but there is not a good correlation between their distribution and the earliest activation during tachycardia.

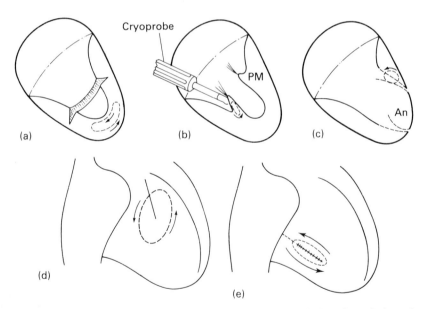

Fig. 14.11 Some of the surgical methods used for ablation or exclusion of ventricular tachycardia. (*a*) An encircling ventriculotomy is shown isolating a ventricular tachycardia circuit. this method is not suitable for foci related to the papillary muscles. (*b*) The cyroprobe is shown applied to a potential circuit on the base of a papillary muscle (PM). (*c*) A left ventricular aneurysm (An) is incised and scar tissue removed. In addition, surrounding endocardium is peeled away and resected. (*d*) A simple ventriculotomy is shown interrupting a right ventricular free wall re-entrant pathway. (*e*) An old right ventriculotomy (e.g. after correction of Fallot's tetralogy) may be the focus of a macrore-entrant circuit. Extension of the scar to the valve ring interrupts the circuit.

Pacemapping can be helpful if activation mapping is not feasible (see Chapter 10). The aim of this method is to mimic the QRS complex morphology by pacing the heart at multiple points in the supposed area of origin of the tachycardia. The resulting QRS morphology is then compared with the spontaneous tachycardia QRS morphology (preferably under identical conditions), and the pacing site resulting in the 'best match' is regarded as the closest to the site of origin. There are several difficulties with this method:

1. Pacing at widely separated points may produce similar QRS shapes.
2. Pacing at closely adjacent points can produce marked differences in the QRS shape.
3. Comparison of intraoperative ECGs with preoperative ECGs is not valid because operative conditions (including an open chest, changing heart position, changing cardiac blood volume, ventriculotomy, etc.) also modify the surface ECG.

Because microre-entrant tachycardias arise from a small area (point source), it is not improbable that pacing at that point could reproduce the tachycardia QRS shape. If, however, the tachycardia involves a macrore-entrant pathway with spread of activation from around the entire pathway, it is difficult to see how pacing at any point can reproduce the tachycardia QRS morphology, unless the tachycardia is entrained and 'driven' (see Chapter 7). Operative pacemapping can be regarded as a useful adjunct to activation mapping, but it is not clear whether or not it is superior to 'blind' procedures or resection of tissue based on visual inspection of abnormal myocardium.

Ablation and exclusion methods

Of the many surgical approaches to ablation and exclusion (Fig. 14.11), the most widely used are:

1. Simple ventriculotomy and disconnection procedures.
2. Encircling partial thickness ventriculotomy.
3. Endocardial resection.
4. Cryothermal ablation.
5. Laser ablation.

A simple transmural ventriculotomy was the first surgical procedure for ventricular tachycardia ablation. It was initially applied to ventricular tachycardias associated with right ventricular dysplasia with some measure of success. The mechanism of the effect is not clear. It was less successful when used for ventricular tachycardias associated with coronary artery disease. These tachycardias arise in the endocardium, and incisions through epicardial breakthrough points may be remote from the endocardial origin. Transmural ventriculotomy was claimed to be successful for the treatment of bundle branch re-entrant tachycardias. This was based on the assumption that the incision was interrupting the re-entry in the bundle branches. It is now known, however, that this mechanism is rare and not responsible the vast majority of tachycardias associated with old myocardial infarction. Because the ventricular arrhythmias in right ventricular dysplasia are often of multiple morphologies, simple incision was not always adequate and more extensive procedures were devised. One such operation, devised by Guiraudon et al. (1983) involves total disconnection of the right ventricular free wall. In this way, continuing ventricular arrhythmias emanating from the right ventricle are isolated from the left ventricle and do not cause haemodynamic upset.

The encircling ventriculotomy was devised to treat tachycardias associated with previous myocardial infarction. It is particularly applicable, therefore, to the left ventricle. The aim of surgery is to isolate the focus of tachycardia, excluding it from the remainder of the heart. The left ventricular cavity is entered through the scar tissue. An encircling incision from the endocardial surface to the subepicardium is made around the scar tissue (Fig. 14.11a). It was thought that this procedure would not cause significant interference with blood supply to viable myocardium in the region of the incision. It is now known, however, that such interference does occur and, in patients with severe left ventricular impairment preoperatively, further deterioration follows encircling ventriculotomy. Tachycardias are controlled in about 75 per cent of patients.

Endocardial resection (Fig. 14.11c) was based on the concept that most ventricular tachycardias associated with previous myocardial infarction arise in the subendocardium on the borders of the scar. It has been applied mostly to left ventricular tachycardias. After operative mapping, an area of 10–25 cm^2 of endocardium is 'peeled' away from the underlying myocardium. The procedure does not appear to cause significant left ventricular impairment. The operation is more likely to be successful in patients with discrete aneurysms and monomorphic tachycardias localized to a small area on the anterolateral free wall. Tachycardias arising from the septum, inferior wall, near the mitral ring and in the papillary muscles are less amenable to ablation by this method. These locations may be more accessible to cryosurgery (see below). Tachycardias are controlled in 75–90 per cent of patients.

Cryothermal ablation is an extension of the method of cryothermal mapping (see above). After electrogram and cryothermal mapping, the cryoprobe is placed on the selected area and the temperature is reduced to $-60°C$ for 2 minutes, sufficient to destroy excitability. There are no large series of this method and it is now used mainly as an adjunct to the other methods described above. The 'encircling cryothermal lesion', designed to ablate potential re-entrant substrates around the borders of an infarction, is a recent modification of cryosurgery.

Laser devices have also been used to treat ventricular tachycardias in man (Saksena et al. 1986). Ciccone et al. (1986) have compared the relative efficacy of continuous and pulsed argon lasers (which emit in the visible part of the spectrum) to vaporise the area of endocardium giving rise to the tachycardia. Gallagher and colleagues (1986) have used a neodymium-YAG laser to photocoagulate (rather than vaporise) endocardium. Although experimental these techniques seem promising and may eventually be capable of transvenous application.

Postoperative evaluation of specific ventricular surgery

In patients with inducible tachycardias before operation, electrophysiological testing can be used after surgery. Failure to induce tachycardia after operation predicts a satisfactory outcome. However, persistently inducible tachycardia after surgery is not always associated with spontaneous recurrences. Another possible indicator of successful surgery is abolition of delayed potentials detected by surface electrocardiographic signal averaging techniques. The presence or absence of ventricular ectopic beats on tape monitoring appears to have no bearing on outcome.

References and further reading

Anderson KP, Stinson EB, Mason JW. (1982) Surgical exclusion of focal atrial tachycardia. *American Journal of Cardiology* **49**, 869

Anderson KP, Mason JW. (1983) Surgical management of ventricular tachyarrythmias. *Clinical Cardiology* **6**, 415

Burchell H, Frye RL, Anderson MW, McGoon DC. (1967) Atrioventricular and ventriculoatrial excitation in Wolff–Parkinson–White syndrome: temporary ablation at surgery. *Circulation* **36**, 663

Camm J, Rees G. (1979) Is the surgical solution to the treatment of tachycardias justified? *Thorax* **34**, 434

Camm AJ, Ward DE, Cory-Pearce R, Rees GM, Spurrell RAJ. (1979) The successful cryosurgical treatment of paroxysmal ventricular tachycardia. *Chest* **75**, 621

Camm AJ, Ward DE, Rees GM, Spurrell RAJ. (1980) Cryothermal mapping and cryoablation in the treatment of refractory cardiac arrhythmias. *Circulation* **62**, 67

Cassidy DM, Vassallo JA, Buxton AE, Doherty JU, Marchlinski FW, Josephson ME. (1984) The value of catheter mapping during sinus rhythm to localize site of origin of ventricular tachycardia. *Circulation* **69**, 1103

Ciccone J, Saksena S, Pantopoulos D. (1986) Comparative efficacy of continuous and pulsed argon laser ablation of human diseased ventricle. *Pacing and Clinical Electrophysiology* **9**, 679

Cobb FR, Blumenschein SD, Sealy WC, Boineau JP, Wagner GS, Wallace AG. (1968) Successful surgical interruption of the bundle of Kent in a patient with Wolff–Parkinson–White syndrome. *Circulation* **38**, 1018

Cox JL. (1985) Status of surgery for cardiac arrhythmias. *Circulation* **71**, 413

Cox JL, Gallagher JJ, Cain ME. (1985) Experience in 118 consecutive patients undergoing operation for the Wolff–Parkinson–White syndrome. *Journal of Cardiovascular Surgery* **90**, 490

Curry PVL, O'Keefe DB, Pitcher D, Sowton E, Deverall PB, Yates AK. (1979) Localization of ventricular tachycardia by a new technique – pace-mapping. *Circulation* **60**, suppl. II, II-25 (abstract)

deBakker JM, Janse MJ, Van Capelle F, Durrer D. (1983) Endocardial mapping by simultaneous recording of endocardial electrograms during cardiac surgery for ventricular aneurysm. *Journal of the American College of Cardiology* **2**, 947

Durrer D, Roos JP. (1967) Epicardial excitation of the ventricles in a patient with Wolff–Parkinson–White (type B). *Circulation* **35**, 15

Fontaine G, Guiraudon G, Frank R. (1980) Ventricular resection for recurrent ventricular tachycardia. *New England Journal of Medicine* **303**, 339

Fontaine G. (1982) Surgery for ventricular tachycardia: the view from Paris. *International Journal of Cardiology* **1**, 351

Fontaine G, Guiraudon G, Frank R, Fillette F, Cabrol C, Grogsgogeat Y. (1982) Surgical management of ventricular tachycardia unrelated to myocardial ischemia or infarction. *American Journal of Cardiology* **49**, 397

Fontaine G, Guiraudon G, Frank R, Tereau Y, Pavie A, Cabrol C, Chomette G, Grosgogeat Y. (1984) Management of ventricular tachycardia not related to myocardial ischemia. *Clinical Progress in Pacing and Electrophysiology* **2**, 193

Gallagher JJ, Gilbert M, Svenson RH, Sealy WC, Kasell J, Wallace AG. (1975) Wolff–Parkinson–White syndrome. The problem, evaluation and surgical correction. *Circulation* **51**, 767

Gallagher JJ, Sealy WC, Anderson RW, Kasell J, Millar R, Campbell RWF, Harrison L, Pritchett ELC, Wallace AG. (1977) Cryosurgical ablation of accessory atrioventricular connections. A method of correction of the preexcitation syndrome. *Circulation* **55**, 471

Gallagher JJ. (1978) Surgical treatment for cardiac arrhythmias: current status and future directions. *American Journal of Cardiology* **41**, 1035

Gallagher JJ, Kasell J, Pritchett ELC, Wallace AG. (1978) Epicardial mapping in the Wolff–Parkinson–White syndrome. *Circulation* **57**, 854

Gallagher JJ, Kasell J, Cox J, Smith WM, Ideker RE, Smith WM. (1982) Techniques of intraoperative electrophysiologic mapping. *American Journal of Cardiology* **49**, 221

Gallagher JJ, Del Rossi AJ, Fernandez J, Maranhao V, Strong MD, White M, Gessman LJ. (1985) Cryothermal mapping of recurrent ventricular tachycardia in man. *Circulation* **71**, 733

Gallagher JJ, Svenson RH, Selle J, Sealy WC, Fedor JM, Zimmern SH, Marroum MC, Robicsek F. (1986) Use of the Nd:YAG laser in the surgical treatment of ventricular tachycardia. *New Trends in Arrhythmias* **2**, 293

Garan H, Ruskin JN, DiMarco JP, McGovern B, Levine FH, Buckley MJ. (1984) Refractory ventricular tachycardia complicating recovery from acute myocardial infarction: treatment with map-guided infarctectomy. *American Heart Journal* **107**, 571

Gessman LJ, Endo T, Egan J, Gallagher JJ, Hastie R, Maroko PR. (1985) Dissociation of the site of origin from the site of cryotermination of ventricular tachycardia. *Pacing and Clinical Electrophysiology* **6**, 1293

Guiraudon G, Fontaine G, Frank R, Escande G, Etevient P, Cabrol C. (1978) Encircling endocardial ventriculotomy: a new surgical treatment for life-threatening ventricular tachycardias resistant to medical treatment following myocardial infarction. *Annals of Thoracic Surgery* **26**, 438

Guiraudon GM, Klein GJ, Gulamhusein SS, Painvin G, Del Campo C, Gonzales JC, Ko P. (1983) Total disconnection of the right ventricular free wall: surgical treatment of right ventricular tachycardia associated with right ventricular dysplasia. *Circulation* **67**, 643

Harken AH, Josephson ME, Horowitz LN. (1979) Surgical endocardial resection for the treatment of malignant ventricular tachycardia. *Annals of Surgery* **190**, 456

Harken AH, Horowitz LN, Josephson ME. (1980) Comparison of standard aneurysmectomy and aneurysmectomy with directed endocardial resection for the treatment of recurrent sustained ventricular tachycardia. *Journal of Thoracic and Cardiovascular Surgery* **80**, 527

Harrison L, Gallagher JJ, Kasell J. (1977) Cryosurgical ablation of the AV node–His bundle. A new method for producing AV block. *Circulation* **55**, 463

Holt PM, Curry PVL, Deverall PB, Yates AK, Sowton E. (1982) Pacemapping in the localisation of sites of ventricular tachycardia. In: *Cardiac Pacing: electrophysiology and pacemaker technology*, p. 323. Ed. by GA Feruglio. Piccin Medical Books: Padova

Holt PM, Smallpeice C, Deverall PB, Yates AK, Curry PVL. (1985) Ventricular arrhythmias: a guide to their localisation. *British Heart Journal* **53**, 417

Horowitz LN, Harken AH, Kastor JA, Josephson ME. (1980a) Ventricular resection guided by epicardial and endocardial mapping for treatment of recurrent ventricular tachycardia. *New England Journal of Medicine* **302**, 589

Horowitz LN, Josephson ME, Harken AH. (1980b) Epicardial and endocardial activation during sustained ventricular tachycardia. *Circulation* **62**, 1227

Josephson ME, Harken AH, Horowitz LN. (1979) Endocardial excision: a new surgical technique for the treatment of recurrent ventricular tachycardia. *Circulation* **60**, 1430

Josephson ME, Horowitz LN, Spielman SR, Greenspan AM, Vandepol C, Harken AH. (1980) Comparison of endocardial catheter mapping with intraoperative mapping of ventricular tachycardia. *Circulation* **61**, 395

Josephson ME, Spear JF, Harken AH, Horowitz LN, Dorio RJ. (1982a) Surgical excision of automatic atrial tachycardia: anatomic and electrophysiologic correlates. *American Heart Journal* **104**, 1076

Josephson ME, Horowitz LN, Spielman SR, Waxman HL, Greenspan AM. (1982b) The role of catheter mapping in the preoperative evaluation of ventricular tachycardia. *American Journal of Cardiology* **49**, 207

Josephson ME, Harken AH, Horowitz LN. (1982c) Long-term results of endocardial resection for sustained ventricular tachycardia in coronary artery disease patients. *American Heart Journal* **104**, 51

Kienzle MG, Martin JL, Horowitz LN, Harken AH, Josephson ME. (1982) Electrocardiographic changes following endocardial resection for ventricular tachycardia. *American Heart Journal* **104**, 753

Kienzle MG, Doherty JU, Roy D, Waxman HL, Harken AH, Josephson ME. (1983) Subendocardial resection for refractory ventricular tachycardia: effects on ambulatory electrocardiogram, programmed stimulation and ejection fraction, and relation to outcome. *Journal of the American College of Cardiology* **2**, 853

Kienzle MG, Miller J, Falcone RA, Harker A, Josephson ME. (1984) Intraoperative endocardial mapping during sinus rhythm: relationship to site of origin of ventricular tachycardia. *Circulation* **70**, 957

Klein H, Karp RB, Kouchoukos NT, Zorn GL, James TN, Waldo AL. (1982) Intraoperative electrophysiologic mapping of the ventricles during sinus rhythm in patients with a previous myocardial infarction. Identification of the electrophysiologic substrate of ventricular arrhythmias. *Circulation* **66**, 847

Klein GJ, Guiraudon GM, Perkins DG, Jones DI, Yee R, Jarvis E. (1984) Surgical correction of the Wolff–Parkinson–White syndrome in the closed heart using cryosurgery: a simplified approach. *Journal of the American College of Cardiology* **3**, 405

Klein GJ, Guiraudon GM, Sharma AD, Milstein S. (1986) Demonstration of macroreentry and feasibility of operative therapy in the common type of atrial flutter. *American Journal of Cardiology* **57**, 587

Kron IL, Lerman BB, DiMarco J. (1985) Extended endocardial resection. A surgical approach to ventricular arrhythmias that cannot be mapped intraoperatively. *Journal of Thoracic and Cardiovascular Surgery* **90**, 586

Martin JL, Untereker WJ, Harken AH, Horowitz LN, Josephson ME. (1982) Aneurysmectomy and endocardial resection for ventricular tachycardia: favorable hemodynamic and antiarrhythmic results in patients with global left ventricular dysfunction. *American Heart Journal* **103**, 960

Mason JW, Stinson EB, Winkle RA, Griffin JC, Oyer PE, Ross DL, Derby G. (1982a) Surgery for ventricular tachycardia: efficacy of left ventricular aneurysm resection compared with operation guided by electrical activation mapping. *Circulation* **65**, 1148

Mason JW, Stinson EB, Winkle RA, Oyer PE, Griffin JC, Ross DL. (1982b) Relative efficacy of blind left ventricular aneurysm resection for the treatment of recurrent ventricular tachycardia. *American Journal of Cardiology* **49**, 421

Mason JW, Stinson EB, Oyer PE, Winkle RA, Hunt S, Anderson KP, Derby GC. (1985) The mechanisms of ventricular tachycardia in humans determined by intraoperative recording of the electrical activation sequence. *International Journal of Cardiology* **8**, 163

Miller JM, Kienzle MG, Harken AH, Josephson ME. (1984a) Subendocardial resection for ventricular tachycardia: predictors of success. *Circulation* **70**, 624

Miller JM, Kienzle MG, Harken AH, Josephson ME. (1984b) Morphologically distinct sustained ventricular tachycardias in coronary artery disease: significance and surgical results. *Journal of the American College of Cardiology* **4**, 1073

Miller JM, Josephson ME. (1985) Intraperative mapping ventricular tachycardia: utility and pitfalls. *International Journal of Cardiology* **8**, 173

Miller JM, Harkon AH, Hargrove C, Josephson ME. (1985) Pattern of endocardial activation during sustained ventricular tachycardia. *Journal of the American College of Cardiology* **6**, 1280

Page PL, Arciniegas JG, Plumb VJ, Henthorn RW, Karp KB, Waldo AL. (1983) Value of early postoperative epicardial programmed ventricular stimulation studied after surgery for ventricular tachycarrythmias. *Journal of the American College of Cardiology* **2**, 1046

Pritchett ELC, Anderson RW, Benditt DG, Kasell J, Harrison L, Wallace AG, Sealy WC, Gallagher JJ. (1979) Reentry within the atrioventricular node: surgical cure with preservation of atrioventricular conduction. *Circulation* **60**, 440

Ross DL, Johnson DC, Denniss AR, Cooper MJ, Richards DA, Uther JB. (1985) Curative surgery for atrioventricular junctional ('AV nodal') reentrant tachycardia. *Journal of the American College of Cardiology* **6**, 1383

Saksena S, Hussain SM, Gielschinsky I, Gadhoke A, Pantopoulos D. (1986) Successful mapping-guided laser ablation of ventricular tachycardia in man. *Circulation* **74**, in press

Sealy WC, Hatter BG, Blumenschein SD, Cobb FR. (1969) Surgical treatment of the Wolff–Parkinson–White syndrome. *Annals of Thoracic Surgery* **8**, 1

Sealy WC, Wallace AG, Ramming KP, Gallagher JJ, Svenson RH. (1974) An improved operation for the definitive treatment of the Wolff–Parkinson–White syndrome. *Annals of Thoracic Surgery* **17**, 107

Spielman SR, Michelson EL, Horowitz LN, Spear JF, Moore EN. (1978) The limitations of epicardial mapping as a guide to the surgical therapy of ventricular tachycardia. *Circulation* **57**, 666

Spurrell RAJ, Sowton E, Deuchar D. (1973) Ventricular tachycardia in four patients evaluated by programmed electrical stimulation of heart and treated in 2 patients by surgical division of anterior radiation of left bundle-branch. *British Heart Journal* **35**, 1014

Spurrell RAJ, Yates AK, Thorburn CW, Sowton E, Deuchar DC. (1975) Surgical treatment of ventricular tachycardia after epicardial mapping studies. *British Heart Journal* **37**, 115

Spurrell RAJ, Camm AJ. (1978) Surgical treatment of ventricular tachycardia. *British Heart Journal* **40**, 38

Waldo AL, Arciniegas JG, Klein H. (1981) Surgical treatment of life-threatening ventricular arrhythmias: role of intraoperative mapping and consideration of presently available surgical techniques. *Progress in Cardiovascular Diseases* **23**, 247

Ward DE, Camm AJ, Cory-Pearce R, Spurrell RAJ, Rees GM. (1979) Incessant atrioventricular tachycardia involving an accessory pathway: preoperative and intraoperative electrophysiologic studies and surgical correction. *American Journal of Cardiology* **44**, 428

Wellens HJJ, Bar FWHM, Vanagt EJDM, Brugada P. (1982) Medical treatment of ventricular tachycardia: considerations in the selection of patients for surgical treatment. *American Journal of Cardiology* **49**, 186

Wiener I, Mindich B, Pitchon R. (1982) Determinants of ventricular tachycardia in patients with ventricular aneurysms: results of intraoperative epicardial and endocardial mapping. *Circulation* **65**, 856

Wiener I, Mindich B, Pitchon R. (1984) Fragmented endocardial electrical activity in patients with ventricular tachycardia: a new guide to surgical therapy. *American Heart Journal* **107**, 86

Wittig JH, Boineau JP. (1975) Surgical treatment of ventricular arrhythmias using epicardial, transmural and endocardial mapping. *Annals of Thoracic Surgery* **20**, 117

Wyndham CRC, Arnsdorf MF, Levitisky MS, Smith TC, Dhingra RC, Denes P, Rosen KM. (1980) Successful surgical excision of focal paroxysmal atrial tachycardia. *Circulation* **62**, 1365

Yee R, Guiraudon GM, Gardner MJ, Gulamhusein SS, Klein GJ. (1984) Refractory paroxysmal sinus tachycardia: management by subtotal right atrial exclusion. *Journal of the American College of Cardiology* **3**, 400

15

Electrical Ablation of Cardiac Conduction Pathways and Ectopic Foci

For various experimental reasons, investigators have for some time sought a simple and effective method of inducing permanent AV block. Among the many techniques used are electrocautery, cryothermal injury and injection of noxious substances such as formalin. As discussed in Chapter 14, the production of permanent AV block is an effective treatment strategy in selected patients, and surgical ablation can also be applied to anomalous pathways and ectopic foci. A non-operative method of achieving these effects would therefore be a considerable advance in the management of refractory tachycardias.

Although some of these methods were used at operative surgery to create therapeutic permanent AV block, none proved suitable for use with a transvascular catheter system. In the late 1970s, however, Beazell and colleagues in the USA devised a needle catheter which could deliver shocks of up to 50 J, and they were able to achieve complete AV block in dogs with this technique. The method was simplified by Gonzalez et al. (1981), who use a standard woven Dacron electrode to deliver high energy shocks of up to 400 J (stored energy) to the region of the His bundle of dogs, causing permanent complete AV block. After experimenting in dogs they used the method successfully in patients with refractory atrial arrhythmias (Scheinman et al., 1982). Since that time the efficacy of the method has been reaffirmed by numerous investigators and is now a standard method of treatment. Indeed, electrical ablation of the AV node–His bundle has superseded the surgical method.

Method of ablation by electrical discharge

A particular advantage of the technique is that no special equipment is needed. Two conventional pacing electrodes are inserted using the usual approaches. One is for temporary ventricular pacing (transient AV block may occur after ablation at any site) and the other is used to deliver the shock to the required site. Most operators have used a new 6F or 7F woven Dacron (USCI) bipolar catheter. It should be noted that these catheters are not purpose built and repeated use may cause internal arcing because of dielectric breakdown. It is recommended that no more than three shocks should be delivered through one catheter. (Furthermore, the catheter should be discarded and not used for bradycardia support pacing.) A conventional external defibrillator is connected, using a simple device, to the electrode (Fig. 15.1).

The procedure is performed under anaesthesia. For ablation of the AV node–His bundle, a short-acting intravenous anaesthetic is sufficient. For the more prolonged procedures involving intracardiac mapping, a full general anaesthetic

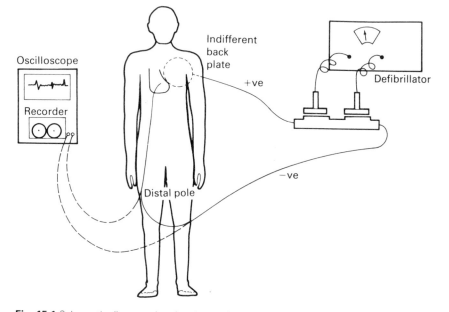

Fig. 15.1 Schematic diagram showing the equipment and connections needed for transvenous ablation electrical procedures.

is preferable. Some operators also use muscle relaxants. An arterial pressure line and a standby ventricular pacemaker are essential for all ablation procedures.

Ablation of the AV node–His bundle

Ablation of the normal AV conduction pathway may be considered in patients with tachycardias which cannot be effectively or safely controlled using another method. For example, refractory atrial fibrillation with a rapid ventricular response is a suitable indication for ablation. Thus, any patient with refractory tachycardias arising above the His bundle is a potential candidate for the procedure. It is usually applied electively, but may also be useful in an emergency where control of the arrhythmia is necessary to prevent further haemodynamic deterioration. The aim of the procedure is to induce permanent AV block, thus removing the ventricles from the influence of supraventricular arrhythmias.

The ablation electrode is positioned in the region of the His bundle (see Chapter 2) and manipulated until a good His potential is recorded. The catheter is then withdrawn until the atrial electrogram is maximal while maintaining the His spike. The reason for this is related to optimal catheter position. It seems that the shock is more likely to cause complete AV block if delivered towards the atrial aspect of the AV node rather than the His bundle aspect. The distal electrode (preferable because the conductor is of lower resistance than that of the proximal electrode) is connected to the defibrillator. Cathodal discharges deliver a higher current and generate less bubble formation than anodal discharges. For these reasons, cathodal discharges are preferable. The anode is connected to a

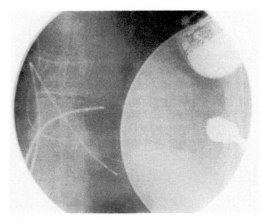

(a)

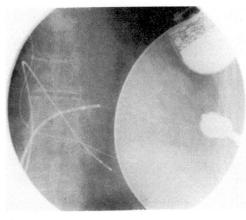

(b)

Fig. 15.2 The position of catheters prior to ablation of the AV node–His bundle (*a*). A 5F pacing electrode is positioned in the apex of the right ventricle and a new 7F bipolar catheter is used to deliver the cathodal discharge to the AV nodal region. The anodal backplate is shown to the right. At the time of the discharge (*b*) a dark halo can be observed surrounding the distal pole.

large backplate (Fig. 15.2). The discharge is synchronized to the QRS complex to avoid provocation of ventricular arrhythmias.

The initial discharge induces permanent AV block in about 75 per cent of patients (Fig. 15.3). In the remainder, conduction block is never achieved or block is transient with conduction resuming within 5 minutes to 48 hours. In these patients a second attempt is successful in about 50 per cent. Thus the procedure is effective in over 85 per cent of patients (Table 15.1). In some patients, a therapeutic result is achieved without causing complete AV block. For example, the response to atrial fibrillation may be much slower after ablation or a mechanism of junctional tachycardia (e.g. dual pathways) may be disturbed without causing permanent block.

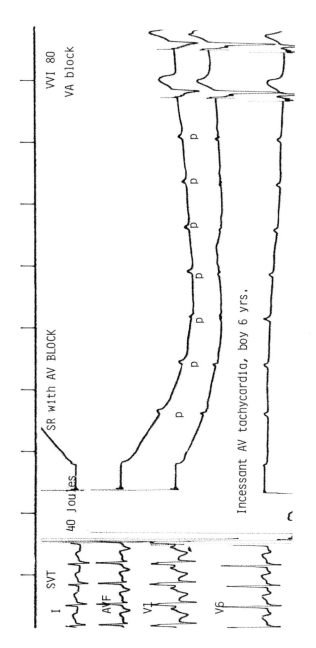

Fig. 15.3 Transvenous electrical ablation of the AV nodal–His bundle in a 6-year-old child with incessant tachycardia. The recordings to the left of the trace show incessant long RP′ tachycardia (see Chapter 9). A discharge of 40 J resulted in complete AV block supported by ventricular pacing during which there was no evidence of retrograde conduction. A permanent pacemaker was implanted and the child was substantially improved. Paper speed 25 mm/sec.

Table 15.1 RESULTS OF AV NODE – HIS BUNDLE ABLATION (M. Scheinman, 1986, personal communication)

Total number of patients	367
Diagnosis:	
Atrial Fibrillation and atrial flutter	220 (60%)
AVNRT	81 (22%)
AVRT	40 (11%)
Automatic atrial tachycardia	48 (13%)
Associated organic heart disease	184 (50%)
Cumulative energy used	50–3500 J
	(mean 600 J)
Results:	
Persistent complete heart block	235 (64%)
Resumption of AVN conduction, but no treatment required	37 (10%)
Resumption of AVN conduction, treatment required	70 (19%)
Completely unsuccessful	25 (7%)

AVNRT = atrioventricular nodal re-entrant tachycardia; AVRT = atrioventricular re-entrant tachycardia.

After the procedure, junctional escape rhythms emerge in most patients (Fig. 15.4). However, this rhythm may be very slow and susceptible to profound overdrive suppression (Fig. 15.5). A permanent pacemaker is implanted in all patients either immediately or after several days.

The complications of the procedure include ventricular arrhythmias induced by the discharge (<2 per cent), transient hypotension (<2 per cent). Tamponade has been reported and may need surgical relief. Later complications include sustained ventricular tachycardia, sudden death, pacing system complications (including infection) and venous thrombosis. The overall complication rate is about 6 per cent (compared with about 25 per cent for surgical ablation). There has been no evidence of myocardial infarction or of valvular or coronary artery damage with this technique. Some patients may require a repeat ablation procedure after the permanent pacemaker has been implanted. There is a risk of damaging the pacing system, but modern units are protected and this risk is minimal.

Preliminary investigations by Narula et al. (1984) have demonstrated that argon laser energy delivered by a transvenous fibreoptic system can effectively modify (induce second first or second degree AV block) or completely interrupt AV conduction in dogs depending on the total energy delivered. Development of such a system may allow human application of this method.

Selective ablation of anomalous conduction tissue

In patients with refractory tachycardias associated with the presence of an anomalous AV connection, surgical division or ablation of the pathway results in a cure (see Chapter 14). The operation has been highly successful, especially for those pathways located on the free wall of the heart. Paraseptal pathways have

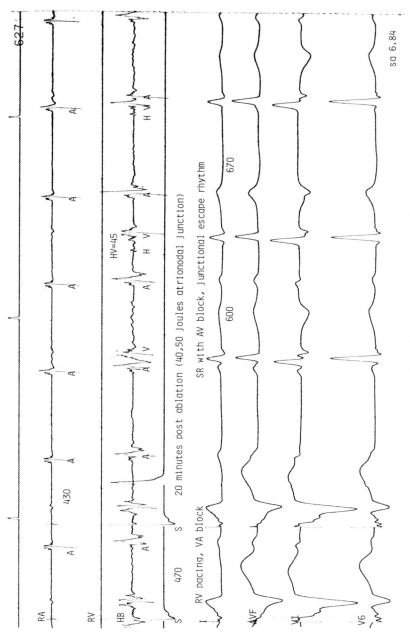

Fig. 15.4 Junctional escape rhythm after AV junctional ablation in a 6-year-old boy with incessant junctional tachycardia. When the ventricular pacing (S) was switched off, complete AV block could be seen. A narrow QRS escape rhythm promptly emerged at a cycle length varying between 600 and 650 msec. Each QRS was preceded by a His potential (HV = 45 msec). Paper speed 100 mm/sec. A = atrial electrogram; RV = right ventricle, disconnected; RA = right atrium; HB = His bundle.

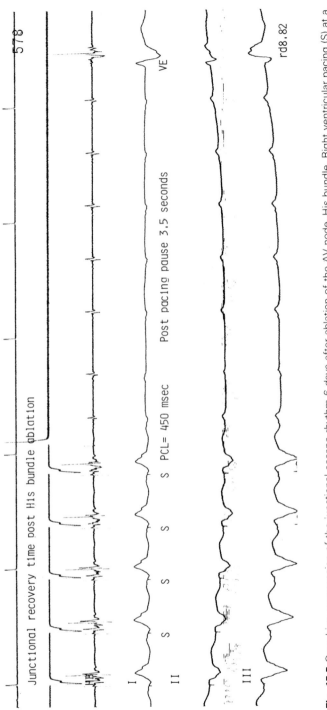

Fig. 15.5 Overdrive suppression of the junctional escape rhythm 6 days after ablation of the AV node–His bundle. Right ventricular pacing (S) at a cycle length (PCL) of 450 msec for 30 seconds resulted in prolonged suppression of the junctional focus. In this particular recording, the escape pause was terminated by a ventricular beat (VE) rather than a junctional beat. This sluggish response reflects the unreliable nature of the escape mechanisms after AV nodal–His bundle ablation. Paper speed 50 mm/sec.

been more difficult to locate and ablate. The principle of electrical ablation of the AV node–His bundle was extended to anomalous pathway conduction by Fisher and colleagues (1982).

The indications for ablation of anomalous conduction have not yet been clearly established and the method must still be regarded as experimental. Nevertheless, there are occasions when patients with refractory or life-threatening arrhythmias associated with anomalous conduction seek a cure but find alternative therapies, such as pacing or surgery, unacceptable.

Accurate localization of the anomalous pathway using standard mapping methods (see Chapters 6 and 9) is a prerequisite to ablation. Coronary arteriography is performed to document coronary artery anatomy and the size of the coronary sinus. If a major artery is close to the intended site of the discharge or if the coronary sinus is of small dimension, the procedure is abandoned. Coronary arteriography may be especially useful in documenting coronary artery spasm after the shock (see below). Because of the risk of delivering high energy shocks in the distal coronary sinus, it is inadvisable to apply the method to free wall pathways in the left AV junction until better techniques are available. A ventricular pacing electrode is positioned to prevent bradycardia due to transient AV nodal block.

The method has been successful in ablating conduction in right free wall and posteroseptal pathways (Table 15.2). The electrode is connected to the defibrillator as described above and an anterior chest wall anode plate is used to complete the external circuit (Fig. 15.6). For pathways located near the ostium of the coronary sinus with this electrode configuration discharges of 50–100 J are used, and for right free wall pathways up to 400 J has been applied. This may result in permanent complete block in the anomalous pathway (Fig. 15.7) with the obvious therapeutic benefit (Fig. 15.8) or modification of the properties of the pathway (longer refractory period, more sensitive to drugs, slower tachycardias) such that disabling arrhythmias no longer occur. Anomalous conduction is abolished in about 20–90 per cent of patients, but the current overall success rate is about 60 per cent (Ward and Camm, 1986).

Table 15.2 ABLATION OF ANOMALOUS CONDUCTION

Number of patients	37
Site of pathway:	
Septal	23
Right free wall	5
Mid coronary sinus	8
Nodoventricular	1
Results:	
No anomalous AV conduction	15
No anomalous VA conduction	10
Modified AV conduction	10
No effect	8

Data from Bardy et al, (1983), Jackman et al. (1983), Weber and Schmitz (1983), Bhandari et al. (1984), Fisher et al. (1984), Kunze and Kuck (1984), Morady (1985), Ward and Camm (1985) and Davies (1986a).

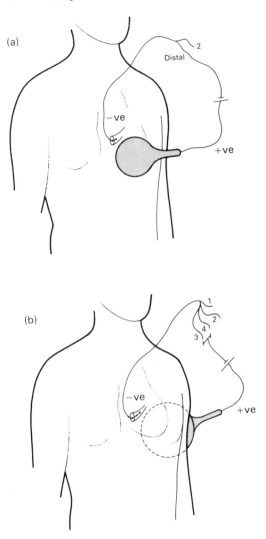

Fig. 15.6 Schematic diagram illustrating two methods which have been used for electrical ablation of posteroseptal anomalous AV pathways. (a) A bipolar catheter in the mouth of the coronary sinus and anterior anodal plate. (b) A quadripolar catheter positioned with poles 3 and 4 (the most proximal poles) straddling the mouth of the coronary sinus, and the anode plate is positioned behind the left scapula.

Serious complications have been uncommon but there are instances of rupture of the coronary sinus causing tamponade and death, possibly related to the energy level and the size of the coronary sinus. Although there is no evidence to suggest a long-term deleterious effect on the coronary circulation, high energy shocks may cause coronary artery spasm (Hartzler et al., 1985).

Morady and collegues (1985) have described a different method for ablation

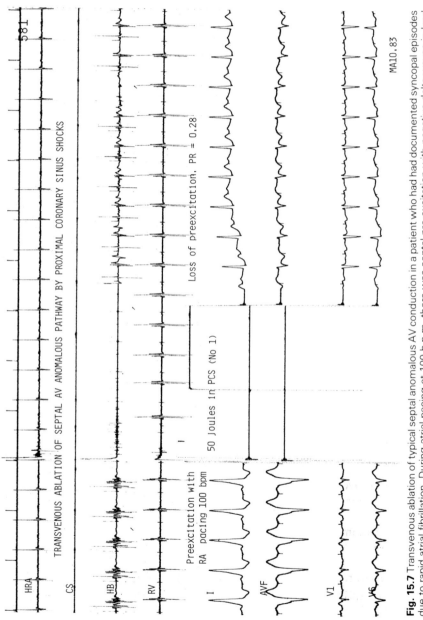

Fig. 15.7 Transvenous ablation of typical septal anomalous AV conduction in a patient who had had documented syncopal episodes due to rapid atrial fibrillation. During atrial pacing at 100 b.p.m. there was septal pre-excitation with negative delta waves in lead AVF. A discharge of 50 J resulted in immediate block in the anomalous pathway. After the shock the PR interval was prolonged at 0.28 sec but gradually returned to normal over a period of minutes. Paper speed 25 mm/sec. CS = coronary sinus; HB = His bundle; HRA = high right atrium; RV = right ventricle.

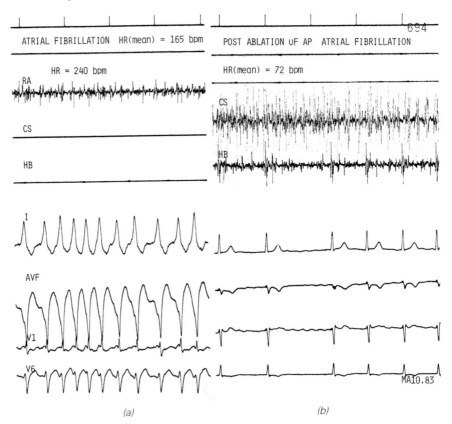

Fig. 15.8 Beneficial effect of ablation of anomalous conduction (same patient as in Fig. 15.7). (*a*) Rapid atrial fibrillation with a mean pre-excited QRS rate of 240 b.p.m. (*b*) After the ablation there was normal AV conduction with a controlled ventricular response. Paper speed 25 mm/ sec.

of posteroseptal pathways. The proximal two poles of a quadripolar electrode catheter are positioned straddling the ostium of the coronary sinus (Fig. 15.6 and 15.9) and connected together to form a single cathode. A discharge of up to 400 J is delivered against an anodal backplate. The primary and long-term success of this method is over 80 per cent. This method, however, is not without serious complications, including rupture of the coronary sinus. A modification suggested in a review article by Scheinman (1986) is positioning of both poles immediately outside the ostium of the coronary sinus. This apparently minor change in the technique originally suggested by this group may have considerable bearing on the safety of the method.

There are few reports of attempts to ablate conduction in anomalous pathways with long conduction times and decremental properties (see Chapter 9). These pathways are situated in the paraseptal region close to the ostium of the coronary sinus and might be expected to be amenable to ablation. Generally, selective ablation of retrograde anomalous conduction in these patients with the long RP′

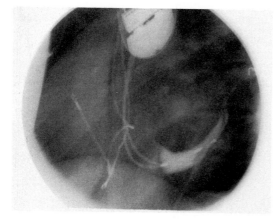

Fig. 15.9 The disposition of electrodes for ablation of posteroseptal anomalous pathways using the technique devised by Morady et al. (1985). The coronary sinus is opacified by retrograde injection (National Institutes of Health catheter shown in the sinus) to delineate the ostium accurately. Electrodes 3 and 4 of a quadripolar catheter are positioned across the ostium and united to form a common cathode for delivery of the electrical discharge.

type of tachycardia using coronary sinus discharges has been unsuccessful (Davies et al., 1986a). In two recently reported cases (Critelli et al., 1985; Gang et al., 1985) selective ablation was achieved.

Transvenous electrical ablation of the AV node–His bundle has been used successfully to treat patients with incessant long RP′ tachycardias. An interesting phenomenon observed in several such patients is the new appearance of ventricular pre-excitation after AV nodal ablation procedure. In most instances there is also prolonged AV conduction (long P–delta interval). It is suggested that retrograde concealed anomalous pathway conduction prevented anterograde anomalous conduction before ablation. With removal of normal AV conduction this mechanism of block is not possible and anterograde anomalous conduction is manifest. This mechanism would not explain the appearance of a short PR interval with septal pre-excitation seen in Fig. 15.10.

In summary, ablation of anomalous conduction is an experimental procedure which has been highly effective in controlling tachycardias associated with some types of Wolff–Parkinson–White (WPW) syndrome. It would seem that pathways located in the right AV junction or in the septum are those most amenable to the technique. For some reason, atypical septal anomalous pathways with long conduction times appear to be more resistant to electrical ablation using current localization methods and ablation techniques.

Ablation of ventricular tachycardia

Endocavitary activation mapping (see Chapter 10) allows accurate localization of the origin of ventricular tachycardias whatever their mechanism. The mapping procedure should include 'pacemapping' (described in Chapter 10). This may reduce the number of induction procedures required to locate accurately the

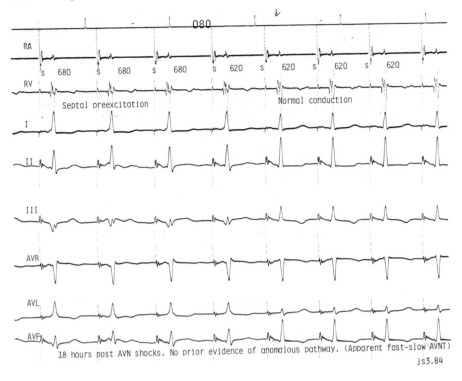

Fig. 15.10 The appearance of pre-excitation within hours of attempted modification of AV nodal conduction in a patient with long RP' tachycardia due to a retrogradely conducting anomalous pathway with a slow conduction time. Ventricular pre-excitation had never been documented prior to the ablation procedure. Twenty-four hours after ablation, atrial pacing at a cycle length of 680 msec (SS) revealed evidence of septal pre-excitation with a short PR interval. When the atrial rate was increased the anomalous pathway became non-conductive and normal AV conduction emerged. Paper speed 50 mm/sec.

tachycardia focus by electrogram mapping. The ablation technique is well suited to the treatment of ventricular tachycardias, especially those of a single QRS morphology (indicating a single mechanism or source) which are stable and sustained (allowing time for mapping). The ablation technique was first applied to the treatment of ventricular tachycardias by Hartzler (1983) in the USA, with dramatic results in three patients. Since that time many more patients have been treated and early results suggest a success rate of about 50 per cent (Ward and Camm, 1986) (Table 15.3). Several methods have been used, including single pole endocardial cathodal discharge with an external anode (Fig. 15.11) and bipolar discharges across the septum for tachycardias emanating from this area.

The complication rate is reputed to be small but has included cardiac rupture, asystole unresponsive to pacemaker stimuli and several deaths. Some of these complications may, however, be related to the fact that many of the patients who underwent treatment were *in extremis*.

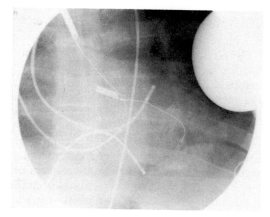

Fig. 15.11 Right oblique view showing position of catheters for endocardial ablation of ventricular tachycardia arising from the anterolateral free wall of the ventricle. This patient, a 55-year-old man, had recurrent monomorphic ventricular tachycardia unresponsive to drug treatment. A right ventricular mapping catheter (introduced via the right subclavian vein), right ventricular pacing electrode (right femoral vein) and left ventricular mapping catheter had been positioned. The discharge was delivered through the left ventricular catheter in the position shown (upper right). A posterior external anode was used.

Table 15.3 CATHETER ABLATION OF VENTRICULAR TACHYCARDIA

Number of patients	69
Results:	
No VT	36
No VT or minimal VT on treatment	22
Recurrence of VT	11
Late deaths	11
Complications:	
None	11
Pulmonary oedema	2
Procedural death	3
Persistent complete AV block	5
Aphasia	1
Asystole (unresponsive to pacing)	1

Data from Hartzler (1983), Steinhaus et al. (1984), Winston et al. (1984), Downar et al. (1985), Huang et al. (1985), Belhassen et al. (1986), Davies et al. (1986b), Fontaine (1986), Touboul et al. (1986).

Ablation of atrial ectopic foci

There is little experience in this application of the ablation method. Preliminary data suggest that automatic atrial tachycardias emanating from the right atrial appendage may be abolished with discharges of 1–2 J/kg (Moak et al., 1985).

Mechanisms and physical aspects

The mechanism whereby ablation achieves abolition of conduction or ablation of ectopic foci is not clear and the physical aspects of fulgurative (spark-producing) and non-fulgurative discharges have not been extensively investigated. Rapid pressure changes and intense current flow have both been suggested as the main instrument of damage. An early study of the phenomena accompanying electrical discharges in water (Tidd et al., 1976) showed rapid development of high pressure and bubble formation. Changes in the current flow and voltage developed during the shock are complex and depend, among other factors, on the energy delivered, the electrode configuration and the amount of gas brought out of solution. Higher resistance to current flow and larger volumes of gas occur with anodal discharges. The volume of gas generated has been the cause of some concern, especially when delivering shocks to the left ventricle. A comprehensive investigation by Bardy and colleagues (1986) has shown that the major determinants are anodal discharges, delivered energy and a smaller electrode surface area. The bubbles are largely composed of nitrogen, oxygen and carbon dioxide. These substances are not generated by electrolysis but are most probably released from solution by shock waves following the discharge (Bardy et al., 1986). Cunningham et al. (1986) have devised a method of delivering the impulse over a shorter time than with a conventional defibrillator. This technique reduces the total energy needed to achieve ablation and therefore reduces the intensity of the shock waves.

As mentioned above, conventional pacing electrodes used for ablation procedures are not designed to withstand high energy electrical discharges, and several mishaps have been reported. These include rupture of the insulation, separation of the connector, complete interruption of the conductor wire and internal arcing. These effects are more likely to occur after several shocks are given in the same catheter. For this reason it is advisable not to use a catheter for more than three discharges.

Histological studies of the AV node–His bundle some months after ablation have shown no scarring or inflammation, whereas in another reported case these findings were noted. It is likely that several complex biophysical and physiological effects are responsible.

In summary, transvenous electrical ablation of the AV node–His bundle has revolutionized the management of refractory supraventricular tachycardias of any type involving conduction through the AV node, and this has now taken the place of operative surgical ablation. It is becoming increasingly clear that both anomalous pathway conduction and ventricular tachycardia foci are amenable to ablation techniques in selected patients. Further developments and improvements are expected. Laser therapy offers the prospect of carefully controlled transvascular endocardial surgery for refractory arrhythmias.

References and further reading

Bardy GH, Ideker R, Kasell J, Worley S, Smith WM, German L, Gallagher JJ. (1983) Transvenous ablation of the atrioventricular conduction system in dogs: electrophysiologic and histologic observations. *American Journal of Cardiology* **51**, 1775

Bardy GH, Poole JE, Coltorti F, Ivey TD, Block TA, Trobaugh GB, Green HL. (1985) Catheter ablation of a concealed accessory pathway. *American Journal of Cardiology* 55, 1366

Bardy GH, Coltorti F, Ivey TD, Alferness C, Rackson M, Hansen K, Stewart R, Greene HL. (1986) Some factors affecting bubble formation with catheter-induced defibrillator pulses. *Circulation* 73, 525

Beazell JW, Adomian GE, Furmanski M, Tan KS. (1982) Experimental production of complete heart block by electrocoagulation in the closed chest dog. *American Heart Journal* 104, 1328

Belhassen B, Miller MI, Geller E, Laniado S. (1986) Transcatheter electrical shock ablation of ventricular tachycardia. *Journal of the American College of Cardiology* 7, 1347

Bhandari A, Morady F, Shen E, Schwartz AB, Botvinick E, Scheinman MM. (1984) Catheter induced His bundle ablation in a patient with reentrant tachycardia associated with a nodoventricular tract. *Journal of the American College of Cardiology* 4, 611

Boyd EGAC, Holt PM. (1985) An investigation into the electrical ablation technique and a method of electrode assessment. *Pacing and Clinical Electrophysiology* 8, 815

Brodman R, Fisher JD. (1983) Evaluation of a catheter technique for ablation of accessory pathways near the coronary sinus ostium using a canine model. *Circulation* 67, 923

Critelli G, Gallagher JJ, Monda V, Coltorti F, Scherillo M, Rossi L. (1984) Anatomic and electrophysiologic substrate of the permanent form of junctional reciprocating tachycardia. *Journal of the American College of Cardiology* 4, 601

Critelli G, Gallagher JJ, Perticone F, Monda V, Scherillo M, Condorelli M. (1985) Transvenous catheter ablation of the accessory pathway in the permanent form of junctional reciprocating tachycardia. *American Journal of Cardiology* 55, 1639

Cunningham AD, Rowland E, Rickards AF. (1986) A low energy power source for ablation and a new index for ablating devices. *Clinical Progress in Electrophysiology* 4, 125 (abstract)

Davies DW, Ward DE, Nathan AN, Camm AJ. (1986a) Fulgurative ablation of accessory atrioventricular pathways in man. In: *Fulguration and Laser in Cardiac Arrhythmias.* Ed. by G Fontaine, MM Scheinman. Futura: Mount Kisco, NY (in press)

Davies DW, Nathan AW, Camm AJ. (1986b) Three deaths after attempted high energy catheter ablation of ventricular tachycardia. *British Heart Journal* 55, 506

Downar E, Parson I, Cameron D, Waxman M, Yao L, Easty A. (1985) Unipolar and bipolar catheter 'ablation' techniques for management of ventricular tachycardia – initial experience. *Journal of the American College of Cardiology* 5, 472 (abstract)

Fisher JD, Brodman R, Kim SG, Matos JA. (1982) Non-surgical Kent bundle ablation via the coronary sinus in patients with the Wolff–Parkinson–White syndrome. *Circulation* 66, suppl. II, 375 (abstract)

Fisher JD, Brodman R, Kim SG, Matos JA, Brodman E. (1984) Attempted nonsurgical ablation of accessory pathways via the coronary sinus in the Wolff–Parkinson–White syndrome. *Journal of the American College of Cardiology* 4, 685

Fisher JD, Kim SG, Matos JA, Waspe LE, Brodman R, Merav A. (1985) Complications of catheter ablation of tachyarrythmias: occurrence, protection and prevention. *Clinical Progress in Electrophysiology and Pacing* 3, 292

Fontaine G. (1986) Fulguration of ventricular tachycardia. In: *Fulguration and Laser in Cardiac Arrhythmias.* Ed. by G Fontaine, MM Scheinman. Futura: Mount Kisco, NY (in press)

Gallagher JJ, Svenson RH, Kasell J, German LD, Bardy GH, Broughton A, Critelli G. (1982) Catheter technique for closed-chest ablation of the atrioventricular conduction system. A therapeutic alternative for the treatment of refractory supraventricular tachycardia. *New England Journal of Medicine* 306, 194

Gallagher JJ, Svenson RH, Kasell J, German LD, Bardy GH, Broughton A, Critelli G. (1982) Catheter technique for closed-chest ablation of the atrioventricular conduction system. A therapeutic alternative for the treatment of refractory supraventricular tachycardia. *New England Journal of Medicine* **306**, 194

Gang ES, Oseran D, Rosenthal M, Mandel WJ, Deng Z, Meesman M, Peter T. (1985a) Closed chest catheter ablation of an accessory pathway in a patient with permanent junctional reciprocating tachycardia. *Journal of the American College of Cardiology* **6**, 1167

Gang ES, Oseran D, Rosenthal M, Mandel WJ, Deng Z, Meesman M, Peter T. (1985b) Closed chest catheter ablation of an accessory pathway in a patient with permanent junctional reciprocating tachycardia. *Journal of the American Colege of Cardiology* **6**, 1167

Gonzalez R, Scheinman MM, Margaretten W, Rubinstein M. (1981) Closed-chest electrode-catheter technique for His bundle ablation in dogs. *American Journal of Physiology* **241**, H283

Gonzalez R, Scheinman MM, Bharati S, Lev M. (1983) Closed chest permanent atrioventricular block in dogs. *American Heart Journal* **105**, 461

Hartzler GO. (1983) Electrode catheter ablation of refractory focal ventricular tachycardia. *Journal of the American College of Cardiology* **2**, 1107

Hartzler GO, Giorgi L, Diehl AM, Hamaker WR. (1985) Right coronary artery spasm complicating electrode catheter ablation of right lateral accessory pathway. *Journal of the American College of Cardiology* **6**, 250

Holt PM, Boyd EGCA, Crick JCP, Sowton E. (1985) Low energies and Helifix electrodes in the successful ablation of atrioventricular conduction. *Pacing and Clinical Electrophysiology* **8**, 639

Holt PM, Boyd EGCA. (1986) Hematologic effects of the high-energy endocardial ablation technique. *Circulation* **73**, 1029

Huang SK, Marcus F, Ewy GA. (1985) Clinical experience with endocardial catheter ablation for ventricular tachycardia. *Journal of the American College of Cardiology* **5**, 473

Jackman WM, Friday KJ, Scherlag BJ, Dehning MM, Schechter E, Reynolds DW, Olsen EG, Berbari EJ, Harrison L, Lazzara R. (1983) Direct endocardial recording from an accessory atrioventricular pathway: localization of the site of block, effect of antiarrhythmic drugs and attempt at non-surgical ablation. *Circulation* **68**, 906

Kunze KP, Kuck KH. (1984) Transvenous ablation of accessory pathways in patients with incessant supraventricular tachycardia. *Circulation* **70**, suppl. II, 412 (abstract)

Levine JH, Spear JF, Weisman HF, Kadish AH, Prood C, Siu CO, Moore EN. (1986) The cellular electrophysiologic changes induced by high-energy electrical ablation in canine myocardium. *Circulation* **73**, 818

Moak JP, Freidman RA, Garson A. (1985) Electrical ablation of atrial muscle: safety assessed in canine atria. *Journal of the American College of Cardiology* **5**, 455

Morady F, Scheinman MM, Winston SA, DiCarlo LA, Davis JC, Griffin JC, Rudler M, Abbott JA, Eldar M. (1985) Efficacy and safety of transcatheter ablation of posteroseptal accessory pathways. *Circulation* **72**, 170

Narula OS, Bharati S, Chan MC, Embi AA, Lev M. (1984) Laser micro transection of the His bundle: a pervenous catheter technique. *Journal of the American College of Cardiology* **3**, 537 (abstract)

Nathan AN, Bennett DH, Ward DE, Camm AJ. (1984) Catheter ablation of atrioventricular conduction. *Lancet* **i**, 1280

Rowland E, Foale R, Nihoyannopoulos P, Perelman M, Krikler DM. (1985) Intracardiac contrast echoes during transvenous His bundle ablation. *British Heart Journal* **53**, 240

Saksena S, Gadhoke A. (1986) Laser therapy for tachyarrhythmias: a new frontier. *Pacing and Clinical Electrophysiology* **9**, 531

Scheinman MM, Morady F, Hess DS, Gonzalez R. (1982) Catheter-induced ablation of the atrioventricular junction to control refractory supraventricular arrhythmias. *Journal of the American Medical Association* **248**, 841

Scheinman MM, Evans-Bell T and the Executive Committee of the Percutaneous Mapping and Ablation Registry. (1984) Catheter ablation of the atrioventricular junction: a report of the percutaneous mapping and ablation registry. *Circulation* **70**, 1024

Scheinman MM. (1986) Catheter ablation for patients with cardiac arrhythmias. *Pacing and Clinical Electrophysiology* **9**, 551

Steinhaus D, Whitford E, Stavens J, Schneller S, McComb J, Carr J. (1984) Percutaneous transcatheter ablation for ventricular tachycardia. *Circulation* **70**, suppl. II, 100 (abstract)

Tidd MJ, Webster J, Cameron Wright H, Harrison IR. (1976) Mode of action of surgical and electronic lithoclast – high speed pressure, cinematographic and Schlieren recordings following an ultrashort underwater electronic discharge. *Biomedical Engineering* **14**, 5

Touboul P, Kirkorian G, Atallah G, Lavaud P, Moleur P, Lamaud M, Mathieu MP. (1986) Bundle branch reentrant tachycardia treated by electrical ablation of the right bundle branch. *Journal of the American College of Cardiology* **7**, 1404

Ward DE, Davies M. (1984) Transvenous high energy shock for ablating atrioventricular conduction in man: observations on the histological effects. *British Heart Journal* **51**, 175

Ward DE, Jones S, Gibson RV. (1984) Emergency transvenous ablation of atrioventricular conduction to control refractory atrial tachycardia. *European Heart Journal* **5**, 126

Ward DE, Camm AJ. (1985) Treatment of tachycardias associated with the Wolff–Parkinson–White syndrome by transvenous electrical ablation of accessory pathways. *British Heart Journal* **53**, 64

Ward DE, Camm AJ. (1986) The current status of ablation of cardiac conduction tissue and ectopic myocardial foci by transvenous electrical discharges. *Clinical Cardiology* **9**, 237, 244

Weber H, Schmitz L. (1983) Catheter technique for closed-chest ablation of an accessory pathway. *New England Journal of Medicine* **308**, 653

Winston SA, Morady F, Davis JC, DiCarlo LA, Waxman M, Scheinman MM. (1984a) Catheter ablation of ventricular tachycardia. *Circulation* **70**, suppl. II, 412 (abstract)

Winston SA, Davis JC, Morady F, DiCarlo LA, Matsubara T, Wexman P, Scheinman MM. (1984b). A new approach to electrode catheter ablation for ventricular tachycardia arising from the interventricular septum. *Circulation* **70**, suppl. II, 412 (abstract)

16

The Place of Electrophysiological Studies in the Management of Arrhythmias in Children

Although invasive electrophysiological testing has made an enormous contribution to the understanding and management of arrhythmias in adults, the role of this technique in the management of arrhythmias in children is not clear. The factors contributing to the generation of arrhythmias in young patients may be different from those in adults, and the indications for electrophysiological studies are also different although their aims are similar – that is, to clarify diagnosis and establish effective therapy. In this chapter we shall examine the usefulness of clinical electrophysiological studies in the managemnt of arrhythmias in infants and children.

Invasive studies in the assessment of bradycardias

The single most common aetiological factor in these disorders is prior corrective or palliative surgery for congenital structural heart defects. Damage to the sinus node or the atrioventricular conduction system may result in symptomatic bradycardias which require pacemaker insertion. Sinoatrial disease or conduction disorders in association with unoperated structural defects or normal hearts are much less common.

Sinoatrial disorders

This type of disorder occurs most commonly after atrial surgery, especially that involved in the physiological correction of ventriculoarterial discordance (complete transposition of the great arteries). Symptomatic sinoatrial disease in children is rare. The decision to implant a permanent pacemaker is often simple, being made on the basis of severe symptoms such as syncope with a proven relationship to prolonged pauses on the electrocardiogram. Invasive studies in this setting do not contribute to the decision to pace although they may help in the selection of a particular pacing system. In the absence of such severe symptoms or where a poor outlook is thought to be determined by sinoatrial disease the decision to pace may be more complex. The utility of invasive electrophysiological studies in this setting has been well studied in adults (see Chapter 4) with disorders of the sinus node of varying severity, and published evidence suggests that the results are of limited value. This is because there is a high incidence of negative results in patients with known disorders. These problems have received limited investigation in children.

Three studies of the electrophysiological assessment of sinoatrial function in

Table 16.1 SINOATRIAL FUNCTION IN CHILDREN

	With SAD (N=41)	With SAD (N=38)
Abnormal SNRT	31	None
Abnormal SACT	20	None

Data from Yabek et al. (1978), Beder et al. (1983), Kugler et al. (1979).

SACT = sinoatrial conduction time; SAD = sinoatrial disorder; SNRT = sinoatrial node recovery time.

children are summarized in Table 16.1. The results suggest that the sinoatrial node recovery time (SNRT) is more specific than the sinoatrial conduction time (SACT) but neither of these is very sensitive. Although these studies embraced a group of children with a wide variety of cardiac disorders (including unoperated disease), it must be concluded that there is little evidence for the value of invasive tests of sinoatrial node function. It should be emphasized, however, that sinoatrial disorders are not infrequently associated with atrial arrhythmias and AV conduction defects. Invasive testing may be of value in these settings. For example, the choice of pacing system (dual chamber or atrial or ventricular) would be influenced by the unmasking of AV conduction disease in a patient with sinoatrial disorder requiring a permanent system.

Several studies have specifically addressed the problem of sinoatrial disorder after atrial surgery. Gillette et al. (1980) noted an abnormal SNRT in 23 children who had undergone Mustard's operation. The proportion of abnormal values in unoperated patients with discordant ventriculoarterial connection, however, is not stated and no long-term data were reported. Only 7 patients were studied pre- and post-operatively and in none was there conclusive electrophysiological evidence of damage to the sinus node. In an earlier study from the same group (El Said et al., 1976) it was noted that a normal recovery time could be found in patients with clinically manifest sinoatrial disorder. Studies of children with atrial septal defect before and after surgery have also shown that a high proportion may have significant abnormalities before the operation. There is also some evidence that similar abnormalities may be present before surgery in children with ventriculoarterial discordance. The small number of patients in these and other studies makes interpretation of the results difficult. Furthermore, no study has documented electrophysiologically determined sinoatrial function before and after surgery and correlated these results with long-term surveillance of sinoatrial performance. Thus, although published reports claim that postoperative electrophysiological testing of sinoatrial node function may be of value in predicting spontaneous failure of the sinus node, the evidence for this claim is not convincing.

Disorders of the atrioventricular conduction

Although a wide variety of atrioventricular conduction defects can be found in children, only two types have been the subject of intense research using electrophysiological techniques: (1) postoperative conduction defects; and (2) congenitally complete AV block.

Postoperative conduction defects

Damage to the AV conduction system during repair of structural congenital heart disease is the most common indication for permanent ventricular pacing in children. Early studies of the problem concluded that the prognosis for patients with complete block after surgery was favourable with 'medical management alone'. More recent information has refuted this view and it is now common practice to pace those children permanently who have persistent complete block after operation. The decision, however, is not a simple one, especially in asymptomatic children. Permanent pacing in children has been accompanied by many problems and, despite recent improvements in techniques, implantation of a permanent system cannot be taken lightly. Furthermore, some children who acquire complete block develop a functionally adequate junctional escape rhythm and may not be dependent on a pacemaker. The origin of the escape rhythm may be located by using intracardiac recordings as described in Chapter 5. Surgically induced block may occur above or below the bundle of His, and Driscoll et al. (1979) have suggested that such localization is useful in that those with distal block should receive a permanent pacemaker. No data to support their contention were presented. No doubt the authors assumed a graver outlook for distal block. Thus, evidence for the value of invasive localization of the site of complete block is tenuous.

Surgically induced bundle branch block and fascicular block after repair or complex defects are common, and have been proclaimed by some to be a harbinger of complete block and by others to carry no additional risk. The association of transient postoperative complete block with right bundle branch block and left axis deviation (Fig. 16.1) probably carries an increased risk of late progression to permanent complete AV block and much attention has been given to the search for a reliable method of predicting this outcome. Measurement of the HV interval (see Chapters 2, 3 and 5) in adults has been used to detect trifascicular damage and select patients for prophylactic permanent pacing. The results of three major studies of this method in children with postoperative AV conduction defects are summarized in Table 16.2. In the study of Godman et al. (1974) none of the patients with a prolonged HV interval received pacemakers and there was no recurrence of complete block during follow-up. Similar results were found by Pahlajani et al. (1975), and after a median of 6.6 years none of

Table 16.2 INTRAVENTRICULAR CONDUCTION IN CHILDREN

	RBBB/LBBB	RBBB+LAD	Normal QRS	Perioperative AV block
Normal HV	32	27	5	10
Long HV	4	16	1	13

Data from Godman et al. (1974), Pahlajani et al. (1975), Yabek et al. (1977).

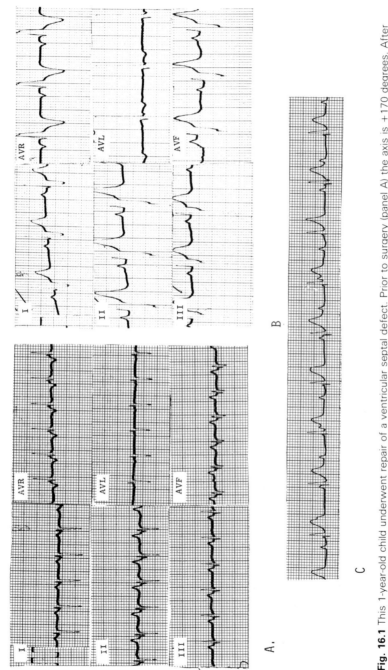
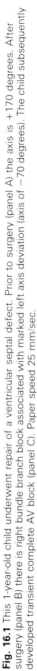

Fig. 16.1 This 1-year-old child underwent repair of a ventricular septal defect. Prior to surgery (panel A) the axis is +170 degrees. After surgery (panel B) there is right bundle branch block associated with marked left axis deviation (axis of −70 degrees). The child subsequently developed transient complete AV block (panel C). Paper speed 25 mm/sec.

the patients had died. Izukawa et al. (1979) have suggested that the association of these conduction defects (HV prolongation, right bundle branch block and left axis deviation) with transient perioperative complete block augurs badly, but Yabek et al. (1977) detected HV prolongation in less than half of all patients who did have perioperative complete block.

Although electrophysiological studies have provided important information about the mechanism and site of block or delay within the AV conduction system, the prognostic value of this information is still unclear. Thus, it must be concluded that the available evidence does not support the notion that such studies are of value in the management of asymptomatic postoperative conduction defects and further prospective studies are needed.

Congenitally complete atrioventricular block

Symptomatic congenitally complete atrioventricular block is an undisputed indication for permanent pacing. Despite extensive debate in the literature, no clear guidelines have emerged for prophylactic pacing in asymptomatic children. The site of block (above or below the His bundle) appears to be of little prognostic value. Measurement of junctional recovery times (see Chapter 5) has also been unhelpful in that prolonged recovery times can be seen in asymptomatic patients and normal results in symptomatic patients. There is some evidence to suggest that the junctional escape mechanism in symptomatic patients is less responsive to atropine. Studies of these phenomena are, however, inconclusive. It seems, therefore, that the decision to implant a permanent pacemaker in a child with congenitally complete AV block must be made on the basis of clinical and electrocardiographic data alone.

Invasive studies in the assessment of tachycardias

Junctional and atrial tachycardias

In adults, the major thrust of electrophysiological investigation in the evaluation and assessment of tachycardias. Gillette and his colleagues (Gillette 1976, 1981b) have been foremost in applying the techniques of clinical cardiac electrophysiology to infants and children with tachycardias. Their studies have shown that the mechanisms of many supraventricular tachycardias in children (especially those involving AV junctional tissues) are identical to those seen in adults. Certain tachycardias are, however, more prevalent in younger age-groups. These include focal His bundle tachycardia (junctional ectopic tachycardia) and incessant AV tachycardia with a long RP′ interval (see Chapter 9). Several mechanisms of tachycardia may coexist and may be distinguished by electrophysiological study. Complex junctional tachycardias may involve several anatomical or functional substrates, and interaction between one mechanism and another is not uncommon.

The information gained by detailed invasive studies has enabled application of non-pharmacological methods of treatment such as pacemakers, surgery and transvascular ablation. All of these have been successfully applied in children, and in this respect electrophysiological studies are essential and of undoubted value in the small minority of children refractory to conventional treatment with drugs. There is little information about electrophysiological drug testing (see Chapter 12) in children. Kugler et al. (1985) used this method in 61 children with a wide variety of arrhythmias, but the study was retrospective and could not be said to demonstrate that invasive drug testing was superior to empirical treatment. Experience with children with refractory supraventricular tachycardias (Ward, 1986) suggests that the number of attacks is significantly reduced (using the patient as his own control) if an 'effective' drug can be identified, but further studies are needed to confirm this impression.

Ventricular tachycardias

The causes of chronic recurrent monomorphic ventricular tachycardias in children are numerous and varied but include:

1. Dilated cardiomyopathy.
2. Intramyocardial tumours.
3. Myocardial infarction.
4. Ventricular surgery, especially for Fallot's tetralogy.
5. Hypertrophic cardiomyopathy.
6. Myocarditis.

Electrophysiological studies in some of these patients have identified features consistent with myocardial re-entrant excitation or abnormally automatic foci. As in adults, further clarification of the method has not been possible. Endocardial mapping during ventricular tachycardia has localized the source of some foci. Thus clinical electrophysiological studies of spontaneous sustained ventricular tachycardia provides information upon which rational therapy could be based, whether it be pharmacological, surgical or electrical. Surgical treatment of incessant ventricular tachycardias based on preoperative and operative electrophysiological findings has been reported by Garson et al. (1984). It is to be expected that antitachycardia pacing and electrical ablation will also be effectively applied to the management of tachycardias in children as they have been in adults.

Of particular interest in children is the role of ventricular surgery in creating a substrate for ventricular tachycardia. Although postoperative complete AV block has been thought to be responsible for a significant proportion of sudden deaths after surgical correction of Fallot's tetralogy, it is now evident that some, possibly a major proportion, of late sudden deaths are caused by ventricular tachycardia. The electrophysiological characteristics of these tachycardias suggest intraventricular re-entry close to the ventricular scar. Other origins remote from sites of the surgical incision or resection have been reported (Kugler et al., 1983; Swerdlow et al., 1986). Several points arising from studies of ventricular tachycardia in this context are worthy of comment (Ward, 1986): firstly, spontaneous tachycardia or any symptom suggestive thereof was noted in a minority of patients; secondly, aggressive burst protocols were used to initiate tachycardia in a significant proportion of patients; thirdly, in only one study

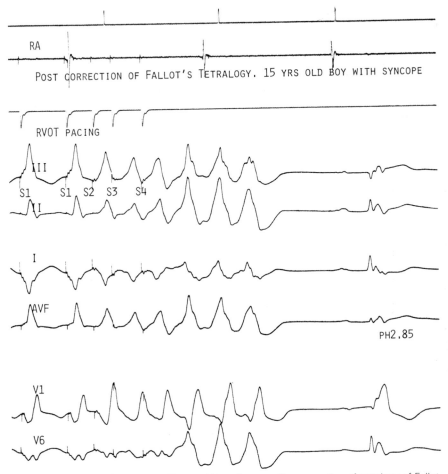

RA

POST CORRECTION OF FALLOT'S TETRALOGY. 15 YRS OLD BOY WITH SYNCOPE

RVOT PACING

II

S1   S1 S2 S3 S4

I

I

AVF

PH2.85

V1

V6

Fig. 16.2 Provocation testing in a 15-year-old boy 2 years after correction of tetralogy of Fallot. The indication for testing was recurrent syncopal episodes. Right ventricular outflow tract pacing (S1S1) and triple extrastimuli (S2S3S4) induced repetitive beats but no sustained tachycardia. This type of response must be regarded as non-specific unless it can be shown that the patient has spontaneous clinical attacks of the same morphology. Paper speed 50 mm/sec.

(Horowitz et al., 1980) was any attempt made to compare the QRS morphology of the induced tachycardia with that of the spontaneous one; lastly, the effect of drugs was formally studied in only a small number of patients. There is very little information about the application of electrophysiological drug testing in this setting. For therapy to be effective, the induced tachycardia must closely resemble the spontaneous one. Induction of non-clinical tachycardias is not uncommon and is misleading (Fig. 16.2). The stringent requirements for meaningful interpretation of these arrhythmias in adults (see Chapter 10) should also apply to children. These considerations are important if provocation testing is to be used to assess the risk of sudden death or collapse regardless of the presence or absence of spontaneous ventricular tachycardias. Byrum et al. (1983)

have advocated the use of 'aggressive burst pacing' in children who have had a ventriculotomy to 'prospectively examine the risk for ventricular tachycardia'. As yet, there is no evidence to support this approach and preventive treatment based on the findings of such studies is not justified.

Because the number of children suffering from ventricular tachycardia is small, it is difficult to conceive of a study of sufficient numbers to ascertain formally whether or not electrophysiological drug testing would offer a better prospect than the empirical approach. Even in adults, data which strongly suggests the superiority of the invasive method are open to criticism because the relevant information allowing derivation of the true specificity, sensitivity and predictive accuracy of the method has not been collected (see Chapters 10 and 12). Nevertheless, until better information is available (whether in adults or in children) it seems medically and ethically justifiable to adopt this approach in selected children with manifest life-threatening or severely symptomatic sustained ventricular tachycardias. With regard to assessment of the risk of such arrhythmias and preventive treatment in children free of spontaneous episodes but with a potential substrate, the role of electrophysiological testing is not known.

References and further reading

Beder S, Gillette P, Garson A, Porter CB, McNamara D. (1983) Symtomatic sick sinus syndrome in children and adolescents as the only manifestation of cardiac abnormality or associated with unoperated congenital heart disease. *American Journal of Cardiology* **51**, 1133

Benson DW, Spach M, Edwards S, Sterba S, Serwer GA, Armstrong BE, Anderson PAW. (1982a) Heart block in children. Evaluation of subsidiary ventricular pacemaker recovery times and ECG tape recordings. *Pediatric Cardiology* **2**, 39

Benson DW, Smith WM, Dunnigan A, Sterba R, Gallagher JJ. (1982b) Mechanisms of regular, wide QRS tachycardia in infants and children. *American Journal of Cardiology* **49**, 1778

Bergdahl DM, Stevenson JG, Kawabori I, Guntheroth W. (1980) Prognosis in primary ventricular tachycardia in the pediatric patient. *Circulation* **62**, 897

Bink-Boelkens MTE, Velvia H, van der Heide JJH, Eygelaar A, Hardjowijono RA. (1983) Dysrhythmias after atrial surgery in children. *American Heart Journal* **108**, 125

Bisset G, Seigel SF, Gaum WE, Kaplan S. (1981) Chaotic atrial tachycardia in childhood. *American Heart Journal* **101**, 268

Butto F, Dunnigan A, Overholt ED, Benditt DG, Benson DW. (1986) Transesophageal study of recurrent atrial tachycardia after atrial baffle procedures for complete transposition of the great arteries. *American Journal of Cardiology* **57**, 1356

Byrum C, Sondheimer H, Kavey R, Blackman M. (1983) Aggressive burst pacing after ventriculotomy: prospective screening for sudden death risk. *Circulation* **68**, II-328 (abstract)

Byrum C, Bove EL, Sondheimer HM, Kavey RW, Blackman MS. (1986) Hemodynamic and electrophysiologic results of the Senning procedure for transposition of the great arteries. *American Journal of Cardiology* **58**, 138

Campbell RM, Disk M, Jenkins JM, Spicer RL, Crowley DC, Rocchini AP, Snider R, Stern AM, Rosenthal A. (1985) Atrial overdrive pacing for conversion of atrial flutter in children. *Pediatrics* **75**, 730

Casta A, Wolff GS, Mehta AV, Tamer DF, Pickoff AS, Gelband H. (1984) Induction of non-sustained atrial flutter by programmed electrical stimulation in children: incidence, mechanisms, and clinical implications. *American Heart Journal* **107**, 444

Clark EB, Kugler JD. (1982) Preoperative secundum atrial septal defect with coexisting sinus node and atrioventricular node dysfunction. *Circulation* **65**, 976

Clarkson PM, Barrat-Boyes BG, Neutze JM. (1976) Late dysrhythmias and disturbances of conduction following Mustard operation for complete transposition of the great arteries. *Circulation* **53**, 519

Coumel P, Fidelle J, Lucet V, Attuel P, Bouvrain Y. (1978) Catecholamine-induced severe ventricular arrhythmias with Adams–Stokes syndrome in children: report of four cases. *British Heart Journal* **40**, (suppl) 28

Deal BJ, Keane JF, Gillette PC, Garson A. (1985) Wolff–Parkinson–White syndrome and supraventricular tachycardia in infancy: management and follow-up. *Journal of the American College of Cardiology* **5**, 130

Driscoll D, Gillette PC, Hallman G, Cooley D, McNamara D. (1979) Management of surgical complete atrioventricular block in children. *American Journal of Cardiology* **43**, 1175

Dunnigan A, Benditt DG, Benson DW. (1986) Modes of onset ('initiating events') for paroxysmal atrial tachycardia in infants and children. *American Journal of Cardiology* **57**, 1280

Duster MC, Bink-Boelkens M, Wampler D, Gillette PC, McNamara DG, Cooley DA. (1985) Long-term follow-up of dysrhythmias following the Mustard procedure. *American Heart Journal* **109**, 1323

El-Said GM, Gillette PC, Cooley DA, Mullins CE, McNamara DG. (1975) Protection of the sinus node in Mustard's operation. *Circulation* **55**, 788

El-Said G, Gillette PC, Mullins C, Nihill M, McNamara DG. (1976) Significance of pacemaker recovery times after the Mustard operation for transposition of the great arteries. *American Journal of Cardiology* **38**, 448

Fulton DR, Chung KJ, Tabakin B, Keane JF. (1985) Ventricular tachycardia in children without heart disease. *American Journal of Cardiology* **44**, 1328

Garson A, Gillette PC. (1979) Junctional ectopic tachycardia in children: electrocardiography, electrophysiology and pharmacologic response. *American Journal of Cardiology* **44**, 298

Garson A. (1981) Evaluation and treatment of chronic ventricular dysrrhythmias in the young. *Cardiovascular Reviews and Reports* **2**, 1164

Garson A, Gillette PC, McNamara DG. (1981) Supraventricular tachycardia in children: clinical features, response to treatment and long-term follow-up in 217 patients. *Journal of Pediatrics* **98**, 875

Garson A, Porter CB, Gillette PC, McNamara DG. (1983) Induction of ventricular tachycardia during electrophysiologic study after repair of tetralogy of Fallot. *Journal of the American College of Cardiology* **1**, 1493

Garson A, Gillette PC, Titus JL, Hawkins E, Kearney D, Ott D, Cooley DA, McNamara DG. (1984) Surgical treatment of ventricular tachycardia in infants. *New England Journal of Medicine* **310**, 1443

Garson A, Bink-Boelkens M, Hesslein PS, Hordof AJ, Keane JF, Neches WH, Porter CB and other investigators of the Pediatric Electrophysiology Society. (1985) Atrial flutter in the young: a collaborative study of 380 cases. *Journal of the American College of Cardiology* **6**, 871

Garson A. (1986) Dosing the newer antiarrhythmic drugs in children: considerations in pediatric pharmacology. *American Journal of Cardiology* **57**, 1405

Gaum WE, Schwartz DC, Kaplan S. (1980) Ventricular tachycardia in infancy: evidence for a reentry mechanism. *Circulation* **62**, 401

Gaum WE, Kaplan S. (1984) Supraventricular tachycardia in infancy. *American Journal of Cardiology* **54**, 664

Gillette PC. (1976) The mechanisms of tachycardia in children. *Circulation* 54, 133

Gillette P, Yeoman M, Mullins C, McNamara D. (1977) Sudden death after repair of tetralogy of Fallot. Electrocardiographic and electrophysiologic abnormalities. *Circulation* 56, 566

Gillette PC, Busch U, Mullins CE, McNamara DG. (1979) Electrophysiological studies in patients with ventricular inversion and 'corrected transposition'. *Circulation* 60, 939

Gillette PC, Kugler JD, Garson A, Gutgesell H, Duff DF, McNamara DG. (1980) Mechanisms of cardiac arrhythmias after the Mustard operation for transposition of the great arteries. *American Journal of Cardiology* 45, 1225

Gillette P. (1981a) Recent advances in mechanisms, evaluation and pacemaker therapy of chronic bradysrhythmias in children. *American Heart Journal* 102, 920

Gillette PC. (1981b) Advances in the diagnosis and treatment of tachydysrhythmias in children. *American Heart Journal* 102, 111

Gillette P, Garson A, Hesslein P, Karpawich PP, Tierney RC, Cooley DA, McNamara D. (1981) Successful surgical treatment of atrial junctional and ventricular tachycardia associated with accessory connexions in children. *American Heart Journal* 102, 984

Gillette PC, Thapar MK. (1984) Repetitive ventricular responses to ventricular extrastimulation studies in children and adolescents. *Texas Heart Journal* 11, 166

Godman MJ, Roberts NK, Izukawa T. (1974) Late post-operative conduction disturbances after repair of ventricular septal defect and tetralogy of Fallot. *Circulation* 49, 214

Greco R, Musto B, Arienzo V, Alborino A, Garofarlo S, Marsico F. (1982) Treatment of paroxysmal tachycardia in infancy with digitalis, adenosine and verapamil: a comparative study. *Circulation* 66, 504

Hayes C, Gersony WM. (1986) Arrhythmias after the Mustard operation for transposition of the great arteries: a long-term study. *Journal of the American College of Cardiology* 7, 133

Hesslein PS, Gutgesell HP, Gillette PC, McNamara DG. (1982) Exercise assessment of sinoatrial node function following the Mustard operation. *American Heart Journal* 103, 351

Horowitz LN, Vetter V, Harken A, Josephson ME. (1980) Electrophysiologic characteristics of sustained ventricular tachycardia occurring after repair of tetralogy of Fallot. *American Journal of Cardiology* 46, 466

Izukawa T, Trusler GA, Williams WG. (1979) Effect of transient heart block occurring at the time of closure of ventricular septal defects on the incidence of late complete heart block. In: *Proceedings of the Sixth World Symposium on Cardiac Pacing*, Chap. 23-5. Ed. by C Meere. Pace Symp: Montreal

Karpawich PP, Gillette PC, Garson A, Hesslein P, Porter CB, McNamara DG. (1981) Congenital complete atrioventricular block: clinical and electrophysiologic precursors of need of pacemaker insertion. *American Journal of Cardiology* 48, 1098

Karpawich P, Antillon J, Carpola P, Agarwal K. (1985) Pre- and postoperative electrophysiologic assessment of children with secundum atrial septal defect. *American Journal of Cardiology* 55, 519

Krongrad E. (1978) Prognosis for patients with congenital heart disease and postoperative intraventricular conduction defects. *Circulation* 57, 867

Krongrad E, Hordof AJ. (1984) Tachycardias in children. In: *Tachycardias*, p. 319. Ed by B Surawicz, CP Reddy, EN Prystowsky. Martinus Nijhoff: Boston, Mass

Kugler J, Gillette P, Mullins C, McNamara D. (1979) Sinoatrial conduction in children: an index of sinoatrial node function. *Circulation* 59, 1266

Kugler J, Pinsky W, Cheatham J, Hofschire P, Mooring P, Fleming W. (1983) Sustained ventricular tachycardia after repair of tetralogy of Fallot: new electrophysiologic findings. *American Journal of Cardiology* 51, 1137

Kugler J, Bansal A, Cheatham J, Pinsky W, Mooring P, Hofschire P. (1985) Drug-electrophysiology studies in children and adolescents. *American Heart Journal* 110, 144

Levy AM, Bonazinga BJ. (1983) Sudden sinus slowing with junctional escape: a common mode of initiation of juvenile supraventricular tachycardia. *Circulation* 67, 84

Lubbers WJ, Losekoot TG, Anderson RH, Wellens HJJ. (1974) Paroxysmal supraventricular tachycardia in infancy and childhood. *European Journal of Cardiology* 2, 91

Murphy DA, Tynan M, Graham R, Bonham-Carter R. (1970) Prognosis of complete atrioventricular dissociation in children after open heart surgery. *Lancet* 1, 750

Pahlajani D, Serrato M, Mehta A, Miller R, Hastreiter A, Rosen KM. (1975) Surgical bifascicular block. *Circulation* 52, 82

Rocchini AP, Chun PO, Dick M. (1981) Ventricular tachycardia in children. *American Journal of Cardiology* 47, 1091

Roguin N, Shapir Y, Zeltzer M, Berand M. (1984) The use of calcium gluconate prior to verapamil in infants with paroxysmal supraventricular tachycardia. *Clinical Cardiology* 7, 613

Rosen KM, Mehta A, Rahimtoola S, Miller R. (1971) Sites of congenital and surgical heart block as defined by His bundle electrocardiography. *Circulation* 44, 833

Rowland TW, Schweiger MJ. (1984) Repetitive paroxysmal ventricular tachycardia and sudden death in a child. *American Journal of Cardiology* 53, 1729

Ruschhaupt D, Khoury L, Thilenius O, Replogle R, Arcilla R. (1984) Electrophysiologic abnormalities of children with ostium seundum atrial septal defect. *American Journal of Cardiology* 53, 1643

Saalouke MG, Rios J, Perry LW, Shapiro SR, Scott LP. (1978) Electrophysiologic studies after Mustard's operation for *d*-transposition of the great vessels. *American Journal of Cardiology* 41, 1104

Sapire DW, O'Riordan AC, Black IFS. (1981) Safety and efficacy of short- and long-term verapamil therapy in children with tachycardia. *American Journal of Cardiology* 48, 1091

Soler-Soler J, Sagrista-Sauleda J, Cabrera A, Sauleda-Pares J, Iglesias-Berengue J, Permanyer-Miralda G, Roca-Llop J. (1978) Effect of verapamil in infants with paroxysmal supraventricular tachycardia. *Circulation* 59, 876

Southall D, Keeton B, Leanage R, Lam J, Joseph MC, Anderson RH, Lincoln CR, Shinebourne EA. (1980) Cardiac rhythm and conduction before and after Mustard's operation for complete transposition of the great arteries. *British Heart Journal* 43, 21

Steeg CN, Krongrad E, Darachi F, Bowman FO, Malm JR, Gersony W. (1975) Post-operative left anterior hemiblock and right bundle branch block following repair of tetralogy of Fallot. Clinical and etiologic considerations. *Circulation* 51, 1026

Swerdlow CD, Oyer PE, Pitlick PT. (1986) Septal origin of sustained ventricular tachycardia in a patient with right ventricular outflow tract obstruction after correction of tetralogy of Fallot. *Pacing and Clinical Electrophysiology* 9, 584

Vetter VL, Josephson ME, Horowitz LN. (1981) Idiopathic recurrent sustained ventricular tachycardia in children and adolescents. *American Journal of Cardiology* 47, 315

Ward DE, Signy M, Oldershaw P, Jones S, Shinebourne E. (1982) Cardiac pacing in children. *Archives of Disease in Childhood* 57, 514

Ward DE, Ho SY, Shinebourne EA. (1984a) Familial atrial standstill and inexcitability in childhood. *American Journal of Cardiology* 53, 965

Ward DE, Rigby M, Dawson P, Collins, M, Shinebourne EA. (1984b) Rapid ventricular pacing to control resistant neonatal atrioventricular reentrant tachycardias. *Pediatric Cardiology* 5, 45

Ward DE, Jones S, Shinebourne EA. (1985) Longterm pacing in congenital heart disease. *Clinical Progress in Electrophysiology and Pacing* 3, 133

Ward DE. (1986) The management of arrhythmias in children. Are electrophysiologic studies of value? *International Journal of Cardiology* 11, 149

Ward DE, Jones S, Shinebourne. (1986) The use of flecainide acetate for refractory junctional tachycardias in children with the Wolff–Parkinson–White syndrome. *American Journal of Cardiology* 57, 787

Wolff GS, Rowland T, Ellison R. (1972) Surgically-induced right bundle branch block with left anterior hemiblock. An ominous sign in post-operative tetralogy of Fallot. *Circulation* 46, 587

Yabek S, Jarmakani J, Roberts N. (1977) Diagnosis of trifascicular damage following tetralogy of Fallot and ventricular septal defect repair. *Circulation* 55, 23

Yabek S. (1978) Evaluation of sinus node automaticity and sinoatrial conduction in children with normal and abnormal sinus node function. *Clinical Cardiology* 1, 136

Index

Italicized numbers refer to tables or figures